LEARNING DISABILITIES
SOURCEBOOK

SEVENTH EDITION

Health Reference Series

LEARNING DISABILITIES
SOURCEBOOK

SEVENTH EDITION

Basic Consumer Health Information about Disabilities That Affect Learning, including Dyslexia; Dyscalculia; Dysgraphia; Speech, Language, and Communication Disorders; Auditory and Visual Processing Disorders; Attention Deficit Hyperactivity Disorder; Down Syndrome and Other Chromosomal Disorders; Fetal Alcohol Spectrum Disorders; Hearing and Visual Impairment; Autism and Other Pervasive Developmental Disorders; and Traumatic Brain Injury

Along with Facts about Learning Disabilities Diagnosis, Early Intervention, Special Education, Assistive Technology Accommodations, Guidelines for Life-Stage Transitions, Suggestions for Coping with Daily Challenges, a Glossary of Related Terms, and a Directory of Additional Resources

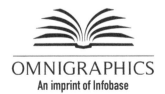

OMNIGRAPHICS
An imprint of Infobase

Bibliographic Note

Because this page cannot legibly accommodate all the copyright notices, the Bibliographic Note portion of the Preface constitutes an extension of the copyright notice.

* * *

OMNIGRAPHICS
An imprint of Infobase
132 W. 31st St.
New York, NY 10001
www.infobase.com
James Chambers, *Editorial Director*

* * *

Copyright © 2023 Infobase
ISBN 978-0-7808-2024-1
E-ISBN 978-0-7808-2025-8

Library of Congress Cataloging-in-Publication Data

Names: Chambers, James (Editor), editor. | Omnigraphics, Inc., issuing body.

Title: Learning disabilities sourcebook / edited by James Chambers.

Description: Seventh edition. | New York, NY: Omnigraphics, an imprint of Infobase, [2023] | Series: Health reference series | Includes index. | Summary: "Provides consumer health information about the signs, symptoms, and diagnosis of learning disabilities and other conditions that impact learning, along with facts about early intervention and the special education process, employment issues guidelines related to learning disabilities, and so on. Includes index, glossary, and other resources"-- Provided by publisher.

Identifiers: LCCN 2022042409 (print) | LCCN 2022042410 (ebook) | ISBN 9780780820241 (library binding ; acid-free paper) | ISBN 9780780820258 (ebook)

Subjects: LCSH: Learning disabilities--United States--Handbooks, manuals, etc. | Learning disabled children--Education--United States--Handbooks, manuals, etc. | Learning disabled--Education--United States--Handbooks, manuals, etc. | Learning disabilities--United States--Diagnosis--Handbooks, manuals, etc.

Classification: LCC LC4705.L434 2023 (print) | LCC LC4705 (ebook) | DDC 371.90903--dc23/eng/20220909

LC record available at https://lccn.loc.gov/2022042409

LC ebook record available at https://lccn.loc.gov/2022042410

Electronic or mechanical reproduction, including photography, recording, or any other information storage and retrieval system for the purpose of resale is strictly prohibited without permission in writing from the publisher.

The information in this publication was compiled from the sources cited and from other sources considered reliable. While every possible effort has been made to ensure reliability, the publisher will not assume liability for damages caused by inaccuracies in the data, and makes no warranty, express or implied, on the accuracy of the information contained herein.

This book is printed on acid-free paper meeting the ANSI Z39.48 Standard. The infinity symbol that appears above indicates that the paper in this book meets that standard.

Printed in the United States

Table of Contents

Preface xi

Part 1. Understanding and Identifying Learning Disabilities
Chapter 1—The Brain and Its Function 3
        Section 1.1—Basics of the Brain: How the Brain Works 5
        Section 1.2—How the Brain Develops............................ 12
        Section 1.3—Early Brain Development and Health................................ 18
        Section 1.4—Executive Function 21
Chapter 2—Early Learning, Speech, and Language Development Milestones..27
        Section 2.1—Speech and Language Development Milestones........................ 29
        Section 2.2—Language and Linguistics: Language Acquisition 32
Chapter 3—Learning Disabilities: An Overview 37
Chapter 4—Diagnosing Learning Disabilities................................39
Chapter 5—Evaluating Children for Learning Disabilities 41
Chapter 6—Other Facts about Learning Disabilities 47

Part 2—Types of Learning Disabilities
Chapter 7—Auditory Processing Disorder 55
Chapter 8—Developmental Dyscalculia 61

Chapter 9—Dysgraphia 67
Chapter 10—Reading Disorders 73
        Section 10.1—Dyslexia............................. 75
        Section 10.2—Hyperlexia.......................... 77
Chapter 11—Nonverbal Learning Disorder 83
Chapter 12—Voice, Speech, and Language Disorders....................89
        Section 12.1—Voice, Speech, and
                       Language Disorders:
                       Quick Statistics................. 91
        Section 12.2—Aphasia............................. 94
        Section 12.3—Apraxia of Speech 97
        Section 12.4—Specific Language
                       Impairment..................... 101
        Section 12.5—Detecting Problems with
                       Language or Speech....... 104
        Section 12.6—Voice, Speech, and
                       Language Program 107
Chapter 13—Visual Processing Disorders 111

Part 3. Other Disorders That Make Learning Difficult

Chapter 14—Attention Deficit Hyperactivity Disorder 119
Chapter 15—Cerebral Palsy..123
Chapter 16—Chromosomal Disorders..137
        Section 16.1—What Are Chromosomal
                       Disorders?...................... 139
        Section 16.2—Down Syndrome............ 144
        Section 16.3—47,XYY Syndrome 148
        Section 16.4—Fragile X Syndrome....... 150
        Section 16.5—Klinefelter Syndrome 154
        Section 16.6—Prader-Willi
                       Syndrome....................... 159
        Section 16.7—Turner Syndrome........... 164
        Section 16.8—Velocardiofacial
                       Syndrome....................... 168
        Section 16.9—Williams Syndrome....... 171

Chapter 17—Epilepsy-Aphasia Spectrum 175
Chapter 18—Fetal Alcohol Spectrum Disorders............................179
   Section 18.1—Alcohol Use and
                 Pregnancy 181
   Section 18.2—Facts about Fetal
                 Alcohol Spectrum
                 Disorders......................... 184
Chapter 19—Gerstmann Syndrome 189
Chapter 20—Hearing Disabilities 191
   Section 20.1—Hearing Loss in
                 Children.......................... 193
   Section 20.2—Hearing Loss Treatment
                 and Intervention
                 Services 196
Chapter 21—Pervasive Developmental Disorders..........................203
   Section 21.1—What Are Pervasive
                 Developmental
                 Disorders?....................... 205
   Section 21.2—Asperger Syndrome 206
   Section 21.3—Autism Spectrum
                 Disorder 208
   Section 21.4—Rett Syndrome................ 209
Chapter 22—Tourette Syndrome..213
   Section 22.1—Tourette Syndrome:
                 Basics 215
   Section 22.2—Co-occurring
                 Conditions of
                 Tourette Syndrome 217
Chapter 23—Traumatic Brain Injury..223
Chapter 24—Visual Impairment in Children.................................235
Chapter 25—Emotional Disturbance 245

Part 4. Learning Disabilities Interventions and Educational Process
Chapter 26—Decoding Learning Disabilities
             Interventions..259

Chapter 27—Early Intervention Strategies 265
    Section 27.1—Early Intervention: An Overview 267
    Section 27.2—Parent Notification and Consent in Early Intervention 269
    Section 27.3—Writing the Individualized Family Service Plan for Your Child 274
    Section 27.4—Providing Early Intervention Services in Natural Environments 278
    Section 27.5—Response to Intervention 283
Chapter 28—The Special Education Process: An Overview 291
Chapter 29—Understanding Your Child's Right to Special Education Services 297
    Section 29.1—Section 504 299
    Section 29.2—The Individuals with Disabilities Education Act 303
    Section 29.3—Every Student Succeeds Act 307
Chapter 30—Individualized Education Programs 311
Chapter 31—Supports, Modifications, and Accommodations for Students with Disabilities 315
Chapter 32—Specialized Teaching Techniques 323
    Section 32.1—Differentiated Instruction 325
    Section 32.2—Speech-Language Therapy 329

Chapter 33—Coping with School-Related Challenges....................333
　　　　　Section 33.1—Building a Good Relationship with Your Child's Teacher................ 335
　　　　　Section 33.2—Parental Involvement in Child's Success in School and Life................ 339
Chapter 34—Alternative Educational Options 343
　　　　　Section 34.1—Homeschooling............... 345
　　　　　Section 34.2—Choosing a Tutor 353
Chapter 35—Transition to High School..361
　　　　　Section 35.1—Transition to High School: An Overview 363
　　　　　Section 35.2—Frequently Asked Questions about Transition to High School............................... 369
Chapter 36—Transition to College and Vocational Programs 381
Chapter 37—Employment and Postsecondary Education............387

Part 5. Living with Learning Disabilities

Chapter 38—Coping with a Learning Disability.............................395
Chapter 39—Self-Esteem and Children with Learning Disabilities..399
Chapter 40—Parenting a Child with a Learning Disability...........405
Chapter 41—Bullying and Learning Disabilities: What Parents Need to Know 411
Chapter 42—Preparing for Adulthood: Tips for Adolescents with Learning Disabilities......................417
Chapter 43—Overview of Independent Living................................423
Chapter 44—Information about Special Needs Trust 427
Chapter 45—Understanding Disability Inclusion..........................435
Chapter 46—Parenting a Child When You Have a Disability.......445
Chapter 47—Employment for People with Learning Disabilities..451

Part 6. Additional Help and Information

Chapter 48—Glossary of Terms Related to Learning
          Disabilities..461
Chapter 49—Sources of College Funding for Students
          with Disabilities..467
Chapter 50—Directory of Resources Related to Learning
          Disabilities..475

Index..**485**

Preface

ABOUT THIS BOOK

Learning disabilities are neurological disorders that affect the brain's ability to process, store, and communicate information. They are widespread, affecting as many as one out of every five people in the United States, according to the U.S. Department of Education. During 2020–2021, the number of students aged 3–21 who received special education services under the Individuals with Disabilities Education Act (IDEA) was 7.2 million, or 15 percent of all public school students. Among students receiving special education services, the most common category of disability was specific learning disabilities (33%). Learning disabilities directly impact many areas in the lives of those affected, making school difficult, affecting employment, complicating day-to-day activities, and even affecting relationships. Yet learning disabilities are invisible obstacles. For this reason, they are often misunderstood, and their impact is often underestimated. Treatment for learning disabilities is mainly based on medications and rehabilitative techniques.

Learning Disabilities Sourcebook, Seventh Edition provides information about dyslexia, dyscalculia, dysgraphia, speech and communication disorders, and auditory and visual processing disorders. It also provides details about other conditions that impact learning, including attention deficit hyperactivity disorder, autism and other pervasive developmental disorders, hearing and visual impairment, and Down syndrome and other chromosomal disorders. The book offers facts about diagnosing learning disabilities, the special education process, and legal protections. Guidelines for life-stage transitions, suggestions for coping with daily challenges, a glossary of related terms, and a directory of resources for additional help and information are also included.

HOW TO USE THIS BOOK

This book is divided into parts and chapters. Parts focus on broad areas of interest. Chapters are devoted to single topics within a part.

Part 1: Understanding and Identifying Learning Disabilities explains how the brain works, defines what learning disabilities are, and describes theories regarding their potential causes. It explains how learning disabilities are evaluated and provides tips on how to choose an evaluation professional.

Part 2: Types of Learning Disabilities describes the most common forms of learning disabilities, including problems with reading, writing, mathematics, speech, language, and communication. It explains what these disorders are, how they are diagnosed, and how they are treated. It also discusses learning disabilities among gifted students, a fairly common—but often unrecognized—phenomenon.

Part 3: Other Disorders That Make Learning Difficult discusses common disorders that have a component that affects a child's ability to learn, including attention deficit hyperactivity disorder, epilepsy, fetal alcohol spectrum disorders, pervasive developmental disorders, visual and hearing disabilities, and chromosomal disorders, such as Down syndrome.

Part 4: Learning Disabilities Interventions and Educational Process provides information about how learning disabilities are accommodated within the schools. It describes early intervention strategies, explains how the special education process works, and details the legal support for students with learning disabilities. Specialized teaching techniques and alternative educational options, such as tutoring and homeschooling, that are used to help learning-disabled students succeed are described, and it also offers guidelines for successfully negotiating the transitions to high school and to college.

Part 5: Living with Learning Disabilities discusses how learning disabilities impact daily life. It includes tips for coping with a learning disability and for parenting a child with a learning disability. The impact of learning disabilities on self-esteem and life skills is discussed, and it offers suggestions to help those with learning disabilities deal with daily tasks, including meal preparation, money management, travel and transportation, and learning to drive. It also provides detailed guidelines for handling the employment issues faced by those with learning disabilities.

Part 6: Additional Help and Information includes a glossary of terms related to learning disabilities, a list of sources of college funding for students with disabilities, and a directory of resources for further help and support.

BIBLIOGRAPHIC NOTE

This volume contains documents and excerpts from publications issued by the following U.S. government agencies: Administration for Children and Families (ACF); Center for Parent Information & Resources (CPIR); Centers for Disease Control and Prevention (CDC); Child Welfare Information Gateway; Early Childhood Learning and Knowledge Center (ECLKC); *Eunice Kennedy Shriver* National Institute of Child Health and Human Development (NICHD); girlshealth.gov; Literacy Information and Communication System (LINCS); MedlinePlus; National Center for Education Statistics (NCES); National Council on Disability (NCD); National Human Genome Research Institute (NHGRI); National Institute of Neurological Disorders and Stroke (NINDS); National Institute on Deafness and Other Communication Disorders (NIDCD); National Science Foundation (NSF); StopBullying.gov; Substance Abuse and Mental Health Services Administration (SAMHSA); U.S. Bureau of Labor Statistics (BLS); U.S. Department of Education (ED); U.S. Department of Health and Human Services (HHS); U.S. Social Security Administration (SSA); United States Census Bureau; USA.gov; and Youth.gov.

It also contains original material produced by Infobase and reviewed by medical consultants.

ABOUT THE *HEALTH REFERENCE SERIES*

The *Health Reference Series* is designed to provide basic medical information for patients, families, caregivers, and the general public. Each volume provides comprehensive coverage on a particular topic. This is especially important for people who may be dealing with a newly diagnosed disease or a chronic disorder in themselves or in a family member. People looking for preventive guidance, information about disease warning signs, medical statistics, and risk factors for health problems will also find answers to their questions in the *Health Reference Series*. The *Series*, however, is not intended to serve as a tool for diagnosing illness, in prescribing treatments, or as a substitute for the physician–patient relationship. All people concerned about medical symptoms or the possibility of disease are encouraged to seek professional care from an appropriate health-care provider.

A NOTE ABOUT SPELLING AND STYLE

Health Reference Series editors use *Stedman's Medical Dictionary* as an authority for questions related to the spelling of medical terms and *The*

Chicago Manual of Style for questions related to grammatical structures, punctuation, and other editorial concerns. Consistent adherence is not always possible, however, because the individual volumes within the *Series* include many documents from a wide variety of different producers, and the editor's primary goal is to present material from each source as accurately as is possible. This sometimes means that information in different chapters or sections may follow other guidelines and alternate spelling authorities. For example, occasionally a copyright holder may require that eponymous terms be shown in possessive forms (Crohn's disease vs. Crohn disease) or that British spelling norms be retained (leukaemia vs. leukemia).

MEDICAL REVIEW

Infobase contracts with a team of qualified, senior medical professionals who serve as medical consultants for the *Health Reference Series*. As necessary, medical consultants review reprinted and originally written material for currency and accuracy. Citations including the phrase "Reviewed (month, year)" indicate material reviewed by this team. Medical consultation services are provided to the *Health Reference Series* editors by:
Dr. Vijayalakshmi, MBBS, DGO, MD
Dr. Senthil Selvan, MBBS, DCH, MD
Dr. K. Sivanandham, MBBS, DCH, MS (Research), PhD

HEALTH REFERENCE SERIES UPDATE POLICY

The inaugural book in the *Health Reference Series* was the first edition of *Cancer Sourcebook* published in 1989. Since then, the *Series* has been enthusiastically received by librarians and in the medical community. In order to maintain the standard of providing high-quality health information for the layperson, the editorial staff felt it was necessary to implement a policy of updating volumes when warranted.

Medical researchers have been making tremendous strides, and it is the purpose of the *Health Reference Series* to stay current with the most recent advances. Each decision to update a volume is made on an individual basis. Some of the considerations include how much new information is available and the feedback we receive from people who use the books. If there is a topic you would like to see added to the update list, or an area of medical concern you feel has not been adequately addressed, please write to: custserv@infobaselearning.com.

Part 1 | Understanding and Identifying Learning Disabilities

Chapter 1 | The Brain and Its Function

Chapter Contents
Section 1.1—Basics of the Brain: How the Brain Works 5
Section 1.2—How the Brain Develops 12
Section 1.3—Early Brain Development and Health 18
Section 1.4—Executive Function 21

Section 1.1 | Basics of the Brain: How the Brain Works

This section includes text excerpted from "Brain Basics: Know Your Brain," National Institute of Neurological Disorders and Stroke (NINDS), September 26, 2022.

The brain is the most complex part of the human body. This three-pound organ is the seat of intelligence, interpreter of the senses, initiator of body movement, and controller of behavior. Lying in its bony shell and washed by protective fluid, the brain is the source of all the qualities that define humanity. The brain is the crown jewel of the human body.

For centuries, scientists and philosophers have been fascinated by the brain until they viewed the brain as nearly incomprehensible. Now, however, the brain is beginning to relinquish its secrets. Scientists have learned more about the brain in the past 10 years than in all previous centuries because of the accelerating pace of research in neurological and behavioral science and the development of new research techniques. As a result, Congress named the 1990s the "decade of the brain." At the forefront of research on the brain and other elements of the nervous system is the National Institute of Neurological Disorders and Stroke (NINDS), which conducts and supports scientific studies in the United States and around the world.

This section is a basic introduction to the human brain. It may help you understand how the healthy brain works, how to keep it healthy, and what happens when the brain is diseased or dysfunctional. The cerebrum, ventricles (with cerebrospinal fluid), cerebellum, brain stem (pons and medulla), and other parts of the brain (refer to Figure 1.1).

THE ARCHITECTURE OF THE BRAIN

The brain is like a committee of experts. All the parts of the brain work together, but each part has its own special properties. The brain can be divided into three basic units: the forebrain, the midbrain, and the hindbrain.

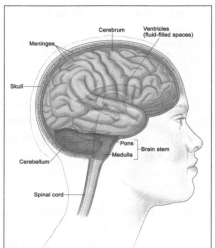
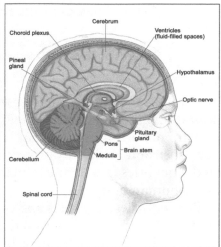

Figure 1.1. Anatomy of Brain *(Source: "Adult Central Nervous System Tumors Treatment (PDQ®)— Patient Version," National Cancer Institute (NCI).)*

The hindbrain includes the upper part of the spinal cord, the brain stem, and a wrinkled ball of tissue called the "cerebellum." The hindbrain controls the body's vital functions, such as respiration and heart rate. The cerebellum coordinates movement and is involved in learned rote movements. When you play the piano or hit a tennis ball, you are activating the cerebellum. The uppermost part of the brainstem is the midbrain, which controls some reflex actions and is part of the circuit involved in the control of eye movements and other voluntary movements. The forebrain is the largest and most highly developed part of the human brain. It consists primarily of the cerebrum and the structures hidden beneath it.

When people see pictures of the brain, it is usually the cerebrum that they notice. The cerebrum sits at the topmost part of the brain and is the source of intellectual activities. It holds your memories, allows you to plan, and enables you to imagine and think. It allows you to recognize friends, read books, and play games.

The cerebrum is split into two halves (hemispheres) by a deep fissure. Despite the split, the two cerebral hemispheres communicate with each other through a thick tract of nerve fibers that lies at the base of this fissure. Although the two hemispheres seem to be mirror images of each other, they are different. For instance, the ability to form words seems to lie primarily in the left hemisphere, while the right hemisphere seems to control many abstract reasoning skills.

For some as-yet-unknown reason, nearly all of the signals from the brain to the body and vice versa cross over on their way to and from the brain. This means that the right cerebral hemisphere primarily controls the left side of the body and the left hemisphere primarily controls the right side. When one side of the brain is damaged, the opposite side of the body is affected. For example, a stroke in the right hemisphere of the brain can leave the left arm and leg paralyzed.

THE GEOGRAPHY OF THOUGHT

Each cerebral hemisphere can be divided into sections, or lobes, each of which specializes in different functions. To understand each lobe and its specialty, take a tour of the cerebral hemispheres, starting with the two frontal lobes, which lie directly behind the forehead. When you plan a schedule, imagine the future, or use reasoned arguments, these two lobes do much of the work. One of the ways the frontal lobes seem to do these things is by acting as short-term storage sites, allowing one idea to be kept in mind while other ideas are considered. In the rearmost portion of each frontal lobe is a motor area, which helps control voluntary movement. A nearby place on the left frontal lobe called "Broca's area" allows thoughts to be transformed into words.

When you enjoy a good meal—the taste, aroma, and texture of the food—two sections behind the frontal lobes called the "parietal lobes" are at work. The forward parts of these lobes, just behind the motor areas, are the primary sensory areas. These areas receive information about temperature, taste, touch, and movement from the rest of the body. Reading and arithmetic are also functions in the repertoire of each parietal lobe.

Most of the time, two areas at the back of the brain are at work. These lobes, called the "occipital lobes," process images from the eyes and link that information with images stored in memory. Damage to the occipital lobes can cause blindness.

The last lobes on the tour of the cerebral hemispheres are the "temporal lobes," which lie in front of the visual areas and nest under the parietal and frontal lobes. Whether you appreciate symphonies or rock music, your brain responds through the activity of these lobes. At the top of each temporal lobe is an area responsible for receiving information from the ears. The underside of each temporal lobe plays a crucial role in forming and retrieving memories, including those associated with music. Other parts of this lobe seem to integrate memories and sensations of taste, sound, sight, and touch.

THE CEREBRAL CORTEX

Coating the surface of the cerebrum and the cerebellum is a vital layer of tissue, the thickness of a stack of two or three dimes. It is called the "cortex," from the Latin word for bark. Most of the actual information processing in the brain takes place in the cerebral cortex. When people talk about "gray matter" in the brain, they are talking about this thin rind. The cortex is gray because nerves in this area lack the insulation that makes most other parts of the brain appear to be white. The folds in the brain add to its surface area and, therefore, increase the amount of gray matter and the quantity of information that can be processed.

THE INNER BRAIN

Deep within the brain, hidden from view, lie structures that are the gatekeepers between the spinal cord and the cerebral hemispheres. These structures not only determine the human emotional state but also modify the perceptions and responses depending on that state and allow us to initiate movements that humans make without thinking about them. Like the lobes in the cerebral hemispheres, the structures come in pairs: each is duplicated in the opposite half of the brain.

The hypothalamus, about the size of a pearl, directs a multitude of important functions. It wakes you up in the morning and gets the adrenaline flowing during a test or job interview. The hypothalamus

The Brain and Its Function

is also an important emotional center, controlling the molecules that make you feel exhilarated, angry, or unhappy. Near the hypothalamus lies the thalamus, a major clearinghouse for information going to and from the spinal cord and the cerebrum.

An arching tract of nerve cells leads from the hypothalamus and the thalamus to the hippocampus. This tiny nub acts as a memory indexer—sending memories out to the appropriate part of the cerebral hemisphere for long-term storage and retrieving them when necessary. The basal ganglia are clusters of nerve cells surrounding the thalamus. They are responsible for initiating and integrating movements. Parkinson disease (PD), which results in tremors, rigidity, and a stiff, shuffling walk, is a disease of nerve cells that lead into the basal ganglia.

MAKING CONNECTIONS

The brain and the rest of the nervous system are composed of many different types of cells, but the primary functional unit is a cell called the "neuron." All sensations, movements, thoughts, memories, and feelings are the result of signals that pass through neurons. Neurons consist of three parts. The cell body contains the nucleus, where most of the molecules that the neuron needs to survive and function are manufactured. Dendrites extend out from the cell body like the branches of a tree and receive messages from other nerve cells. Signals then pass from the dendrites through the cell body and may travel away from the cell body down an axon to another neuron, a muscle cell, or cells in some other organ. The neuron is usually surrounded by many support cells. Some types of cells wrap around the axon to form an insulating sheath. This sheath can include a fatty molecule called "myelin," which provides insulation for the axon and helps nerve signals travel faster and farther. Axons may be very short, such as those that carry signals from one cell in the cortex to another cell less than a hair's width away. Or axons may be very long, such as those that carry messages from the brain all the way down the spinal cord.

Scientists have learned a great deal about neurons by studying the synapse—the place where a signal passes from the neuron to another cell. When the signal reaches the end of the axon, it stimulates the release of tiny sacs. These sacs release chemicals known as "neurotransmitters" into the synapse. The neurotransmitters cross the synapse and attach to receptors on the neighboring cell. These receptors can change the properties of the receiving cell. If the receiving cell is also a neuron, the signal can continue the transmission to the next cell. Here is an illustration of the structure of a typical neuron (refer to Figure 1.2).

SOME KEY NEUROTRANSMITTERS AT WORK

Neurotransmitters are chemicals that brain cells use to talk to each other. Some neurotransmitters make cells more active (called "excitatory"), while others block or dampen a cell's activity (called "inhibitory").

Acetylcholine is an excitatory neurotransmitter because it generally makes cells more excitable. It governs muscle contractions and causes glands to secrete hormones. Alzheimer disease (AD), which initially affects memory formation, is associated with a shortage of acetylcholine.

Glutamate is a major excitatory neurotransmitter. Too much glutamate can kill or damage neurons and has been linked to disorders including PD, stroke, seizures, and increased sensitivity to pain.

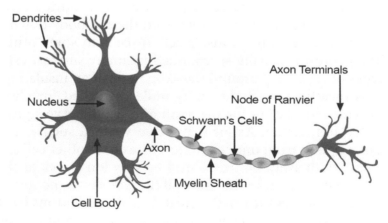

Figure 1.2. Typical Neuron *(Source: "Nerve Tissue," Surveillance, Epidemiology, and End Results (SEER) Program, National Cancer Institute (NCI).)*

The Brain and Its Function

Gamma-aminobutyric acid (GABA) is an inhibitory neurotransmitter that helps control muscle activity and is an important part of the visual system. Drugs that increase GABA levels in the brain are used to treat epileptic seizures and tremors in patients with Huntington disease (HD).

Serotonin is a neurotransmitter that constricts blood vessels and brings on sleep. It is also involved in temperature regulation. Low levels of serotonin may cause sleep problems and depression, while too much serotonin can lead to seizures.

Dopamine is an inhibitory neurotransmitter involved in mood and the control of complex movements. The loss of dopamine activity in some portions of the brain leads to the muscular rigidity of PD. Many medications used to treat behavioral disorders work by modifying the action of dopamine in the brain.

NEUROLOGICAL DISORDERS

The brain is one of the hardest-working organs in the body. When the brain is healthy, it functions quickly and automatically. But, when problems occur, the results can be devastating. Some 100 million Americans suffer from devastating brain disorders at some point in their lives. The NINDS supports research on more than 600 neurological diseases. Some of the major types of disorders include neurogenetic diseases (such as HD and muscular dystrophy), developmental disorders (such as cerebral palsy (CP)), degenerative diseases of adult life (such as PD and AD), metabolic diseases (such as Gaucher disease (GD)), cerebrovascular diseases (such as stroke and vascular dementia), trauma (such as spinal cord and head injury), convulsive disorders (such as epilepsy), infectious diseases (such as acquired immunodeficiency syndrome (AIDS)), dementia, and brain tumors. Knowing more about the brain can lead to the development of new treatments for diseases and disorders of the nervous system and improve many areas of human health.

Learning Disabilities Sourcebook, Seventh Edition

Section 1.2 | How the Brain Develops

This section includes text excerpted from "Understanding the Effects of Maltreatment on Brain Development," Child Welfare Information Gateway, U.S. Department of Health and Human Services (HHS), April 2015. Reviewed November 2022.

Learning about the process of brain development helps us understand more about the roles both genetics and the environment play in human development. It appears that genetics predispose us to develop in certain ways, but experiences, including interactions with other people, have a significant impact on how human predispositions are expressed. In fact, research now shows that many capacities thought to be fixed at birth are actually dependent on a sequence of experiences combined with heredity. Both factors are essential for the optimum development of the human brain.

EARLY BRAIN DEVELOPMENT

The raw material of the brain is the nerve cell, called the "neuron." During fetal development, neurons are created and migrate to form the various parts of the brain. As neurons migrate, they also differentiate or specialize in governing specific functions in the body in response to chemical signals. This process of development occurs sequentially from the "bottom up," that is, from areas of the brain controlling the most primitive functions of the body (e.g., heart rate, breathing) to the most sophisticated functions (e.g., complex thought).

The first areas of the brain to fully develop are the brainstem and midbrain; they govern the bodily functions necessary for life, called the "autonomic functions." At birth, these lower portions of the nervous system are very well developed, whereas the higher regions (the limbic system and cerebral cortex) are still rather primitive. Higher-function brain regions involved in regulating emotions, language, and abstract thought grow rapidly in the first three years of life.

THE GROWING CHILD'S BRAIN

Brain development, or learning, is actually the process of creating, strengthening, and discarding connections among the neurons; these connections are called "synapses." Synapses organize the brain by forming pathways that connect the parts of the brain governing everything humans do—from breathing and sleeping to thinking and feeling. This is the essence of postnatal brain development because, at birth, very few synapses have been formed. The synapses present at birth are primarily those that govern human bodily functions such as heart rate, breathing, eating, and sleeping. The development of synapses occurs at an astounding rate during a child's early years in response to that child's experiences. At its peak, the cerebral cortex of a healthy toddler may create two million synapses per second. By the time children are two years old, their brains have approximately 100 trillion synapses, many more than they will ever need. Oriented on the child's experiences, some synapses are strengthened and remain intact, but many are gradually discarded. This process of synapse elimination—or pruning—is a normal part of development. By the time children reach adolescence, about half of their synapses have been discarded, leaving the number they will have for most of the rest of their lives.

Another important process that takes place in the developing brain is myelination. Myelin is the white fatty tissue that forms a sheath to insulate mature brain cells, thus ensuring the clear transmission of neurotransmitters across synapses. Young children process information slowly because their brain cells lack the myelin necessary for fast, clear nerve impulse transmission. Like other neuronal growth processes, myelination begins in the primary motor and sensory areas (the brain stem and cortex) and gradually progresses to the higher-order regions that control thought, memories, and feelings. Also, like other neuronal growth processes, a child's experiences affect the rate and growth of myelination, which continues into young adulthood.

By three years of age, a baby's brain has reached almost 90 percent of its adult size. The growth in each region of the brain largely depends on receiving stimulation, which spurs activity in that region. This stimulation provides the foundation for learning.

ADOLESCENT BRAIN DEVELOPMENT
Studies using magnetic resonance imaging (MRI) techniques show that the brain continues to grow and develop into young adulthood

(at least to the mid-twenties). White matter, or brain tissue, volume has been shown to increase in adults as old as 32. Right before puberty, adolescent brains experience a growth spurt that occurs mainly in the frontal lobe, which is the area that governs planning, impulse control, and reasoning. During the teenage years, the brain goes through a process of pruning synapses—somewhat like the infant and toddler brain—and also sees an increase in white matter and changes in neurotransmitter systems. As the teenager grows into young adulthood, the brain develops more myelin to insulate the nerve fibers and speed neural processing, and this myelination occurs last in the frontal lobe. MRI comparisons between the brains of teenagers and the brains of young adults have shown that most of the brain areas were the same—that is, the teenage brain had reached maturity in the areas that govern such abilities as speech and sensory capabilities. The major difference was the immaturity of the teenage brain in the frontal lobe and in the myelination of that area.

Normal puberty and adolescence lead to the maturation of a physical body, but the brain lags behind in development, especially in the areas that allow teenagers to reason and think logically. Most teenagers act impulsively at times, using a lower area of their brains—their "gut reaction"—because their frontal lobes are not yet mature. Impulsive behavior, poor decisions, and increased risk-taking are all part of the normal teenage experience. Another change that happens during adolescence is the growth and transformation of the limbic system, which is responsible for emotions. Teenagers may rely on their more primitive limbic system in interpreting emotions and reacting since they lack the more mature cortex that can override the limbic response.

PLASTICITY—THE INFLUENCE OF THE ENVIRONMENT

Researchers use the term plasticity to describe the brain's ability to change in response to repeated stimulation. The extent of a brain's plasticity is dependent on the stage of development and the particular brain system or region affected. For instance, the lower parts of the brain, which control basic functions such as breathing and heart rate, are less flexible, or plastic, than the higher

The Brain and Its Function

functioning cortex, which controls thoughts and feelings. While cortex plasticity decreases as a child gets older, some degree of plasticity remains. In fact, this brain plasticity is what allows us to keep learning into adulthood and throughout human lives.

The developing brain's ongoing adaptations are the result of both genetics and experience. Human brains prepare us to expect certain experiences by forming the pathways needed to respond to those experiences. For example, human brains are "wired" to respond to the sound of speech; when babies hear people speaking, the neural systems in their brains responsible for speech and language receive the necessary stimulation to organize and function. The more babies are exposed to people speaking, the stronger their oriented synapses become. If the appropriate exposure does not happen, the pathways developed in anticipation may be discarded. This is sometimes referred to as the concept of using it or losing it. It is through these processes of creating, strengthening, and discarding synapses that human brains adapt to a unique environment.

The ability to adapt to the human environment is a part of normal development. Children growing up in cold climates, on rural farms, or in large sibling groups learn how to function in those environments. Regardless of the general environment, though, all children need stimulation and nurturance for healthy development. If these are lacking (e.g., if a child's caretakers are indifferent, hostile, depressed, or cognitively impaired), the child's brain development may be impaired. Because the brain adapts to its environment, it will adapt to a negative environment just as readily as it will adapt to a positive one.

SENSITIVE PERIODS

Researchers believe that there are sensitive periods for the development of certain capabilities. These refer to windows of time in the developmental process when certain parts of the brain may be most susceptible to particular experiences. Animal studies have shed light on sensitive periods, showing, for example, that animals that are artificially blinded during the sensitive period for developing a vision may never develop the capability to see, even if the blinding mechanism is later removed.

It is more difficult to study human-sensitive periods, but if certain synapses and neuronal pathways are not repeatedly activated, they may be discarded, and their capabilities may diminish. For example, infants have a genetic predisposition to form strong attachments to their primary caregivers, but they may not be able to achieve strong attachments, or trusting, durable bonds if they are in a severely neglectful situation with little one-on-one caregiver contact. Children from Romanian institutions that had been severely neglected had a much better attachment response if they were placed in foster care—and thus received more stable parenting—before they were 24 months old. This indicates that there is a sensitive period for attachment, but it is likely that there is a general sensitive period rather than a true cutoff point for recovery.

While sensitive periods exist for development and learning, the plasticity of the brain also often allows children to recover from missing certain experiences. Both children and adults may be able to make up for missed experiences later in life, but it is likely to be more difficult. This is especially true if a young child was deprived of certain stimulation, which resulted in the pruning of synapses (neuronal connections) relevant to that stimulation and the loss of neuronal pathways. As children progress through each developmental stage, they will learn and master each step more easily if their brains have built an efficient network of pathways to support optimal functioning.

MEMORIES

The organizing framework for children's development is oriented toward the creation of memories. When repeated experiences strengthen a neuronal pathway, the pathway becomes encoded, and it eventually becomes a memory. Children learn to put one foot in front of the other to walk. They learn words to express themselves. And they learn that a smile usually brings a smile in return. At some point, they no longer have to think much about these processes—their brains manage these experiences with little effort because the memories that have been created allow for a smooth, efficient flow of information.

The Brain and Its Function

The creation of memories is part of human adaptation to the environment. The human brains attempt to understand the world around us and fashion their interactions with that world in a way that promotes human survival, and hopefully growth, but if the early environment is abusive or neglectful, human brains may create memories of these experiences that adversely color the view of the world throughout their life.

Babies are born with the capacity for implicit memory, which means that they can perceive their environment and recall it in certain unconscious ways. For instance, they recognize their mother's voice from an unconscious memory. These early implicit memories may have a significant impact on a child's subsequent attachment relationships.

In contrast, explicit memory, which develops around age two, refers to conscious memories and is tied to language development. Explicit memory allows children to talk about themselves in the past and future or in different places or circumstances through the process of conscious recollection.

Sometimes, children who have been abused or suffered other trauma may not retain or be able to access explicit memories of their experiences; however, they may retain implicit memories of the physical or emotional sensations, and these implicit memories may produce flashbacks, nightmares, or other uncontrollable reactions. This may be the case with very young children or infants who suffer abuse or neglect.

RESPONDING TO STRESS

Humans experience different types of stress throughout their lives. The type of stress and the timing of that stress determine whether and how there is an impact on the brain. The National Scientific Council on the Developing Child (NSCDC) outlines the following three classifications of stress:

- **Positive stress**. It is moderate, brief, and generally a normal part of life (e.g., entering a new childcare setting). Learning to adjust to this type of stress is an essential component of healthy development.

- **Tolerable stress.** It includes events that have the potential to alter the developing brain negatively but occur infrequently and give the brain time to recover (e.g., the death of a loved one).
- **Toxic stress.** It includes strong, frequent, and prolonged activation of the body's stress response system (e.g., chronic neglect).

Healthy responses to typical life stressors (i.e., positive and tolerable stress events) are very complex and may change depending on individual and environmental characteristics, such as genetics, the presence of a sensitive and responsive caregiver, and past experiences.

A healthy stress response involves a variety of hormone and neurochemical systems throughout the body, including the sympathetic-adrenomedullary (SAM) system, which produces adrenaline, and the hypothalamic-pituitary-adrenocortical (HPA) system, which produces cortisol. Increases in adrenaline help the body engage energy stores and alter blood flow. Increases in cortisol also help the body engage energy stores and can also enhance certain types of memory and activate immune responses. In a healthy stress response, the hormonal levels will return to normal after the stressful experience has passed.

Section 1.3 | Early Brain Development and Health

This section includes text excerpted from "Early Brain Development and Health," Centers for Disease Control and Prevention (CDC), March 25, 2022.

The early years of a child's life are very important for later health and development. One of the main reasons is how fast the brain grows, starting before birth and continuing into early childhood. Although the brain continues to develop and change into adulthood, the first eight years can build a foundation for future learning, health, and

The Brain and Its Function

life success. How well a brain develops depends on many factors in addition to genes, such as:
- Proper nutrition during pregnancy
- Exposure to toxins or infections
- The child's experiences with other people and the world

Nurturing and responsive care for the child's body and mind is the key to supporting healthy brain development. Positive or negative experiences can add up to shape a child's development and can have lifelong effects. To nurture their child's body and mind, parents and caregivers need support and the right resources. The right care for children, starting before birth and continuing through childhood, ensures that the child's brain grows well and reaches its full potential. The Centers for Disease Control and Prevention (CDC) is working to protect children so that their brains have a healthy start.

THE IMPORTANCE OF EARLY CHILDHOOD EXPERIENCES FOR BRAIN DEVELOPMENT

Children are born ready to learn and have many skills to learn over many years. They depend on parents, family members, and other caregivers as their first teachers to develop the right skills to become independent and lead healthy and successful lives. How the brain grows is strongly affected by the child's experiences with other people and the world. Nurturing care for the mind is critical for brain growth. Children grow and learn best in a safe environment where they are protected from neglect and from extreme or chronic stress, with plenty of opportunities to play and explore.

Parents and other caregivers can support healthy brain growth by speaking to, playing with, and caring for their children. Children learn best when parents take turns when talking and playing and build on their child's skills and interests. Nurturing a child by understanding their needs and responding sensitively helps protect children's brains from stress. Speaking with children and exposing them to books, stories, and songs helps strengthen children's language and communication, which puts them on a path toward learning and succeeding in school.

Exposure to stress and trauma can have long-term negative consequences for the child's brain, whereas talking, reading, and playing can stimulate brain growth. Ensuring that parents, caregivers, and early childhood care providers have the resources and skills to provide safe, stable, nurturing, and stimulating care is an important public health goal.

When children are at risk, tracking their development and making sure they reach developmental milestones can help ensure that any problems are detected early and children can receive the intervention they may need.

A HEALTHY START FOR THE BRAIN

To learn and grow appropriately, a baby's brain has to be healthy and protected from diseases and other risks. Promoting the development of a healthy brain can start even before pregnancy. For example, a healthy diet and the right nutrients, such as sufficient folic acid, will promote a healthy pregnancy and a healthy nervous system in the growing baby. Vaccinations can protect pregnant women from infections that can harm the brain of the unborn baby.

During pregnancy, the brain can be affected by many types of risks, such as infectious diseases such as cytomegalovirus or Zika virus; exposure to toxins, including from smoking or alcohol; or when pregnant mothers experience stress, trauma, or mental health conditions such as depression. Regular health care during pregnancy can help prevent complications, including premature birth, which can affect the baby's brain. Newborn screening can detect conditions that are potentially dangerous to the child's brain, such as phenylketonuria (PKU).

Healthy brain growth in infancy continues to depend on the right care and nutrition. Because children's brains are still growing, they are especially vulnerable to traumatic head injuries, infections, or toxins, such as lead. Childhood vaccines, such as the measles vaccine, can protect children from dangerous complications such as swelling of the brain. Ensuring that parents and caregivers have access to healthy foods and places to live and play that are healthy and safe for their children can help them provide more nurturing care.

The Brain and Its Function

Section 1.4 | Executive Function

This section contains text excerpted from the following sources: Text beginning with the heading "What Is Executive Function?" is excerpted from "Executive Function," Administration for Children and Families (ACF), U.S. Department of Health and Human Services (HHS), January 11, 2017. Reviewed November 2022; Text beginning with the heading "A Common Feature of Many Disabilities and Disorders That Impair Learning" is excerpted from "Executive Function: Implications for Education," U.S. Department of Education (ED), 2016. Reviewed November 2022.

WHAT IS EXECUTIVE FUNCTION?

Executive function (EF) or self-regulation is the foundation for lifelong functioning in critical thinking and problem-solving, planning, decision-making, and executing tasks. The EF or self-regulatory capacities are the building blocks for many important skills. These skills mature at different rates and develop over time. Working memory and self-control are among the first set of EF that develop (typically during early childhood), setting the stage for attentional capacities and goal-directed behavior during the preteens years, better planning and refined goal-directed behavior during adolescence, and more efficient problem-solving, decision-making, and cognitive flexibility in adulthood.

The experience of trauma, especially when it is prolonged, can disrupt executive functioning skills. Children who have experienced prolonged or pronounced stress and adversity, including poverty and trauma experiences, may struggle more than other children to regulate their thoughts, feelings, and behaviors. Severe childhood stress appears to have lasting effects, with EF or self-regulation-related difficulties seen into adulthood. In addition, adolescents who report having experienced trauma, such as maltreatment or exposure to a parent's intimate partner violence, are less effective than their peers at controlling their attention, regulating their emotions, and planning. Adults whose overall functioning has been compromised by adversity and continued stress are less likely to engage in intentional self-regulation and have difficulty with problem-solving and impulse control. Less is known about the effects of trauma in adulthood on executive functioning and related skills.

WHY IS THE CONCEPT OF EXECUTIVE FUNCTION IMPORTANT TO HUMAN SERVICES?

Executive functions involve regions of the brain associated with information processing (including attention and working memory), regulating emotions and behavior (including impulse control and suppressing inappropriate responses), creativity, and some aspects of personality. Individuals with executive functions in childhood or adulthood may have difficulty with social appropriateness, planning projects, working independently, remembering details, paying attention, or starting and completing tasks.

Human service agencies can strive to build and enhance executive functioning skills for their programs' children, youth, and adults. Improving executive functioning skills will be needed to promote engagement and participation in human service programs for individuals who are also impacted by toxic stress, trauma, and other adverse experiences. Children and adults who can develop these skills may be better able to benefit from programs and services provided by human services agencies.

It is important for human service agencies to keep in mind that executive functioning skills change across development from infancy through late life. For example, programs serving infants from birth to three years may be designed to support the child's ability to maintain focus and attention, show persistence in actions, and demonstrate flexibility in actions and behavior. Preschool programs may target increasing the child's ability to control impulses, maintain focus, persist in tasks, hold information, and demonstrate flexibility in thinking and behavior. Programs serving older children may target additional developmentally appropriate skills and abilities, including planning, problem-solving, and organizing. Programs may address reasoning, goal-setting, and decision-making in adolescence and adulthood. Agencies focused on supportive care for older adults may offer cognitive health promotion programs that enhance cognition, memory, and inhibitory control.

RELEVANT INTERVENTIONS AND APPROACHES

A wide range of activities requires executive functioning skills, and targeted interventions may foster these skills. Interventions to improve executive functions include training working memory, mindfulness programs to help address focus and attention, routine structure and organization to facilitate task completion, and coaching to motivate behavior. However, it is important to consider carefully how executive functioning and other regulation-related skills are defined and measured in research and evaluation. Programs that improve one specific skill will not necessarily improve other related skills.

Human services agencies offer various social services and support for individuals, children and families, and adults throughout their life spans. While the programs may differ regarding the target population, services provided, and expected outcomes, a general understanding of how executive functioning and self-regulation skills can foster optimal health, development, and well-being will be important for all programs and staff. Human services agencies are well-positioned to use information about the importance of executive functioning skills in program planning, design, implementation, staff development, and family engagement efforts.

A COMMON FEATURE OF MANY DISABILITIES AND DISORDERS THAT IMPAIR LEARNING

Given the important role that EF plays in learning and the robust association between EF and academic achievement, it is perhaps not surprising that difficulties with EF, particularly in working memory, are associated with learning difficulties and specific learning disabilities. Difficulties with EF are also associated with autism spectrum disorder (ASD), conduct disorder, obsessive-compulsive disorder (OCD), and attention deficit hyperactivity disorder (ADHD). Different aspects of EF may be implicated in each disorder. Still, there are also reasons to believe that the same EF difficulties may result from many different forms of atypical cognitive development.

The EF difficulty may then be expected to interfere with learning directly through the ability to process complex information and indirectly through behaviors related to learning. Several studies have found EF is also implicated in specific learning disabilities such as reading disabilities. Working memory, in particular, is related to specific language impairment.

Difficulties with different aspects of EF may be implicated in different forms of a single disorder. Because of the multiple influences on and pathways that interact with EF, researchers are working to identify the heterogeneity in disorders characterized by EF difficulty. They are also exploring the heterogeneity of psychological functioning in typically developing populations to better understand the etiology, diagnosis, and treatment of disorders. For example, although models of ADHD have focused on EF deficits as a core feature of the disorder, there is evidence that ADHD is a heterogeneous disorder, with different subtypes, and that several pathways can lead to ADHD, including increased sensitivity to rewards, particularly in adolescence. Castellanos and colleagues have proposed that while inattention symptoms are due to cool EF deficits, hyperactivity/impulsivity symptoms depend on more difficulties with hot EF. Empirical studies suggest that measures of hot EF (e.g., delay aversion or the motivation to escape or avoid delay) and measures of cool EF (e.g., the stop-signal task that measures inhibitory control) are independent predictors of ADHD status. Furthermore, even after controlling for working memory, hot EF is associated with symptoms of hyperactivity/impulsivity but not with inattention.

It is currently unclear to what extent difficulties with EF contribute to the broad category of emotional and behavioral disorders (EBDs; Individuals with Disabilities Education Act (IDEA) Regulations, Section 300.8 c 4). However, several studies have found EF to be associated with conduct problems in preschool-aged children. Others have found EF to relate to parent reports of social competence and social skills in elementary school. This is an area for future research, and it will be of interest to examine the role of hot versus cool EF in EBDs and the role of bottom-up influences such as stress and arousal.

EXECUTIVE FUNCTION AND LEARNING
The executive function provides a valuable lens for looking at the challenges that learners may face in mastering specific academic

content, such as those aspects of mathematics and reading that make substantial demands on EF. The distinction between EF and knowledge-based aspects of ability and learning is important for education. Both are vitally important, but effective approaches to fostering EF skills are particularly important in the early stages of development because these skills allow children to acquire content knowledge more easily. There are currently some good examples of programs and approaches that effectively promote EF skills. A growing body of intervention studies has established that the acquisition of EF skills can be enhanced through repeated practice in reflecting upon and using specific EF skills. This research suggests that it is important to keep children motivated to practice EF skills and to challenge those skills continually using a graduated series of exercises that vary in difficulty. However, much more work is needed to develop and refine promising approaches and extend these programs to the later elementary and secondary grades. Although the acquisition of EF skills may be especially important in early childhood, these skills continue to be necessary for learning and adaptation across the life span. Programs focusing on EF in education have been developed primarily for early childhood. However, the principles on which these programs are based also apply to learning and achievement throughout the elementary and secondary grades. An important direction for future research is to develop programs to foster EF that are applicable throughout the school years.

A related point is a need for continued research on the measurement of EF skills and the typical course of EF development in childhood. Although there is ongoing psychometric and longitudinal developmental research is needed for increasingly well-established measures of EF appropriate for longitudinal use. A central goal of this research will be to develop measures that can be used in formative assessments of school-based programs designed to foster self-regulation. This is highly relevant to developing and refining programs for children with or at risk for specific learning disabilities and other developmental disorders that interfere with learning, including ADHD and EBDs. Assessment of EF before kindergarten and during the school years would provide for more rapid detection of potential EF difficulties, potentially leading to earlier and more effective intervention and remediation. In addition, information about developmental and individual differences in EF may support the tailoring of individual and classroom-based instruction, as when teachers scaffold children's EF skills when introducing new concepts.

Chapter 2 | Early Learning, Speech, and Language Development Milestones

Chapter Contents
Section 2.1—Speech and Language Development
　　　　　Milestones 29
Section 2.2—Language and Linguistics: Language
　　　　　Acquisition 32

Section 2.1 | Speech and Language Development Milestones

This section includes text excerpted from "Speech and Language Developmental Milestones," National Institute on Deafness and Other Communication Disorders (NIDCD), October 13, 2022.

WHAT ARE VOICE, SPEECH, AND LANGUAGE?

Voice, speech, and language are the tools we use to communicate with each other.

Voice is the sound we make as air from our lungs is pushed between vocal folds in our larynx, causing them to vibrate.

Speech is talking, which is one way to express language. It involves the precisely coordinated muscle actions of the tongue, lips, jaw, and vocal tract to produce the recognizable sounds that make up language.

Language is a set of shared rules that allow people to express their ideas in a meaningful way. Language may be expressed verbally or by writing, signing, or making other gestures, such as eye blinking or mouth movements.

HOW DO SPEECH AND LANGUAGE DEVELOP?

The first three years of life, when the brain is developing and maturing, is the most intensive period for acquiring speech and language skills. These skills develop best in a world that is rich with sounds, sights, and consistent exposure to the speech and language of others.

There appear to be critical periods for speech and language development in infants and young children when the brain is best able to absorb language. If these critical periods are allowed to pass without exposure to language, it will be more difficult to learn.

WHAT ARE THE MILESTONES FOR SPEECH AND LANGUAGE DEVELOPMENT?

The first signs of communication occur when an infant learns that a cry will bring food, comfort, and companionship. Newborns also begin to recognize important sounds in their environment, such as the voice of their mother or primary caretaker. As they grow, babies begin to sort out the speech sounds that compose the words of their language. By six months of age, most babies recognize the basic sounds of their native language.

Children vary in their development of speech and language skills. However, they follow a natural progression or timetable for mastering the skills of language. A checklist of milestones for the normal development of speech and language skills in children from birth to five years of age is included below. These milestones help doctors and other health professionals determine if a child is on track or if she or he may need extra help. Sometimes, a delay may be caused by hearing loss, while other times, it may be due to a speech or language disorder.

WHAT IS THE DIFFERENCE BETWEEN A SPEECH DISORDER AND A LANGUAGE DISORDER?

Children who have trouble understanding what others say (receptive language) or difficulty sharing their thoughts (expressive language) may have a language disorder. Specific language impairment (SLI) is a language disorder that delays the mastery of language skills. Some children with SLI may not begin to talk until their third or fourth year.

Children who have trouble producing speech sounds correctly or who hesitate or stutter when talking may have a speech disorder. Apraxia of speech is a speech disorder that makes it difficult to put sounds and syllables together in the correct order to form words.

WHAT SHOULD BE DONE IF A CHILD'S SPEECH OR LANGUAGE APPEARS TO BE DELAYED?

Talk to your child's doctor if you have any concerns. Your doctor may refer you to a speech-language pathologist, who is a health professional trained to evaluate and treat people with speech or language disorders. The speech-language pathologist will talk to you about your child's communication and general development. She or he will also use special spoken tests to evaluate your child. A hearing test is often included in the evaluation because a hearing problem can affect speech and language development. Depending on the result of the evaluation, the speech-language pathologist may suggest activities you can do at home to stimulate your child's development. They might also recommend a group or individual therapy or suggest further evaluation by an audiologist (a health-care professional trained to identify and measure hearing loss) or a developmental psychologist (a health-care professional with special expertise in the psychological development of infants and children).

WHAT RESEARCH IS BEING CONDUCTED ON DEVELOPMENTAL SPEECH AND LANGUAGE PROBLEMS?

The National Institute on Deafness and Other Communication Disorders (NIDCD) sponsors a broad range of research to better understand the development of speech and language disorders, improve diagnostic capabilities, and fine-tune more effective treatments. An ongoing area of study is the search for better ways to diagnose and differentiate among the various types of speech delay. A large study following approximately 4,000 children is gathering data as the children grow to establish reliable signs and symptoms for specific speech disorders, which can then be used to develop accurate diagnostic tests. Additional genetic studies are looking for matches between different genetic variations and specific speech deficits.

Researchers sponsored by the NIDCD have discovered one genetic variant, in particular, that is linked to SLI, a disorder that delays children's use of words and slows their mastery of language skills throughout their school years. The finding is the first to tie the presence of a distinct genetic mutation to any kind of inherited language impairment. Further research is exploring the role this genetic variant may also play in dyslexia, autism, and speech-sound disorders.

A long-term study looking at how deafness impacts the brain is exploring how the brain "rewires" itself to accommodate deafness. So far, the research has shown that adults who are deaf react faster and more accurately than hearing adults when they observe objects in motion. This ongoing research continues to explore the concept of "brain plasticity"—the ways in which the brain is influenced by health conditions or life experiences—and how it can be used to develop learning strategies that encourage healthy language and speech development in early childhood.

A workshop convened by the NIDCD drew together a group of experts to explore issues oriented to a subgroup of children with autism spectrum disorders (ASDs) who do not have functional verbal language by the age of five. Because these children are so different from one another, with no set of defining characteristics or patterns of cognitive strengths or weaknesses, the development of standard assessment tests or effective treatments has been difficult. The workshop featured a series of presentations to familiarize participants with the challenges facing these children and helped them identify a number of research gaps and opportunities that could be addressed in future research studies.

Section 2.2 | Language and Linguistics: Language Acquisition

This section includes text excerpted from "Language and Linguistics: Introduction | NSF—National Science Foundation," National Science Foundation (NSF), December 30, 2019.

Almost all human beings acquire a language (and sometimes more than one), to the level of native competency, before age five. How do children accomplish this remarkable feat in such a short amount of time? Which aspects of language acquisition are biologically programmed into the human brain, and which are oriented on experience? Do adults learn language differently from children? Researchers have long debated the answers to these questions, but there is one thing they agree on: language acquisition is a complex process.

Most researchers agree that children acquire language through an interplay of biology and environmental factors. A challenge for linguists is to figure out how nature and nurture come together to influence language learning.

Early Learning, Speech, and Language Development Milestones

EMPHASIS ON NATURE

Some researchers theorize that children are born with an innate biological "device" for understanding the principles and organization common to all languages. According to this theory, the brain's "language module" gets programmed to follow the specific grammar of the language a child is exposed to early in life. Yet the language rules and grammar children use in their speech often exceed the input to which they are exposed. What accounts for this discrepancy?

That is where the theory of universal grammar comes in. This theory posits that all languages have the same basic structural foundation. While children are not genetically "hardwired" to speak a particular language such as Dutch or Japanese, universal grammar lets them learn the rules and patterns of these languages—including those they were never explicitly taught. Some linguists believe that universal grammar and its interaction with the rest of the brain is the design mechanism that allows children to become fluent in any language during the first few years of life. In fact, childhood may be a critical period for the acquisition of language capabilities. Some scientists claim that if a person does not acquire any language before the teenage years, they will never do so in a functional sense. Children may also have a heightened ability, compared to adults, to learn second languages—especially in natural settings. Adults, however, may have some advantages in the conscious study of a second language in a classroom setting.

NO NONSENSE: BABIES RECOGNIZE SYLLABLES

Babies are born into a world buzzing with new noises. How do they interpret sounds and make sense of what they hear? At the University of Wisconsin-Madison, researcher Dr. Jenny Saffran, Ph.D., strives to answer these types of questions by studying the learning abilities "that babies bring to the table" for language acquisition. "Studying learning gives us the chance to see the links between nature and nurture," says Saffran.

One thing babies must learn about language is where words begin and end in a fluid stream of speech. This is not an easy task because the spaces perceived between words in sentences are obvious only if it is familiar with the language being spoken. It is difficult to recognize word boundaries in foreign speech. Yet, according to Saffran, by seven or eight months of age, babies can pluck words out of sentences.

In her studies, Saffran introduced babies to a simple nonsense language of made-up, two-syllable words spoken in a stream of monotone speech. There are no pauses between the "words," but the syllables are presented in a particular order. If the babies recognize the pattern, they can use it to identify word boundaries in subsequent experiments. To test this, Saffran plays new strings of speech where only some parts fit the previous pattern, then records how long the babies pay attention to the familiar versus novel "words." Since babies consistently pay attention to unfamiliar sounds for longer periods than familiar ones, a difference in attention times indicates what the babies learned from their initial exposure to nonsense language.

Saffran's research suggests babies readily identify patterns in speech and can even evaluate the statistical probability that a string of sounds represents a word. Her research reveals the sophisticated learning capabilities involved in language acquisition and demonstrates how these skills evolve as an infant matures.

EMPHASIS ON EXPERIENCE AND USAGE

Not all linguists believe that innate capacities are most important in language learning. Some researchers place greater emphasis on the influence of usage and experience in language acquisition. They argue that adults play an important role in language acquisition by speaking to children—often in a slow, grammatical, and repetitive way. In turn, children discern patterns in the language and experiment with speech gradually—uttering single words at first and eventually stringing them together to construct abstract expressions. At first glance, this may seem reminiscent of how language is traditionally taught in classrooms. But most scientists think children and adults learn language differently.

Early Learning, Speech, and Language Development Milestones

While they may not do it as quickly and easily as children seem to, adults can learn to speak new languages proficiently. However, few would be mistaken for a native speaker of a non-native tongue. Childhood may be a critical period for mastering certain aspects of language, such as proper pronunciation. What factors account for the different language learning capabilities of adults and children? Researchers suggest that accumulated experience and knowledge could change the brain over time, altering the way language information is organized and/or processed.

Chapter 3 | Learning Disabilities: An Overview

WHAT IS A LEARNING DISABILITY?
Learning disabilities are conditions that affect the ability to learn. They can cause problems with the following:
- Understanding what people are saying.
- Speaking.
- Reading.
- Writing.
- Doing math.
- Paying attention.

Often, children have more than one kind of learning disability. They may also have another condition, such as attention deficit hyperactivity disorder (ADHD), which can make learning even more of a challenge.

WHAT CAUSES LEARNING DISABILITIES?
Learning disabilities do not have anything to do with intelligence. They are caused by differences in the brain, and they affect the way the brain processes information. These differences are usually present at birth. But there are certain factors that can play a role in the development of a learning disability, including:
- Genetics
- Environmental exposures (such as lead)
- Problems during pregnancy (such as the mother's drug use)

This chapter includes text excerpted from "Learning Disabilities," MedlinePlus, National Institutes of Health (NIH), September 24, 2019.

HOW TO IDENTIFY IF A CHILD HAS LEARNING DISABILITY
The earlier you can find and treat a learning disability, the better. Unfortunately, learning disabilities are usually not recognized until a child is in school. If you notice that your child is struggling, talk to your child's teacher or health-care provider about an evaluation for a learning disability. The evaluation may include a medical exam, a discussion of family history, and intellectual and school performance testing.

WHAT ARE THE TREATMENTS FOR LEARNING DISABILITIES?
The most common treatment for learning disabilities is special education. A teacher or other learning specialist can help your child learn skills by building on strengths and finding ways to make up for weaknesses. Educators may try special teaching methods, make changes to the classroom, or use technologies that can assist your child's learning needs. Some children also get help from tutors or speech or language therapists.

A child with a learning disability may struggle with low self-esteem, frustration, and other problems. Mental health professionals can help your child understand these feelings, develop coping tools, and build healthy relationships.

If your child has another condition, such as ADHD, she or he will need treatment for that condition as well.

Chapter 4 | Diagnosing Learning Disabilities

Learning disabilities are often identified once a child is in school. The school may use a process called "response to intervention" (RTI) to help identify children with learning disabilities. Special tests are required to make a diagnosis.

RESPONSE TO INTERVENTION
Response to intervention usually involves the following:
- Monitoring all students' progress closely to identify possible learning problems.
- Providing children who are having problems with help on different levels or tiers.
- Moving children to tiers that provide increasing support if they do not show sufficient progress.

Students who are struggling in school can also have individual evaluations. An evaluation can:
- Identify whether a child has a learning disability.
- Determine a child's eligibility under federal law for special education services.
- Help develop an individualized education plan (IEP) that outlines help for a child who qualifies for special education services.
- Establish benchmarks to measure the child's progress.

This chapter includes text excerpted from "How Are Learning Disabilities Diagnosed?" *Eunice Kennedy Shriver* National Institute of Child Health and Human Development (NICHD), September 11, 2018. Reviewed November 2022.

A full evaluation for a learning disability includes the following:
- A medical exam, including a neurological exam, that is to rule out other possible causes of the child's difficulties. These might include emotional disorders, intellectual and developmental disabilities, and brain diseases.
- Reviewing the child's developmental, social, and school performance.
- A discussion of family history.
- Academic and psychological testing.

Usually, several specialists work as a team to do the evaluation. The team may include a psychologist, a special education expert, and a speech-language pathologist. Many schools also have reading specialists who can help diagnose a reading disability.

ROLE OF SCHOOL PSYCHOLOGISTS
School psychologists are trained in both education and psychology. They can help diagnose students with learning disabilities and help the student and her or his parents and teachers come up with plans to improve learning.

ROLE OF SPEECH-LANGUAGE PATHOLOGISTS
All speech-language pathologists are trained to diagnose and treat speech and language disorders. A speech-language pathologist can do a language evaluation and assess the child's ability to organize her or his thoughts and possessions. The speech-language pathologist may evaluate the child's learning skills, such as understanding directions, manipulating sounds, and reading and writing.

Chapter 5 | Evaluating Children for Learning Disabilities

THE PURPOSE OF EVALUATION
Many children have trouble in school. Some have trouble learning to read or write. Others have a hard time remembering new information. Still, others may have trouble behaving themselves. Children can have all sorts of problems.

It is important to find out why a child is not doing well in school. The child may have a disability. By law, schools must provide special help to eligible children with disabilities. This help is called "special education" and "related services."

You may ask the school to evaluate your child, or the school may ask you for permission to do an evaluation. If the school thinks your child may have a disability and may need special education and related services, the school must evaluate your child before providing your child with these services. This evaluation is at no cost to you.

Once you give your informed written permission for the evaluation, the school has 60 days to evaluate your child. (If your state has set its own time frame for conducting evaluations, then the school will follow the state's time frame.) The evaluation will tell you and the school:
- If your child has a disability
- What kind of special help your child needs in school

This chapter includes text excerpted from "Your Child's Evaluation," Center for Parent Information & Resources (CPIR), U.S. Department of Education (ED), April 2022.

STEP 1: USING WHAT IS KNOWN

A team of people, including you, will be involved in evaluating your child. This team will begin by looking at what is already known about your child. The team will look at your child's school file and recent test scores. You and your child's teacher(s) may provide information to be included in this review.

The evaluation team needs enough information to decide if your child has a disability. It also needs to know what kind of special help your child needs. Is there enough information about your child to answer these questions? If your child is being evaluated for the first time, maybe not.

STEP 2: COLLECTING MORE INFORMATION

The team of people involved in your child's evaluation, including you, will identify what additional information about your child is needed in order to answer the questions that are just mentioned. Before the school may conduct additional testing to collect that information, school personnel must ask you for permission. They must explain to you what the evaluation of your child will involve. This includes describing the tests they will use with your child and the other ways they will collect information about your child.

The school will collect additional information about your child in many different ways and from many different people, including you.

Tests are an important part of an evaluation, but they are only one part. The evaluation should also include the following:
- The observations and opinions of professionals who have worked with your child
- Your child's medical history when it is relevant to her or his performance in school
- Your observations about your child's experiences, abilities, needs, and behavior in school and outside of school and her or his feelings about school

Professionals will observe your child. They may give your child tests. They are trying to get a picture of the "whole child." It is important that the school evaluate your child in all areas where she

Evaluating Children for Learning Disabilities

or he might have a disability. For example, they will want to know more about the following:
- How well does your child speak and understand language, and how does your child think and behave?
- How well does your child adapt to change?
- What has your child achieved in school?
- How well does your child function in areas such as movement, thinking, learning, seeing, and hearing?
- What job-related and other postschool interests and abilities does your child have (important when your child is nearing 16 years old, or sooner, if appropriate)?

Evaluating your child completely will help you and the school decide if your child has a disability. The information will also help you and the school plan instruction for your child.

STEP 3: DECIDING IF YOUR CHILD IS ELIGIBLE FOR SPECIAL EDUCATION

The next step is to decide if your child is eligible for special education and related services. This decision will be oriented on the results of your child's evaluation and the policies in your area about eligibility for these special services.

It is important that your child's evaluation results be explained to you in a way that is easy to understand. The school will discuss your child's scores on tests and what they mean. Is your child doing as well as other children her or his age? What does your child do well? Where is your child having trouble? What is causing the trouble?

If you do not understand something in your child's evaluation results, be sure to speak up and ask questions. This is your child. You know your child very well. Do the results make sense, considering what you know about your child? Share your special insights. Your knowledge of your child is important.

Oriented on your child's evaluation results, a group of people will decide if your child is eligible for special education and related services. Under the Individuals with Disabilities Education Act (IDEA), you have the right to be part of any group that decides your child's eligibility for special education and related services.

This decision is oriented in part on IDEA's definition of a "child with a disability." You should also be aware that:
- The disability must affect the child's educational performance. (Your child does not have to be failing school, however, and maybe moving from grade to grade.)
- A child may not be identified as having a disability primarily because she or he speaks a language other than English and does not speak or understand English well. A child may not be identified as having a disability just because she or he has not had enough appropriate instruction in math or reading.
- The Center for Parent Information and Resources (CPIR) offers fact sheets about the disability categories listed in the law.

As a parent, you have the right to receive a copy of the evaluation report on your child at no cost to you. You also have the right to receive a copy of the paperwork about your child's eligibility for special education and related services.

If your child is eligible for special education and related services (such as speech therapy) and you agree with this determination, then you and the school will meet and talk about your child's special educational needs. However, you can disagree with the decision and refuse special education and related services for your child.

If your child is not eligible for special education and related services, the school must tell you so in writing. You must also receive information about what to do if you disagree with this decision. If this information is not in the materials the school gives you, ask for it. You have the right to disagree with the eligibility decision and be heard. Also, ask how the school will help your child if she or he will not be getting special education services.

STEP 4: DEVELOPING YOUR CHILD'S EDUCATIONAL PROGRAM
If, however, your child is found eligible for special education and related services and you agree, the next step is to write an

Evaluating Children for Learning Disabilities

individualized education program (IEP) for your child. This is a written document that you and your school personnel develop together. The IEP will describe your child's educational program, including the special services your child will receive.

Chapter 6 | Other Facts about Learning Disabilities

HOW COMMON ARE LEARNING DISABILITIES?

Very common! As many as one out of every five people in the United States has a learning disability. Almost one million children (aged 6–21) have a learning disability and receive special education in school. One-third of all children who receive special education have a learning disability.

THE INDIVIDUALS WITH DISABILITIES EDUCATION ACT'S DEFINITION OF SPECIFIC LEARNING DISABILITY

Not surprisingly, the Individuals with Disabilities Education Act (IDEA) includes a definition of specific learning disabilities as follows:

- **General**. A specific learning disability means a disorder in one or more of the basic psychological processes involved in understanding or in using language, spoken or written, that may manifest itself in the imperfect ability to listen, think, speak, read, write, spell, or do mathematical calculations, including conditions such

---

This chapter contains text excerpted from the following sources: Text beginning with the heading "How Common Are Learning Disabilities?" is excerpted from "Learning Disabilities (LD)," Center for Parent Information & Resources (CPIR), U.S. Department of Education (ED), July 15, 2015. Reviewed November 2022; Text under the heading "How Many Students with Disabilities Receive Services?" is excerpted from "Students with Disabilities," U.S. Department of Education (ED), May 8, 2007. Reviewed November 2022.

as perceptual disabilities, brain injury, minimal brain dysfunction, dyslexia, and developmental aphasia.
- **Disorders not included.** A specific learning disability does not include learning problems primarily resulting from visual, hearing, or motor disabilities; intellectual disability; emotional disturbance; or environmental, cultural, or economic disadvantage.

The IDEA also lists evaluation procedures that must be used at a minimum to identify and document that a child has a specific learning disability.

ADDITIONAL EVALUATION PROCEDURES FOR LEARNING DISABILITIES

Now for the confusing part! How children are identified as having a learning disability has changed over the years. Until recently, the most common approach was to use a severe discrepancy formula. This referred to the gap, or discrepancy, between the child's intelligence or aptitude and her or his actual performance. However, the 2004 reauthorization of IDEA of how learning disability is determined has been expanded. IDEA now requires that states adopt criteria that:
- Must not require the use of a severe discrepancy between intellectual ability and achievement in determining whether a child has a specific learning disability.
- Must permit local educational agencies (LEAs) to use a process oriented on the child's response to scientific, research-based intervention and may permit alternative research-based procedures for determining whether a child has a specific learning disability.

This means that instead of using a severe discrepancy approach to determining learning disability, school systems may provide the student with a research-based intervention and keep close track of the student's performance. Analyzing the student's response to intervention (RTI) may be considered by school districts in identifying a child with a learning disability.

Other Facts about Learning Disabilities

There are also other aspects required when evaluating children for learning disabilities. These include observing the student in her or his learning environment (including the regular education setting) to document academic performance and behavior in the areas of difficulty.

WHAT ABOUT SCHOOL?

Once a child is evaluated and found eligible for special education and related services, school staff and parents meet and develop what is known as an "individualized education program," or "IEP." This document is very important in the educational life of a child with learning disabilities. It describes the child's needs and the services the public school system will provide to address them.

Supports or changes in the classroom (called "accommodations") help most students with learning disabilities. Accessible instructional materials (AIM) are among the most helpful to students whose learning disability affects their ability to read and process printed language.

Assistive technology can also help many students work around their learning disabilities. Assistive technology can range from "low-tech" equipment such as tape recorders to high-tech tools such as reading machines (which read books aloud) and voice recognition systems (which allow the student to "write" by talking to the computer).

HOW MANY STUDENTS WITH DISABILITIES RECEIVE SERVICES?

Enacted in 1975, the IDEA, formerly known as the "Education for All Handicapped Children Act," mandates the provision of a free and appropriate public school education for eligible students aged 3–21. Eligible students are those identified by a team of professionals as having a disability that adversely affects academic performance and needs special education and related services. Data collection activities to monitor compliance with IDEA began in 1976. From 2009–2010 through 2020–2021, the number of students aged 3–21 who received special education services under IDEA increased from 6.5 million, or 13 percent of total public school enrollment, to 7.2 million, or 15 percent of total public school enrollment. In the fall of 2020, after the beginning of the coronavirus pandemic, overall enrollment in public schools was three percent lower than in the fall of 2019. Meanwhile, the number of students receiving IDEA services was about one percent lower in 2020–2021 than in 2019–2020. This was the first drop in the number of students receiving IDEA services since 2011–2012. However, the percentage of students served under IDEA was higher in 2020–2021 (15 percent) than in 2019–2020 (14 percent), continuing the upward trend.

Among students who received special education services under IDEA in the school year 2020–2021, the category of disabilities with the largest reported percentage of students was "specific learning disabilities." A specific learning disability is a disorder in one or more basic psychological processes involved in understanding or using spoken or written language. It may manifest in an imperfect ability to listen, think, speak, read, write, spell, or do mathematical calculations. Thirty-three percent of all students who received special education services had specific learning disabilities; 19 percent had speech or language impairments; and 15 percent had other health impairments (including having limited strength, vitality, or alertness due to chronic or acute health problems such as a heart condition, tuberculosis, rheumatic fever, nephritis, asthma, sickle cell anemia, hemophilia, epilepsy, lead poisoning, leukemia, or diabetes). Students with autism, developmental delays, intellectual disabilities, and emotional disturbances each accounted for between 5 and 12 percent of students served under IDEA. Students with multiple disabilities, hearing impairments, orthopedic impairments, visual impairments, traumatic brain injuries, and deaf-blindness accounted for two percent or less of those served under IDEA. For the percentage distribution of students aged 3–21 with selected disabilities served under the IDEA in 2020–2021, refer to Table 6.1.

Other Facts about Learning Disabilities

Table 6.1. Percentage Distribution of Students Served under the IDEA by Selected Disability

Disability Type	Percent
Specific learning disability	33
Speech or language impairment	19
Other health impairment[1]	15
Autism	12
Development delay	7
Intellectual disability	6
Emotional disturbance	5
Multiple disabilities	2
Hearing impairment	1

[1]*Other health impairments include having limited strength, vitality, or alertness due to chronic or acute health problems such as a heart condition, tuberculosis, rheumatic fever, nephritis, asthma, sickle cell anemia, hemophilia, epilepsy, lead poisoning, leukemia, or diabetes.*
Note: *Data are only for the 50 states and the District of Columbia (DC). Orthopedic impairment, visual impairment, traumatic brain injury, and deaf-blindness are not shown because they account for less than 0.5 percent of students served under IDEA. Due to categories not being shown, detail does not sum to 100 percent. Although rounded numbers are displayed, the figures are based on unrounded data.*

Part 2 | Types of Learning Disabilities

Chapter 7 | **Auditory Processing Disorder**

Children who have difficulty using information they hear in academic and social situations may have central auditory processing disorder (CAPD), later termed "auditory processing disorder" (APD). These children typically can hear information but have difficulty attending to, storing, locating, retrieving, and/or clarifying that information to make it useful for academic and social purposes. This can have a negative impact on both language acquisition and academic performance.

WHAT IS CENTRAL AUDITORY PROCESSING?

When the ears detect sound, the auditory stimulus travels through the structures of the ears, or the peripheral auditory system, to the central auditory nervous system that extends from the brain stem to the temporal lobes of the cerebral cortex. The auditory stimulus travels along the neural pathways where it is "processed," allowing the listener to determine the direction from which the sound comes, identify the type of sound, separate the sound from background noise, and interpret the sound. The listener builds upon what is heard by storing, retrieving, or clarifying the auditory information to make it functionally useful.

WHAT IS A DISORDER OF AUDITORY PROCESSING?

Auditory processing disorder is an impaired ability to attend to, discriminate, remember, recognize, or comprehend information

---

This chapter includes text excerpted from "ED474303 2002-12-00 Auditory Processing Disorders: An Overview. Eric Digest," U.S. Department of Education (ED), December 2002. Reviewed November 2022.

presented auditorily in individuals who typically exhibit normal intelligence and normal hearing. This definition has been expanded to include the effects that peripheral hearing loss may contribute to auditory processing deficits. Auditory processing difficulties become more pronounced in challenging listening situations, such as noisy backgrounds or poor acoustic environments, great distances from the speaker, speakers with fast speaking rates, or speakers with foreign accents.

WHAT ARE THE BEHAVIORS OF CHILDREN WITH AUDITORY PROCESSING DISORDER?

Children who have auditory processing disorders may behave as if they have hearing loss. While not all children present all behaviors, the following are examples of behaviors that may be displayed by children who have APD:
- Inconsistent response to speech
- Frequent requests for repetition (What? Huh?)
- Difficulty listening or paying attention in noisy environments
- Often misunderstanding what is said
- Difficulty following long directions
- Poor memory for information presented verbally
- Difficulty discerning the direction from which sound is coming
- History of middle ear infection

WHAT ARE ACADEMIC CHARACTERISTICS OF CHILDREN WHO HAVE AUDITORY PROCESSING DISORDER?

In addition to the preceding behaviors, children may also present a variety of academic characteristics that may lead teachers and parents to suspect APD. Dr. Jane A. Baran, Ph.D., working as a professor, Department of Communication Disorders, University of Massachusetts, Amherst, Massachusetts, offers the following characteristics. Again, all children will not present all characteristics.
- Poor expressive and receptive language abilities
- Poor reading, writing, and spelling

Auditory Processing Disorder

- Poor phonics and speech sound discrimination
- Difficulty taking notes
- Difficulty learning foreign languages
- Weak short-term memory
- Behavioral, psychological, and/or social problems resulting from poor language and academic skills

HOW IS AUDITORY PROCESSING DISORDER DIAGNOSED?

Given the complexity of auditory processing disorders, it is important to involve a multidisciplinary team, including psychologists, physicians, teachers, parents, and, of course, audiologists and speech-language pathologists. Audiologists diagnose the presence of APD (hearing and processing problems), and speech-language pathologists evaluate a child's perception of speech and receptive-expressive language use. Other team members conduct additional assessments to determine a child's educational strengths and weaknesses. Checklists that ask teachers and parents to observe the child's auditory behaviors may be used to determine a need for an APD evaluation. The parent's description of the child's auditory behavior at home is an especially important contribution to the diagnosis of APD.

WHAT DOES THE AUDIOLOGIST DO?

The audiologist assesses the peripheral and central auditory systems using a battery of tests, which may include both electrophysiological and behavioral tests. Peripheral hearing tests determine if the child has a hearing loss and, if so, the degree to which the loss is a factor in the child's learning problems. Assessment of the central auditory system evaluates the child's ability to respond under different conditions of auditory signal distortion and competition. It is oriented on the assumption that a child with an intact auditory system can tolerate mild distortions of speech and still understand it, while a child with APD will encounter difficulty when the auditory system is stressed by signal distortion and competing messages. The test results allow the audiologist to identify strengths and weaknesses in the child's auditory system that can be used to develop educational and remedial intervention strategies.

HOW SHOULD TEST RESULTS BE INTERPRETED?

As with any kind of evaluation, test results should be interpreted with caution. The effects of neurological maturation may influence test results for children under the age of 12 years. A true diagnosis of APD cannot be determined until that time. However, there are much younger children whose auditory behaviors, language, and academic characteristics indicate that APD is a strong possibility, and even without a formal diagnosis, these children would benefit from intervention. Remediation should address their strengths and areas of need oriented on available speech-language and psycho-educational testing.

IS THERE A RELATIONSHIP BETWEEN AUDITORY PROCESSING DISORDER AND ATTENTION DEFICIT HYPERACTIVITY DISORDER?

The behaviors of children with APD and attention deficit hyperactivity disorder (ADHD) may be very similar, especially with regard to distractibility. Given what is presently known as "APD" and "ADHD" do not appear to be a single developmental disorder. Each can occur independently, or they can coexist. This is a prime example of where the team approach to evaluation is critical, as the team can rule out the presence of ADHD or determine its contribution to the potential educational impact on the child.

WHAT CAN BE DONE TO HELP CHILDREN WITH AUDITORY PROCESSING DISORDER IN THE CLASSROOM?

Traditional educational and therapeutic approaches can be employed to remediate areas of need in language, reading, and writing. Many techniques that have shown to be effective with children with APD would be beneficial to all children, with and without APD, if the strategies employed are specific to the child's areas of need. Some of these are described below:

- Modify the environment by reducing background noise and enhancing the speech signal to improve access to auditory information:
  - Eliminate or reduce sources of noise in the classroom (air vent, street traffic, playground, hallway, furniture noises, etc.).

- Use assistive listening devices (ALDs) such as a sound field amplification system or a frequency-modulated (FM) auditory trainer.
- Allow preferential or roving seating to ensure that the child is seated as close to the speaker as possible.
- Allow the child to use a tape recorder and/or a peer notetaker.
- Ensure that the speaker gets the child's attention before speaking and considers using a slower speaking rate, repeating directions, allowing time for the child to respond to questions, pausing to allow the child to catch up, and presenting information in a visual format through overheads, illustrations, and print.
- Teach the child to use compensatory strategies, "meta" strategies, or executive functions to teach how to listen actively. The child should:
  - Learn to identify and resolve difficult listening situations.
  - Develop skills to understand the demands of listening: attending, memory, identifying important parts of the message, self-monitoring, clarifying, and problem-solving.
  - Develop memory techniques: verbal rehearsal (reauditorization) and mnemonics (chunking, cueing, chaining).
  - Encourage the use of external organizational aids: checklist, notebook, calendar, and so on.
  - Develop vocabulary, syntax, and pragmatic skills to facilitate language comprehension.
- Provide auditory training to remediate specific auditory deficits:
  - Children who have poor reading, writing, and spelling skills may benefit from phonological awareness activities.
  - Auditory closure activities may assist children in filling in or predicting the information they are listening to in the classroom and in conversations.

- Instruction in interpreting intonation, speaking rate, vocal intensity, and the relationship between syllable and word may assist children in determining important parts of the message.
- When the child has demonstrated success on the above tasks in a quiet environment, give the child practice engaging in the same tasks in an environment that includes background noise.
- Explore the use of commercially available computer programs designed to develop the child's attention to the phonological aspects of speech. These should be recommended by a professional who can determine their applicability to the child's needs.

Chapter 8 | Developmental Dyscalculia

WHAT IS DEVELOPMENTAL DYSCALCULIA?

It is not new to have learners in a primary class who experience significant challenges in learning arithmetic while having no problems learning other curriculum areas. Developmental dyscalculia (DD) was coined as a term to describe this condition and was defined several decades ago by Dr. Ladislav Kosc, Ph.D., Head of the Department of Child Pathopsychology in Bratislava, Czechoslovakia, as DD is a structural disorder of mathematical abilities that originates in a genetic or congenital disorder of those parts of the brain that are the direct anatomical-physiological substrate of the maturation of the mathematical abilities adequate to age, without a simultaneous disorder of general mental functions.

Dr. Kucian and Dr. von Aster, M.D., defined DD as a specific learning disability affecting the development of arithmetic skills and a heterogeneous disorder resulting from individual deficits in numerical or arithmetic functioning at behavioral, cognitive/neuropsychological, and neuronal levels. DD is described in the *Diagnostic and Statistical Manual* (*DSM*) of mental disorders as a specific learning disorder that inadequate learning opportunities cannot explain and is characterized by problems processing numerical information, learning arithmetic facts, and performing accurate or fluent calculations. There is a high incidence of comorbidities with DD, such as attention deficit hyperactivity disorder (ADHD). Some researchers suggest this could be due to the broad functional and structural differences across the brain observed in

---

This chapter includes text excerpted from "Hypothesis of Developmental Dyscalculia and Down Syndrome: Implications for Mathematics Education," U.S. Department of Education (ED), 2017. Reviewed November 2022.

individuals with DD. Down syndrome may be another disability paired with DD.

Consensus is emerging from neuroimaging and other behavioral evidence that DD has a basis in neurological impairment. Early evidence for highly specialized areas of the brain performing various aspects of quantity, calculation, and other mathematics came from observations of people who had experienced brain injuries.

DIAGNOSING DEVELOPMENTAL DYSCALCULIA

Growing evidence of the neurobiological basis of DD would suggest diagnosis could be made using neuroimaging techniques. Philipp Johannes Dinkel, a researcher from RWTH Aachen University, Aachen, Germany, and his colleagues describe using functional magnetic resonance imaging (fMRI) to diagnose DD; however, this technique's research is in its infancy. Some fMRI studies of people with Down syndrome have been undertaken; however, it appears no calculation studies have occurred to this point.

Without reliable imaging techniques, a diagnosis of DD has been made oriented on clinical assessments of arithmetic skills. Timed tests are commonly used because the answer alone will not provide evidence of DD; very laborious or inefficient strategies may eventually find correct answers. For example, in determining the bigger of two sets of objects, people with DD would count both sets of objects to compare rather than being able to know at a glance (subitize). Diagnosis of DD is considered when the performance in arithmetic is significantly lower than expected for the child's aptitude.

ARITHMETICAL DEVELOPMENT OF LEARNERS WITH DOWN SYNDROME

The mathematical development of learners with Down syndrome remains an emerging field of research. Most studies in the area have investigated basic arithmetic, the area of interest in a discussion of DD, and these studies indicate considerable difficulties. Of significance, the areas of difficulty in arithmetic almost completely match the areas of impairment in DD where the evidence exists.

Perhaps due to the pervasive view of mathematics as hierarchical, with the attainment of basic arithmetic considered a prerequisite for further study, research on the mathematical development of learners with Down syndrome into areas beyond calculation is rare. Some research has emerged, reporting success in areas such as algebra and coordinate geometry.

The research literature on the mathematics attainment of learners with Down syndrome indicates universal difficulties with basic arithmetic. Studies report a range of achievements. However, in none is the achievement on par with matched participants without Down syndrome. In addition, studies indicate that arithmetic is a specific difficulty, over and above other difficulties, such as language.

THE HYPOTHESIS OF DEVELOPMENTAL DYSCALCULIA
The hypothesis proposed here is that people with Down syndrome experience DD. While occurring in 3–6 percent of the general population, in the subset of Down syndrome the hypothesis is that DD is comorbid and likely to affect the majority.

Evidence
Down syndrome is a chromosomal pattern marked by the triplication of some or all of chromosome 21. While it is known that Down syndrome affects the brain in several areas, such as decreased brain volume, including in frontal and occipital lobes, and different brain activation patterns, this remains an area of research. With the invention of less invasive analysis techniques, such as fMRI, there is potential for advances in understanding the neurobiology of people with Down syndrome.

There is no direct evidence from brain imaging studies of DD in Down syndrome. Indirect evidence, however, abounds. Psychology research studies have begun exploring mathematical cognition in Down syndrome. These fine-grained studies are beginning to shed light on the subskills involved in representing quantity and give a clear indication of aspects of the nonverbal mechanism that are not operating as they should—that is, there is evidence of DD.

Dr. Carmen Belacchi, Ph.D., associate professor, Faculty of Humanities and Social Sciences, University of Queensland, and her colleagues studied approximate additions and working memory.

The model of number cognition would suggest approximate additions would be part of the approximate number system (ANS) and, therefore, undertaken by the intraparietal sulcus (IPS). Working memory is part of the verbal mechanism and uses the brain's frontal cortex. Their study observed impairment of the ANS with significant impairment of numerosity estimation involving one set. When participants were able to use working memory resources (the verbal system), they successfully estimated the numerosity of additions.

Another research team has studied a numerical estimation. Dr. Silvia Lanfranchi, Ph.D., associate professor, Department of Developmental Psychology and Socialisation, University of Padova, and her colleagues researched the ability of people with Down syndrome and two groups matched either by mental or chronological age to estimate the location of numbers on number lines. This would be a feature of the ANS. Their results suggest that this aspect is within the expected findings for the participants' developmental stage. The paper also reported findings from numerical intelligence and arithmetic knowledge measures, including statistically significant poorer performance on nonverbal calculations. Participants had to add or subtract one or more dots from a given set. The operands were in the single-digit range. This would involve the object tracking system (OTS) if four or fewer. Greater than four would imply the ANS was activated. Their results indicate impairment of the nonverbal mechanism, a marker of DD. The research team had previously reported findings from related data, studying enumeration skills. They note evidence for a specific deficit in the OTS for individuals with Down syndrome, which would again suggest DD. Number acuity (the ability to distinguish the larger of two numbers) and the understanding of cardinality were in keeping with mental age.

The work of this research team noted that the groups matched on mental age were much younger (DS mean age was 14 years; MA matched mean age was five years). The superior lexical performance of individuals with Down syndrome was suggested due to their long experience with number words and symbols. This finding would appear to indicate the importance and value of education. Dehaene emphasizes the critical role of teaching the cultural tools necessary for moving from the nonverbal to the verbal mechanism, which is essential for exact arithmetic. Several studies have indicated that children with Down syndrome can use the verbal system, which employs other parts of the brain than the IPS.

The challenge in this hypothesis is that scientific understandings of DD are still emerging, and there continues to be definitional confusion about the condition, its causes, symptoms, and its impact on learners. A further challenge relates to the diagnosis of DD in learners with Down syndrome. Timed arithmetic tests are problematic as the results can be confounded by difficulties completing the tests—understanding what is being asked, recording responses, and so on, all of which take time. Observational tests or task-based interviews may provide evidence of inefficient strategies, such as counting small sets rather than subitizing. The key here would be the discrepancy between arithmetical achievement and the learner's general achievement profile.

IMPLICATIONS OF THE HYPOTHESIS FOR EDUCATION

Researchers in DD have considered the implications of the diagnosis for learners, and some propose cognitive training to attempt to rewire the brain. Many also assume that calculation and number sense are essential prerequisites for a further mathematics study. These positions are problematic for learners with Down syndrome (and perhaps others as well).

Some evidence for the efficacy of cognitive training in ameliorating the symptoms of DD is emerging though an intense effort is needed to achieve this improvement. If DD is a person's only cognitive impairment, the learner may be well motivated, and the potential gains are significant enough to justify the effort. For learners with Down syndrome with many other challenges, devotion to brain training may not be a feasible intervention.

The second implication proposed by others is that calculation is a precursor to further study in mathematics; therefore, learners with DD will have limitations in further mathematics study. Even though this has been the accepted and rarely questioned view in mathematics education until recent times, there is growing evidence to suggest this is not the case; it is possible for learners with

DD to learn other mathematics. Indeed, evidence is available in the work of researchers in DD.

As noted earlier, some learners with Down syndrome have accomplished mathematics in several areas, including algebra, trigonometry, and percentages. Each of these students, it must be noted, could not calculate without the support of an electronic calculator.

For learners with Down syndrome, the following are alternative implications:
- Learners should use an electronic calculator as a prosthetic device, that is, a device that replaces the function of a part of the body. In this case, a calculator is used to overcome the impaired calculation functions of the brain.
- Explicit and lifelong attention to supporting conceptions of numbers must be made, using various visual supports such as number lines. This encourages and reinforces alternative neural activity.
- Previously, so-called functional mathematics programs for learners with Down syndrome needs to be fundamentally changed to focus on prosthetic devices such as calculators and electronic banking methods in finance and measurement.
- Learners should not be required to demonstrate accomplishment on basic number work before they are taught mathematics from across the discipline. The content should be from the curriculum of their schooling level and adjusted as needed.

TESTING THE HYPOTHESIS

The indirect evidence for the hypothesis of DD being a feature of Down syndrome lies in the pervasive nature of calculation difficulties for this population worldwide and over decades of research in the field. Direct evidence to confirm the hypothesis is needed and may come from fMRI studies, particularly to examine if the IPS is affected. Alternatively, clinical assessment tools, such as task-based interviews, need to be designed for learners with Down syndrome and explicitly probe areas of number development by observing strategy use.

Chapter 9 | Dysgraphia

WHAT IS DYSGRAPHIA?[1]

Dysgraphia is a neurological disorder characterized by writing disabilities. Specifically, the disorder causes a person's writing to be distorted or incorrect. In children, the disorder generally emerges when they are first introduced to writing. They make inappropriately sized and spaced letters or write wrong or misspelled words despite thorough instruction.

Children with the disorder may have other learning disabilities; however, they usually have no social or other academic problems. Cases of dysgraphia in adults generally occur after some trauma. In addition to poor handwriting, dysgraphia is characterized by wrong or odd spelling and the production of words that are not correct (i.e., using "boy" for "child"). The cause of the disorder is unknown, but in adults, it is usually associated with damage to the parietal lobe of the brain.

PERFORMANCE OF STUDENTS' HANDWRITING AND DYSGRAPHIA[2]

Writing is a skill highly valued in our society, even in a time of computers and technology. In the past, handwriting was prized because it was a primary form of communication; people needed to get notes to others that were legible. Now that typewriters and computers are used to communicate between people, handwriting has become a rare form of communication. However, handwriting is still a critical skill and is needed for many reasons that people

---

This chapter includes text excerpted from documents published by two public domain sources. Text under the headings marked 1 is excerpted from "Dysgraphia," National Institute of Neurological Disorders and Stroke (NINDS), July 25, 2022; Text under the heading "Performance of Student Handwriting and Dysgraphia" is excerpted from "Dysgraphia: How It Affects a Student's Performance and What Can Be Done about It?" U.S. Department of Education (ED), 2007. Reviewed November 2022.

might not readily recognize. Writing notes, recipes, prescriptions, messages, checks, and filling out applications are a few reasons why the development and teaching of handwriting skills need to be continued in schools and at home. Additionally, research has shown that handwriting is causally related to writing and that explicit and supplemental instructions of handwriting are important elements in an elementary program to prevent writing difficulties.

Unfortunately, many students struggle in school because of dysgraphia, a problem with expressing thoughts in written form. Dysgraphia can hurt the success of a child in school. Many children with dysgraphia cannot keep up with written assignments, cannot put coherent thoughts together on paper, or write legibly. This disability must be recognized and remediated before it creates long-lasting negative consequences for the child.

Characteristics of Dysgraphia

The following are some of the common characteristics of dysgraphia:
- Cramped fingers on the writing tool
- Odd wrist, body, and paper positions
- Excessive erasures
- A mixture of uppercase and lowercase letters
- A mixture of printed and cursive letters
- Inconsistent letter formations and slant
- Irregular letter sizes and shapes
- Unfinished cursive letters
- Misuse of line and margin
- Poor organization on the page
- Inefficient speed in copying
- Decreased speed of writing
- General illegibility
- Inattentiveness about details when writing
- Frequent need for verbal cues and use of subvocalizing
- Heavy reliance on vision to monitor what the hand is doing during the writing
- Slow implementation of verbal directions that involve sequencing and planning

Dysgraphia

Dysgraphia can be categorized into four subtypes. The first subtype is phonological dysgraphia, which is "writing and spelling disturbances in which the spelling of unfamiliar words, nonwords, and phonetically irregular words are impaired." These students tend to have trouble spelling by sounds and rely on the visual aspect of letters; therefore, because spelling is an auditory task, they will have trouble with spelling tests. The second subtype is surface dysgraphia, where students have trouble with orthographic representations of words, which makes the student rely too heavily on sound patterns, the opposite of phonological dysgraphia. Mixed dysgraphia is the third subtype of dysgraphia. This type refers to students having trouble with mixing up letter formations and trouble with spelling tasks, a combination of the first two types. Recalling letter formations is hard for these students because there are so many instructions or rules that they get confused and have inconsistent spellings of words. Finally, semantic/syntactic dysgraphia is a grammatical problem in which students struggle with how words can be combined to make complete and comprehensive phrases.

In addition, children with dysgraphia usually have some type of problem with automaticity that interferes with the retrieval of letter formation. Concentrating on how to form the letter overwhelms the child to the degree that the letter is written poorly. The incorrect letter or word formation can also exceed margins or lines. Letter formation is automatic for most students after initial skill attainment. When letter formation is automatic, students can concentrate on spelling, grammar, sentence structure, and other aspects of written language. However, for many students with dysgraphia, letter formation is a cognitive task that leaves little mental capacity to devote to these other aspects. Children with dysgraphia can become frustrated, leading to low motivation to use and practice written language.

Students concentrating too hard on letter formation may develop problems gripping the pencil. Gripping the pencil in the "wrong" way can interfere with performance because the child focuses on holding the pencil instead of writing the letter. Richards suggested a proper pencil grip that included placing the fingers about one inch above the tip of the pencil, maintaining a 45-degree angle with the paper, and using moderate pressure. Teachers should be aware of a child improperly holding the pencil and aim to correct the grip.

Strategies to Use

There are two different approaches to addressing dysgraphia. The first is using systematic techniques that improve function, referred to as remedial treatment. Remedial treatments seek to correct handwriting through direct handwriting instruction or a fine motor program. The second strategy is using bypass strategies, such as technology, to find a way around handwriting difficulties. Compensatory techniques or ways to alleviate the problem would be bypass strategies. For the purpose of this strategy review, only remedial treatments were included.

One such remedial treatment is using drills and practice. The teacher provides a clear example of good handwriting, and then the children practice and drill using the teacher's model. People with dysgraphia struggle with the display of letters because often the letter asked for in the brain is not the letter that is retrieved and produced. Repetitive practice, correct position, and pencil grip can help with this process.

Another remedial treatment that has empirical evidence is building fine motor skills. Drills that build the muscles used for fine motor activities can help improve hand functioning, leading to better handwriting. Dr. Keller, Ph.D., used such activities in a club she created to help the handwriting of students with dysgraphia.

In a doctor of education practicum report, Nova Southeastern University, Davie, Florida, Timothy J. Dikowski, a psychology researcher, studied children's visual–motor skills related to handwriting. He found schools offered little help to students with handwriting or visual–motor disabilities. He observed that when children had visual–motor integration problems, this led to problems with hand-eye coordination. Since the brain, hand, and eye all work together to perform anything written, Dikowski believes that it is important to work on both fine and gross motor strengthening to increase the ability to stabilize the hand when writing.

Discussion

The need to have clear, neat handwriting is of utmost importance in nowadays society. Communicating ideas, writing and signing checks, signing legal agreements, and other daily activities need clear handwriting that is legible to others. One may argue that technology can replace the need for handwriting. For example, paying bills is now available online. However, computers cannot be relied on for everything. One factor to consider is the technology gap. Many homes and workplaces do not have computers, and there are many other instances in daily life when a computer is not readily available.

Furthermore, as young children learn the writing process and how to formulate thoughts in writing, the use of technology may not be practical. The physical act of writing down one's thoughts is part of the cognitive process of learning to communicate through writing. A young child who has not yet learned these skills would not be able to transfer the skills to a word processing program.

TREATMENT OF DYSGRAPHIA[1]

Treatment for dysgraphia varies and may include treatment for motor disorders to help control writing movements. Other treatments may address impaired memory or other neurological problems. Some physicians recommend that individuals with dysgraphia use computers to avoid the problems of handwriting.

PROGNOSIS OF DYSGRAPHIA[1]

Some individuals with dysgraphia improve their writing ability, but for others, the disorder persists.

Chapter 10 | Reading Disorders

Chapter Contents
Section 10.1—Dyslexia 75
Section 10.2—Hyperlexia 77

Section 10.1 | **Dyslexia**

This section contains text excerpted from the following sources: Text beginning with the heading "What Are Reading Disorders?" is excerpted from "What Are Reading Disorders?" Eunice Kennedy Shriver National Institute of Child Health and Human Development (NICHD), March 5, 2020; Text under the heading "What Is Dyslexia?" is excerpted from "Dyslexia," National Institute of Neurological Disorders and Stroke (NINDS), July 25, 2022.

WHAT ARE READING DISORDERS?

Reading disorders occur when a person has trouble reading words or understanding what they read. Dyslexia is one type of reading disorder. It generally refers to difficulties reading individual words and can lead to problems understanding text.

Most reading disorders result from specific differences in the way the brain processes written words and text. Usually, these differences are present from a young age. But a person can develop a reading problem from an injury to the brain at any age.

People with reading disorders often have problems recognizing words they already know and understanding the text they read. They also may be poor spellers. Not everyone with a reading disorder has every symptom.

Reading disorders are not a type of intellectual or developmental disorder, and they are not a sign of lower intelligence or unwillingness to learn. People with reading disorders may have other learning disabilities, too, including problems with writing or numbers.

Types of Reading Disorders

The following are two types of reading disorders:
- Dyslexia
- Hyperlexia

Other people may have normal reading skills but have problems understanding written words. Reading disorders can also involve problems with specific skills:
- **Word decoding**. People who have difficulty sounding out written words struggle to match letters to their proper sounds.

- **Fluency**. People who lack fluency have difficulty reading quickly, accurately, and with proper expression (if reading aloud).
- **Poor reading comprehension**. People with poor reading comprehension have trouble understanding what they read.

WHAT IS DYSLEXIA?

Dyslexia is a brain-based type of learning disability that specifically impairs a person's ability to read. These individuals typically read at levels significantly lower than expected despite having normal intelligence. Although the disorder varies from person to person, common characteristics among people with dyslexia are difficulty with phonological processing (the manipulation of sounds), spelling, and/or rapid visual–verbal responding.

In individuals with adult onset of dyslexia, it usually occurs as a result of brain injury or in the context of dementia; this contrasts with individuals with dyslexia who simply were never identified as children or adolescents. Dyslexia can be inherited in some families, and recent studies have identified a number of genes that may predispose an individual to develop dyslexia.

TREATMENT OF DYSLEXIA

The main focus of treatment should be on the specific learning problems of affected individuals. The usual course is to modify teaching methods and the educational environment to meet the specific needs of the individual with dyslexia.

PROGNOSIS OF DYSLEXIA

For those with dyslexia, the prognosis is mixed. The disability affects such a wide range of people and produces such different symptoms and varying degrees of severity that predictions are hard to make. The prognosis is generally good, however, for individuals whose dyslexia is identified early, who have supportive family and friends and a strong self-image, and who are involved in a proper remediation program.

Section 10.2 | Hyperlexia

"Hyperlexia," © 2022 Infobase. Reviewed November 2022.

WHAT IS HYPERLEXIA?
Hyperlexia is the ability of a child to recognize and read words beyond their age level without being trained to do so. A child with hyperlexia has an intense interest in letters and numbers, allowing them to outperform other children their age in recognizing and reading letters, numbers, and words. A hyperlexic child may quickly learn to decode or sound out words, but they may not comprehend or grasp most of what they read. This can result in communication or speaking disabilities.

Studies show that around 84 percent of children with hyperlexia have autism. It has also been observed that hyperlexic children often have underdeveloped social skills because many have problems speaking and communicating.

SIGNS OF HYPERLEXIA
Most children with hyperlexia exhibit the following four distinct characteristics:
- **Quick learning ability**. They learn to read rapidly without much instruction and may even teach themselves.
- **Ardent readers**. Books and other reading materials appeal to children with hyperlexia more than other toys and activities. Some hyperlexic children are captivated by numbers as much as words and letters.
- **Communication difficulty**. Despite their ability to read effectively, hyperlexic children may have difficulty talking or be unable to communicate with other children their age.
- **Low comprehension**. Children with hyperlexia have excellent reading skills but poor comprehension and learning abilities and have a hard time doing tasks such as putting together puzzles.

WHAT ARE THE DIFFERENT TYPES OF HYPERLEXIA?
Hyperlexia is classified into the following three types:
- **Hyperlexia I.** This type is transitory and occurs in neurotypical children who learn to read at an early age but later develop on par with other children their age as they grow.
- **Hyperlexia II.** This type occurs in autistic children. These children typically exhibit symptoms of autism, such as avoidance of eye contact and affection. They are frequently preoccupied with numbers and letters and might prefer books and magnetic letters over other toys. They may also have excellent recall of numbers such as birth dates and phone numbers. They demonstrate very early reading as a splinter skill.
- **Hyperlexia III.** Children of this type are early readers and are often sociable and affectionate. These children have a strong memory and exceptional reading comprehension, but their vocal language development may lag behind their age group.

CAUSES OF HYPERLEXIA
Researchers have not yet identified a cause for hyperlexia. Future studies using functional MRI imaging and genetics may provide insight into what leads to hyperlexia. A change in the brain's neurological structure may indicate the presence of hyperlexia in the context of other developmental deficits.

SYMPTOMS OF HYPERLEXIA
The symptoms listed below are frequently used to make a diagnosis of hyperlexia. Their intensity can vary from child to child.
- Preoccupation with numbers or letters
- An unusual ability to read words beyond what is expected of the child's age
- Difficulty socializing and connecting with others

Reading Disorders

- Difficulty speaking and understanding spoken language
- Compromised comprehensive skills
- Repeating a word or phrase that another person speaks (echolalia)

DIAGNOSIS OF HYPERLEXIA

Hyperlexia does not frequently occur as a standalone condition but is generally observed with a combination of other behavioral and learning difficulties. This disorder is difficult to identify because there are no specific tests or guidelines for diagnosing it. Doctors rely on the signs and symptoms to diagnose hyperlexia.

To confirm a hyperlexia diagnosis, the doctor will consult with additional medical professionals such as a speech therapist, child psychologist, or behavioral therapist.

Some specific tests, such as solving a puzzle, arranging blocks, or just having a conversation, may be carried out to determine language comprehension. Medical professionals may also examine a child's hearing, vision, and reflexes to rule out hearing difficulties that can often limit or delay speaking and communication abilities. Other health specialists, such as occupational therapists, exceptional education instructors, and social workers, are consulted for additional opinions on a hyperlexia diagnosis.

TREATMENT OF HYPERLEXIA

A correct diagnosis made early is the first step in the effective treatment of hyperlexia. When a child presents with hyperlexia, a multidisciplinary team experienced with autism spectrum disorder (ASD) and hyperlexia assesses the patient and prescribes focused therapy.

Usually, children with hyperlexia I do not require therapy, while those with hyperlexia II and III may benefit from various treatment modalities. Treatment approaches for hyperlexia depend on the learning style of the child. Some children may require treatment with learning assistance for only a few years, while others require treatment that lasts to adulthood or sometimes lifelong.

In the United States, individualized education plans (IEPs) are developed for young children who require extra help in particular areas. Sessions with a child psychologist and an occupational therapist may also be beneficial.

- **Speech and language therapy.** Speech and language therapy can assist children with hyperlexia develop their language and social abilities, including social interaction and comprehension. Some of the effective methods used by therapists to improve these skills are:
  - Visual approaches to aid comprehension
  - Word association games for teaching word relationships
  - Storytelling
- **Occupational therapy (OT).** This approach is tailored to supporting the patient's needs in activities such as:
  - Sleeping
  - Feeding
  - Self-care
  - Participating in social and school activities
  - Writing

Every child is unique and has varied learning styles and distinct communication style and learns at their own pace. Still, all children with hyperlexia benefit from learning through written language. This allows them to leverage their abilities, gain confidence, and reduce stress while learning. As with any learning impairment, getting a diagnosis and starting treatment as early as possible is critical. A child will have every opportunity to thrive if a strategy for continuous learning achievement is in place.

References

"Hyperlexia," CHAT Life Changing Speech Therapy, October 26, 2019.

"Hyperlexia," Disorders.org, March 18, 2012.

"Hyperlexia: Signs, Diagnosis, and Treatment," Healthline, May 27, 2020.

Reading Disorders

"Hyperlexia: What It Means, What the Symptoms Are, and More," WebMD LLC, October 25, 2021.

Kupperman, Phyllis; Bligh, Sally; and Barouski, Kathy, "Hyperlexia," Center for Speech and Language Disorders, 1998.

Midivelly, Srinivas, MBBS, DNB, "Hyperlexia—Causes, Symptoms, Treatment, and Therapy," Yashoda Hospitals, August 27, 2021.

Chapter 11 | Nonverbal Learning Disorder

WHAT IS NONVERBAL LEARNING DISORDER?

Nonverbal learning disorders (NVLD) are less common than the typical language-based learning disabilities identified by school staff. Appropriate intervention is highly dependent on the accurate diagnosis of this disorder. Emphasis on performance and behavior management often obscures the etiology of a child's difficulties and leads to ineffective treatment approaches. The differential diagnosis can be confusing. As a result, many children do not receive adequate intervention, and teachers cannot develop appropriate techniques for their education and management.

It is important to understand the cognitive, academic, and neuropsychological characteristics of students with NVLD and how these attributes translate into behavior and performance in the classroom. The focus of this paper is to clarify the diagnosis of NVLD, differentiate them from other learning disorders, and introduce effective educational intervention strategies. This knowledge will enable school psychologists, teachers, parents, and clinicians to understand the characteristics of a child with an NVLD, identify these children earlier, and initiate effective remedial programs.

DIAGNOSIS AND MANAGEMENT OF NONVERBAL LEARNING DISORDERS

Historically, school psychologists have been encouraged to identify students with learning disabilities generally, emphasizing the

This chapter includes text excerpted from "Diagnosis and Management of Nonverbal Learning Disorders," U.S. Department of Education (ED), April 2000. Reviewed November 2022.

discrepancy between cognitive ability and academic performance. There has been little focus on the nature and clinical assessment of the specific disability. With new practices emerging, it is imperative to develop a knowledge base that allows interpretation of the diagnostic information presented and results in the development of appropriate and effective intervention strategies.

Language-based learning disabilities comprise the majority of disabilities identified and are reflected in the development and expression of reading and writing skills. A subtype of learning disorder called "nonverbal learning disabilities" includes approximately 20 percent of students with learning disabilities. NVLD is not well understood, and the differential diagnosis can be confusing. As a result, many children do not receive adequate intervention.

Individuals with nonverbal learning disabilities display strengths in verbal and auditory skills but may have profound deficits in visual perception, visual motor coordination, and spatial organization. Academic difficulties are noted in math computation, reasoning, science, writing, and reading comprehension. The mechanisms that result in these deficits are quite different for nonverbal learning disabilities than for language-based disabilities; therefore, the strategies needed for remediation also differ. Due to the inability to accurately read nonverbal social cues, overreliance on verbal expression, impaired appreciation of humor, and spatial disorientation, children with these disorders may have related problems with social skills and psychological adjustment.

Adequate treatment, from a psychiatric and academic viewpoint, depends highly on accurate diagnosis. There is a significant correlation between these learning disorders and specific types of developmental disorders. Clinical staff may identify the psychiatric or developmental difficulties with little attention to the educational ramifications. It is also evident that school staff focus on academic and social deficiencies with inadequate treatment of the underlying developmental disorder. Collaboration between those involved in treatment is necessary to bridge this gap and provide the most effective treatment plan. For this to be accomplished, it is critical for school psychologists to have a thorough understanding of the characteristics of NVLD and the categories of developmental

Nonverbal Learning Disorder

disorders (as per the diagnostic and statistical manual of mental disorders (*DSM-IV*)). This knowledge will bolster the collaborative effort and provide the basis for effective communication.

Most individuals with nonverbal learning disabilities demonstrate strengths in areas that rely on auditory processing and language ability. These individuals exhibit verbal fluency, a strong rote verbal capacity, and well-developed auditory memory. The ability may demonstrate this to product descriptions, which sound like memorization of large tracts of the encyclopedia or movie dialog. Attention to verbal information may be acute, and receptive language tends to be well-developed. These areas of strength may produce the effect of verbal precocity when, in fact, the skills tend to be rote in nature and do not reflect any depth of comprehension.

Cognitive weaknesses are noted in visual perceptual and spatial skills. A child with NVLD may struggle with attention to visually presented information, nonverbal memory, and concept formation. Nonverbal reasoning tasks may appear confusing and difficult to process novel visual stimuli accurately. Visuospatial organizational skills are weak. These weaknesses translate to difficulty with a wide variety of tasks. Individuals speak of problems ranging from difficulty reading maps, driving, and operating appliances to an inability to manage their time, remember faces, or organize materials.

Inherent in NVLD is also a weakness in understanding the intent of visual information. The expression of facial and body language may be meaningless. There may be little appreciation of physical humor although puns and wordplay are well understood. Individuals with NVLD may violate the boundaries and personal space of others. While a stern look on a parent's face may elicit a particular behavior or cessation of behavior in a nondisabled child, the child with nonverbal problems may fail to understand the look and notice the expression. This leads to identifying defiance in a child who simply does not comprehend and may be mystified when punishment ensues.

Difficulties in the development of social skills and relationships are common. Nonverbal cues are essential to effective communication. Failure to comprehend the meaning of these cues alters our understanding of the intent of the communication. Individuals with

NVLD are noted to display inappropriate social behaviors, which may include interruption of conversation, abrupt changes of topic, and failure to respond to the communication of others. Excessive talking is common, and reciprocal conversation is impaired. An individual may fail to make eye contact or walk away from the speaker. If there is some development of social skills, the individual may make eye contact, speak about a subject of interest to her/him, wait while the other person is speaking, and then return to a monologue without responding to the speaker's statement. Pragmatic use of language may be impaired.

Academically, NVLD translates to difficulty with reading comprehension, mathematical reasoning, computation, science, and writing. Strengths may be seen in decoding, spelling, and content subjects that require the retention of factual information presented orally. Although acquiring fine motor skills may initially be difficult, the rote skills are eventually secured, becoming a strength. However, the more complex skills necessary for written language are difficult to master and may continue to be problematic.

Difficulties with reading comprehension appear to be related to weakness in visual imagery. Strong visual imagery allows us to connect to incoming language and link it to prior knowledge. It assists in the process of accessing background experiences. Imagery also enhances the ability to store information in memory. Individuals with NVLD have difficulty producing visual images in response to verbal input. Normally functioning individuals produce these images without effort. As one hears a story, for example, the mental visual scene shifts in response to changes in the narrative. Therefore, it is not necessary to recall all the verbal detail. One need only "view" the shifting image. A child with NVLD and deficits in visual imagery may frantically attempt to remember the verbal sequence of information and quickly becomes lost in the rush of information presented. The recall is compromised without the visual image accompanying the verbiage, negatively impacting comprehension.

Difficulties with visual imagery are then characterized by poor comprehension in the presence of excellent decoding ability. This produces a situation where the individual may appear to be a competent reader; however, understanding and recall are limited. The child may be able to read fluently, well beyond the level of understanding. Frequent rereading is noted. Although this may enhance comprehension of a portion of the text, it interferes with the continuity of thought.

Math, which essentially comprises spatial tasks, also presents difficulty and often is the primary academic deficit. The spatial concepts are difficult to understand, and the mode of instruction further inhibits learning. Unlike many academic tasks that rely on oral presentation, math is taught through demonstration, particularly at the primary levels. Manipulatives display the computations, and the student is asked to solve the problem by demonstration. While rarely heard in other classes, math teachers are frequently noted to say, "Let me show you how to do this problem."

Difficulties in math can be found at several levels. There may be an inability to grasp the basic concepts and reasoning involved. The student may have difficulty with number formation and organization on paper. Their work is characterized by various sizes of numbers, inaccurate vertical alignment, and slanted horizontal positioning. Students may also struggle with computational skills and cannot recall a series of steps. Finally, the student may have difficulty with the fine motor and motor planning skills necessary to complete the problems.

Reading skills are put to practical use in content areas as students continue in school. Students with NVLD tend to have difficulty with classes in the general area of science. Biology, botany, zoology, anatomy, and similar areas involve the discrimination, recall, and integration of visual images. Physics and chemistry involve visual processing skills as well as upper-level math. Of course, difficulties are prevalent in art, physical education, and drama classes.

As a result of NVLD, individuals may display behaviors that alienate them from others. There may be an overreliance on talk. It may be necessary for them to "talk themselves" through tasks in a way that irritates other students. Thinking may become rigid with an intense focus on detail. Poor comprehension of nonverbal cues impairs understanding. These deficiencies may lead to problems in the development of satisfactory peer relationships. A reliance and dependency on adults with whom they tend to relate more effectively may develop. Poor motor coordination limits participation in sports or the typical outdoor play of other children.

Although NVLD is not easily or quickly remediated, some strategies help students cope and learn. The key to remediation is the use of language. Individualized instruction that relies on verbal strengths is essential. Teaching verbal self-direction can be of significant value. Analyzing tasks and clarifying concepts in a verbal format are necessary. Teachers must always accompany demonstration and visual information with extensive verbal instruction and description. The student with difficulties in visual imaging may benefit from direct instruction in building visual images beginning with actual pictures of events taking place in the text. Children with communication problems may need direct instruction in the rules of conversation and pragmatic language.

When considering the possibility of NVLD in a student, it is important to rule out other possible causes of the difficulties seen. Depression, anxiety, or obsessive-compulsive disorders (OCD) can mimic some of the manifestations of NVLD. The presence of a psychotic process must be considered. Assessment should also focus on attention problems, developmental disorders, and substance abuse. Although there is a significant overlap of NVLD with developmental disorders such as pervasive developmental disorder (PDD) and Asperger syndrome (AS), NVLD can exist in isolation; therefore, the symptoms do not mandate the diagnosis of a developmental disorder. Careful assessment, often involving multiple professionals, must make these distinctions.

Students with NVLD struggle on multiple levels. Academic, cognitive, communication, and social skills may affect various degrees. Some individuals face social isolation, and withdrawal can lead to a higher incidence of depression, anxiety, and frustration. The student may become even more rigid and less available to intervention efforts to cope. Early intervention is, therefore, critical before the secondary issues of psychological maladjustment develop. Only the collaborative and often intense effort of teachers, parents, and clinicians allows the development of an effective remedial program for individuals with NVLD.

Chapter 12 | Voice, Speech, and Language Disorders

Chapter Contents
Section 12.1—Voice, Speech, and Language Disorders:
  Quick Statistics 91
Section 12.2—Aphasia 94
Section 12.3—Apraxia of Speech.................................... 97
Section 12.4—Specific Language Impairment............................ 101
Section 12.5—Detecting Problems with Language
  or Speech 104
Section 12.6—Voice, Speech, and Language Program 107

Section 12.1 | **Voice, Speech, and Language Disorders: Quick Statistics**

This section includes text excerpted from "Quick Statistics about Voice, Speech, Language," National Institute on Deafness and Other Communication Disorders (NIDCD), May 19, 2016. Reviewed November 2022.

OVERALL STATISTICS OF VOICE, SPEECH, LANGUAGE, AND SWALLOWING PROBLEMS AMONG U.S. CHILDREN

- Nearly one in 12 (7.7%) U.S. children aged 3–17 have had a disorder oriented to voice, speech, language, or swallowing in the past 12 months.
- Among children with a voice, speech, language, or swallowing disorder, 34 percent of those aged 3–10 have multiple communication or swallowing disorders, while 25.4 percent of those aged 11–17 have multiple disorders.
- Boys aged 3–17 are more likely than girls to have a voice, speech, language, or swallowing disorder (9.6% compared to 5.7%).
- The prevalence of voice, speech, language, or swallowing disorders is highest among children aged 3–6 (11.0%), compared to children aged 7–10 (9.3%) and children aged 11–17 (4.9%).
- Nearly one in 10, or 9.6 percent, of Black children (aged 3–17) has a voice, speech, language, or swallowing disorder, compared to 7.8 percent of White children and 6.9 percent of Hispanic children.
- More than half (55.2%) of U.S. children aged 3–17 with a voice, speech, language, or swallowing disorder received intervention services in the past year. White children (aged 3–17) with a voice, speech, language, or swallowing disorder are more likely to have received intervention services in the past 12 months, compared to Hispanic and Black children, at 60.1, 47.3, and 45.8 percent, respectively.
- Boys (aged 3–17) with a voice, speech, language, or swallowing disorder are more likely than girls to receive intervention services, at 59.4 and 47.8 percent, respectively.

- Among children aged 3–17 who have a voice, speech, language, or swallowing disorder, those with speech or language problems, 67.6 and 66.8 percent, respectively, are more likely to receive intervention services compared to those who have a voice disorder (22.8%) or swallowing problems (12.7%).

STATISTICAL INFORMATION ABOUT VOICE
- An estimated 17.9 million U.S. adults aged 18 or older, or 7.6 percent, report having had a problem with their voice in the past 12 months. Approximately 9.4 million (4.0%) adults report having a problem using their voice that lasted one week or longer during the last 12 months.
- About 1.4 percent of U.S. children have a voice disorder that lasted for a week or longer during the past 12 months.
- Spasmodic dysphonia, a voice disorder caused by involuntary movements of one or more larynx muscles (voice box), can affect anyone. The first signs of this disorder are found most often in people aged 30–50. More women than men appear to be affected.

STATISTICAL INFORMATION ABOUT SPEECH
- Five percent of U.S. children aged 3–17 have a speech disorder that has lasted for a week or longer during the past 12 months.
- The prevalence of speech sound disorders (articulation disorders or phonological disorders) in young children is 8–9 percent. By the first grade, roughly five percent of children have noticeable speech disorders, including stuttering, speech sound disorders, and dysarthria; most have no known cause.
- More than three million Americans (about 1%) stutter. Stuttering can affect individuals of all ages but occurs most frequently in young children between the ages of two and six. Boys are 2–3 times more likely than girls to stutter. Although most children who stutter outgrow

Voice, Speech, and Language Disorders

the condition while young, as many as one in four will continue to stutter for the rest of their lives, a condition known as "persistent developmental stuttering."

STATISTICAL INFORMATION ABOUT LANGUAGE
- About 3.3 percent of U.S. children aged 3–17 have a language disorder that lasted for a week or longer during the past 12 months.
- Research suggests that the first six months of life are the most crucial to a child's development of language skills. For a person to become fully competent in any language, exposure must begin as early as possible, preferably before school age.
- Anyone can acquire aphasia (a loss of the ability to use or understand language), but most people with aphasia are in their middle to late years. Men and women are equally affected. Nearly 180,000 Americans acquire the disorder each year. About one million persons in the United States have aphasia.

STATISTICAL INFORMATION ABOUT SWALLOWING
- About 0.9 percent of U.S. children aged 3–17 have a swallowing disorder that lasted for a week or longer during the past 12 months.

Section 12.2 | Aphasia

This section includes text excerpted from "Aphasia," MedlinePlus, National Institutes of Health (NIH), May 3, 2022.

WHAT IS APHASIA?

Aphasia is a language disorder that makes it hard for you to read, write, and say what you mean to say. Sometimes, it makes it hard to understand what other people are saying, too. Aphasia is not a disease. It is a symptom of damage to the parts of the brain that control language.

The signs of aphasia depend on which part of the brain is damaged. There are four main types of aphasia:
- **Expressive aphasia** is when you know what you want to say but have trouble saying or writing your thoughts.
- **Receptive aphasia** affects your ability to read and understand speech. You can hear what people say or can see words on a page, but you have trouble making sense of what they mean.
- **Global aphasia** is the loss of almost all language ability. You cannot speak, understand speech, read, or write.
- **Anomic or amnesia aphasia** is when you have trouble using the right words for certain things, people, places, or events.

In some cases, aphasia may get better on its own. But it can be a long-term condition. There is no cure, but treatment may help improve language skills.

WHAT CAUSES APHASIA?

Aphasia happens from damage to one or more parts of the brain involved with language. The damage may be from:
- Stroke, which is the most common cause of aphasia
- Brain tumor
- Brain infection or inflammation

Voice, Speech, and Language Disorders

- Brain injury
- Other brain disorders or neurologic diseases that affect the brain and get worse over time, such as dementia

WHO IS MORE LIKELY TO DEVELOP APHASIA?
Anyone can have aphasia at any age, but most people with aphasia are middle-aged or older. Most aphasia happens suddenly from a stroke or brain injury. Aphasia from a brain tumor or other brain disorder may develop slowly over time.

HOW IS APHASIA DIAGNOSED?
If a health-care provider sees signs of aphasia, the provider will usually:
- Test the person's ability to understand language and speech. This includes asking questions and checking to see if the person can follow simple commands.
- Order an imaging scan to see if there is a brain injury and what part of the brain is damaged. Possible tests include:
  - Magnetic resonance imaging (MRI)
  - Computerized tomography (CT) scan

If imaging shows signs of aphasia, more tests may be needed. These tests measure how much the brain damage has affected the ability to talk, read, write, and understand. In most cases, the tests are done by a speech-language pathologist or speech therapist (a specialist who treats speech and communication disorders).

WHAT ARE THE TREATMENTS FOR APHASIA?
Some people fully recover from aphasia without treatment. But most people should begin speech-language therapy to treat aphasia as soon as possible.

Treatment may be one-on-one with a speech therapist or in a group. Therapy using a computer may also be helpful.

The specific therapy depends on the type of language loss that a person has. It may include exercises in reading, writing, following directions, and repeating what the therapist says. Therapy may also include learning how to communicate with gestures, pictures, smartphones, or other electronic devices.

Family participation may be an important part of speech therapy. Family members can learn to help with recovery in many ways, such as:
- Using simpler language.
- Including the person with aphasia in conversations.
- Repeating or writing down keywords to help communicate more clearly.

Language abilities may continue to improve over many years. In general, people recover their ability to understand language more fully than their ability to speak.

How much a person recovers depends on many things, including:
- What caused the brain injury
- What part of the brain was hurt
- How badly and how much of the brain was hurt
- The age and health of the person

CAN APHASIA BE PREVENTED?

You can help prevent aphasia by:
- Making heart-healthy lifestyle changes to lower your chance of having:
  - A stroke
  - Heart disease
  - Vascular disease (problems with your blood vessels)
- Protecting your brain from injury:
  - Wearing the right helmet for sports safety, such as when riding a bike.
  - Taking action to prevent falls.
  - Always wearing your seat belt and driving safely.

Section 12.3 | Apraxia of Speech

This section includes text excerpted from "Apraxia of Speech," National Institute on Deafness and Other Communication Disorders (NIDCD), October 31, 2017. Reviewed November 2022.

WHAT IS APRAXIA OF SPEECH?

Apraxia of speech (AOS)—also known as "acquired apraxia of speech," "verbal apraxia," or "childhood apraxia of speech" (CAS) when diagnosed in children—is a speech sound disorder. Someone with AOS has trouble saying what she or he wants to say correctly and consistently. AOS is a neurological disorder that affects the brain pathways involved in planning the sequence of movements involved in producing speech. The brain knows what it wants to say but cannot properly plan and sequence the required speech sound movements.

The AOS is not caused by weakness or paralysis of the speech muscles (the muscles of the jaw, tongue, or lips). Weakness or paralysis of the speech muscles results in a separate speech disorder known as "dysarthria." Some people have dysarthria and AOS, which can make diagnosing the two conditions more difficult.

The severity of AOS varies from person to person. It can be so mild that it causes trouble with only a few speech sounds or pronouncing words with many syllables. In the most severe cases, someone with AOS might not be able to communicate effectively by speaking and may need the help of alternative communication methods.

WHAT ARE THE TYPES AND CAUSES OF APRAXIA OF SPEECH?

There are two main types of AOS they are acquired apraxia of speech and childhood apraxia of speech.

- **Acquired AOS can affect someone at any age although it typically occurs in adults**. Acquired AOS is caused by damage to the parts of the brain involved in speaking and involves the loss or impairment of existing speech abilities. It may result from a stroke, head injury, tumor, or other illness affecting the brain. Acquired AOS may occur together with other

conditions caused by damage to the nervous system. One of these is dysarthria, as mentioned earlier. Another is aphasia, which is a language disorder.
- **Childhood AOS is present from birth.** This condition is also known as "developmental apraxia of speech," "developmental verbal apraxia," or "articulatory apraxia." Childhood AOS is not the same as developmental delays in speech, in which a child follows the typical path of speech development but does so more slowly than usual. The causes of childhood AOS are not well understood. Imaging and other studies have not found evidence of brain damage or differences in the brain structure of children with AOS. Children with AOS often have family members who have a history of a communication disorder or a learning disability. This observation and research findings suggest that genetic factors may play a role in the disorder. Childhood AOS appears to affect more boys than girls.

WHAT ARE THE SYMPTOMS OF APRAXIA OF SPEECH?

People with either form of AOS may have several different speech characteristics or symptoms:
- **Distorting sounds.** People with AOS may have difficulty pronouncing words correctly. Sounds, especially vowels, are often distorted. Because the speaker may not place the speech structures (e.g., tongue, jaw) in the right place, the sound comes out wrong. Longer or more complex words are usually harder to say than shorter or simpler words. Sound substitutions might also occur when AOS is accompanied by aphasia.
- **Making inconsistent errors in speech.** For example, someone with AOS may say a difficult word correctly but then have trouble repeating it or may be able to say a particular sound one day and have trouble with the same sound the next day.

Voice, Speech, and Language Disorders

- **Groping for sounds**. People with AOS often appear to be groping for the right sound or word and may try saying a word several times before they say it correctly.
- **Making errors in tone, stress, or rhythm**. Another common characteristic of AOS is the incorrect use of prosody. Prosody is the rhythm and inflection of speech that is used to help express meaning. Someone who has trouble with prosody might use equal stress, segment syllables in a word, omit syllables in words and phrases, or pause inappropriately while speaking.

Children with AOS generally understand language much better than they can use it. Some children with the disorder may also have other speech, expressive language, or motor-skill problems.

HOW IS APRAXIA OF SPEECH DIAGNOSED?

Professionals known as "speech-language pathologists" play a key role in diagnosing and treating AOS. Because no single symptom or test can be used to diagnose AOS, the person making the diagnosis generally looks for the presence of several of a group of symptoms, including those described earlier. Ruling out other conditions, such as muscle weakness or language production problems (e.g., aphasia), can help with the diagnostic process.

In formal testing for both acquired and childhood AOS, a speech-language pathologist may ask the patient to perform speech tasks such as repeating a particular word several times or repeating a list of words of increasing length (e.g., love, loving, lovingly). A speech-language pathologist may also examine the patient's ability to converse, read, write, and perform nonspeech movements for acquired AOS. To diagnose childhood AOS, parents and professionals may need to observe a child's speech over a period of time.

HOW IS APRAXIA OF SPEECH TREATED?

In some cases, people with acquired AOS recover some or all of their speech abilities independently. This is called "spontaneous recovery."

Children with AOS will not outgrow the problem on their own. They also do not acquire the basics of speech just by being around other children, such as in a classroom. Therefore, speech-language therapy is necessary for children with AOS and people with acquired AOS who do not spontaneously recover all of their speech abilities.

Speech-language pathologists use different approaches to treat AOS, and no single approach has been proven to be the most effective. Therapy is tailored to the individual and is designed to treat other speech or language problems that may occur together with AOS. Frequent, intensive, one-on-one speech-language therapy sessions are needed for children and adults with AOS. In parallel with normal schooling, children with severe AOS may need intensive speech-language therapy for years to obtain adequate speech abilities.

In severe cases, adults and children with AOS may need other ways to express themselves. These might include formal or informal sign language, a notebook with pictures or written words that can be pointed to and shown to other people, or an electronic communication device—such as a smartphone, tablet, or laptop computer—that can be used to write or produce speech. Such assistive communication methods can also help children with AOS learn to read and better understand spoken language by stimulating areas of the brain involved in language and literacy.

Some adults and children will make more progress during treatment than others. Support and encouragement from family members and friends and extra practice in the home environment are important.

Section 12.4 | Specific Language Impairment

This section includes text excerpted from "Specific Language Impairment," National Institute on Deafness and Other Communication Disorders (NIDCD), July 2019.

WHAT IS SPECIFIC LANGUAGE IMPAIRMENT?

Specific language impairment (SLI) is a communication disorder that interferes with the development of language skills in children who have no hearing loss. SLI can affect a child's speaking, listening, reading, and writing. SLI is also called "developmental language disorder" (DLD), "language delay," or "developmental dysphasia." It is one of the most common developmental disorders, affecting approximately 7–10 percent of children in kindergarten. Of those children with language impairment, approximately 2–3 percent also have an existing medical condition and/or intellectual disability. The impact of SLI usually persists into adulthood.

WHAT CAUSES SPECIFIC LANGUAGE IMPAIRMENT?

The cause of SLI is unknown, but some of the discoveries suggest that it has a strong genetic link. Children with SLI are more likely than those without SLI to have parents and siblings who have also had difficulties and delays in speaking. In fact, 50–70 percent of children with SLI have at least one family member with the disorder. Learning more than one language at a time does not cause SLI. The disorder can, however, affect both multilingual children and children who speak only one language.

WHAT ARE THE SYMPTOMS OF SPECIFIC LANGUAGE IMPAIRMENT?

A child with SLI often has a history of being a late talker (reaching spoken language milestones later than peers).

Preschool-aged children with SLI may:
- Be late to put words together into sentences.
- Struggle to learn new words and make conversation.

- Have difficulty following directions, not because they are stubborn but because they do not fully understand the words spoken to them.
- Make frequent grammatical errors when speaking.

Although some late talkers eventually catch up with peers, children with SLI have persistent language difficulties. Symptoms common in older children and adults with SLI include the following:
- Limited use of complex sentences
- Difficulty finding the right words
- Difficulty understanding figurative language
- Reading problems
- Disorganized storytelling and writing
- Frequent grammatical and spelling errors

HOW IS SPECIFIC LANGUAGE IMPAIRMENT DIAGNOSED?

If a doctor, teacher, or parent suspects that a child has SLI, a speech-language pathologist (a professional trained to assess and treat people with speech or language problems) can evaluate the child's language skills. The type of evaluation depends on the child's age and the concerns that led to the evaluation. In general, an evaluation includes:
- Direct observation of the child
- Interviews and questionnaires that were completed by parents and/or teachers
- Assessments of the child's learning ability
- Standardized tests of current language performance

These tools allow the speech-language pathologist to compare the child's language skills to those of same-age peers, identify specific difficulties, and plan for potential treatment targets.

IS SPECIFIC LANGUAGE IMPAIRMENT A LIFELONG CONDITION?

Specific language impairment is a developmental disorder, which means that its symptoms first appear in childhood. This does not mean that as children develop, they grow out of the problem.

Instead, the problem is apparent in early childhood and will likely continue but change with development.

For instance, a young child with SLI might use ungrammatical sentences in conversation, while a young adult with SLI might avoid complex sentences in conversations and struggle to produce clear, concise, well-organized, and grammatically accurate writing.

Early treatment during the preschool years can improve the skills of many children with language delays, including those with SLI. Children who enter kindergarten with significant language delays are likely to continue having problems, but they and even older children can still benefit from treatment. Many adults develop strategies for managing SLI symptoms. This can improve their daily social, family, and work lives.

WHAT TREATMENTS ARE AVAILABLE FOR SPECIFIC LANGUAGE IMPAIRMENTS?

Treatment services for SLI are typically provided or overseen by a licensed speech-language pathologist. Treatment may be provided in homes, schools, university programs for speech-language pathology, private clinics, or outpatient hospital settings.

Identifying and treating children with SLI early in life is ideal, but people can respond well to treatment regardless of when it begins. Treatment depends on the age and needs of the person. Starting treatment early can help young children to:
- Acquire missing elements of grammar.
- Expand their understanding and use of words.
- Develop social communication skills.

For school-age children, treatment may focus on understanding instruction in the classroom, including helping with issues such as:
- Following directions.
- Understanding the meaning of the words that teachers use.
- Organizing information.
- Improving speaking, reading, and writing skills.

Adults entering new jobs, vocational programs, or higher education may need help learning technical vocabulary or improving workplace writing skills.

Section 12.5 | **Detecting Problems with Language or Speech**

This section includes text excerpted from "Language and Speech Disorders in Children," Centers for Disease Control and Prevention (CDC), May 11, 2022.

Children are born ready to learn a language, but they need to learn the language or languages that their family and environment use. Learning a language takes time, and children vary in how quickly they master language and speech development milestones. Typically developing children may have trouble with some sounds, words, and sentences while learning. However, most children can use language easily around five years of age.

HELPING CHILDREN LEARN LANGUAGE

Parents and caregivers are the most important teachers during a child's early years. Children learn language by listening to others speak and by practicing. Even young babies notice when others repeat and respond to the noises and sounds they make. Children's language and brain skills strengthen when they hear many different words. Parents can help their children learn in many ways, such as:

- Responding to the first sounds, gurgles, and gestures a baby makes.
- Repeating what the child says and adding to it.
- Talking about the things that a child sees.
- Asking questions and listening to the answers.
- Looking at or reading books.
- Telling stories.
- Singing songs and sharing rhymes.

This can happen both during playtime and during daily routines. Parents can also observe the following:

- How their child hears and talks and compares it with typical milestones for communication skills
- How their child reacts to sounds and has their hearing tested if they have concerns

Voice, Speech, and Language Disorders

EVALUATING PROBLEMS WITH LANGUAGE OR SPEECH
If a child has a language or speech development problem, talk to a health-care provider about an evaluation. An important first step is determining if the child may have hearing loss. Hearing loss may be difficult to notice, particularly if a child has hearing loss only in one ear or has partial hearing loss, which means they can hear some sounds but not others.

A language development specialist, such as a speech-language pathologist, will conduct a careful assessment to determine what type of problem with language or speech the child may have.

Overall, learning more than one language does not cause language disorders, but children may not follow exactly the same developmental milestones as those who learn only one language. Developing the ability to understand and speak in two languages depends on how much practice the child has using both languages and the kind of practice. If a child learning more than one language has difficulty with language development, careful assessment by a specialist who understands the development of skills in more than one language may be needed.

WHAT TO DO IF THERE ARE CONCERNS
Some children struggle with understanding and speaking and need help. They may not master the language milestones simultaneously as other children, which may be a sign of a language or speech delay or disorder. Language development has different parts, and children might have problems with one or more of the following:
- **Understanding what others say (receptive language).** This could be due to the following:
  - Not hearing the words (hearing loss).
  - Not understanding the meaning of the words.
- **Communicating thoughts using language (expressive language).** This could be due to the following:
  - Not knowing the words to use.
  - Not knowing how to put words together.
  - Knowing the words to use but not being able to express them.

Language and speech disorders can exist together or by themselves. Examples of problems with language and speech development include the following:
- **Speech disorders**:
  - Difficulty with forming specific words or sounds correctly
  - Difficulty making words or sentences flow smoothly, such as stuttering or stammering
- **Language delay**. The ability to understand and speak develops more slowly than is typical.
- **Language disorders**:
  - Aphasia (difficulty understanding or speaking parts of language due to a brain injury or how the brain works)
  - Auditory processing disorder (difficulty understanding the meaning of the ear's sounds to the brain)

Language or speech disorders can occur with other learning disorders that affect reading and writing. Children with language disorders may feel frustrated that they cannot understand others or make themselves understood, and they may act out, act helpless, or withdraw. Language or speech disorders can also be present with emotional or behavioral disorders, such as attention deficit hyperactivity disorder (ADHD) or anxiety. Children with developmental disabilities, including autism spectrum disorder (ASD), may also have difficulties with speech and language. The combination of challenges can make it difficult for a child to succeed in school. Properly diagnosing a child's disorder is crucial so each child can get the right help.

TREATMENT FOR LANGUAGE OR SPEECH DISORDERS AND DELAYS

Children with language problems often need extra help and special instruction. Speech-language pathologists can work directly with children and their parents, caregivers, and teachers.

Having a language or speech delay or disorder can qualify a child for early intervention (for children up to three years of age) and special education services (for children aged three years and older). Schools can do their own testing for language or speech disorders to see if a child needs intervention. An evaluation by a health-care professional is needed if there are other concerns about the child's hearing, behavior, or emotions. Parents, health-care providers, and the school can work together to find the right referrals and treatment.

WHAT SHOULD EVERY PARENT KNOW?

Children with specific learning disabilities, including language or speech disorders, are eligible for special education services or accommodations at school under the Individuals with Disabilities in Education Act (IDEA) and Section 504, an antidiscrimination law.

THE ROLE OF HEALTH-CARE PROVIDERS

Health-care providers can play an important part in collaborating with schools to help a child with speech or language disorders, delays, or other disabilities get the special services they need. The American Academy of Pediatrics (AAP) has created a report describing health-care providers' roles in helping children with disabilities, including language or speech disorders.

Section 12.6 | Voice, Speech, and Language Program

This section includes text excerpted from "Voice, Speech, and Language Program," National Institute on Deafness and Other Communication Disorders (NIDCD), October 13, 2022.

Disorders involving voice, speech, or language can overwhelmingly affect an individual's health and quality of life. These disorders affect people of all ages with or without hearing impairment, including children with autism, those who stutter, and adults with aphasia or speech disorders.

The voice, speech, and language program of the National Institute on Deafness and Other Communication Disorders (NIDCD) uses a wide range of research approaches to develop effective diagnostic and intervention strategies for individuals with communication impairments.

Research in voice and speech includes studies to determine the nature, causes, treatment, and prevention of disorders of motor speech production throughout the life span.

- Researchers are learning how reflux from the stomach to the throat and vocal fold tissue harms the larynx. They have demonstrated that reflux significantly alters the expression of 27 genes associated with malignant changes in the larynx. Understanding how changes in gene expression lead to laryngeal injury provides a comprehensive model for identifying novel diagnostic and therapeutic targets to treat reflux-oriented injury.
- Investigators are working to provide a direct means of producing speech to people with locked-in syndrome (LIS)—near-total paralysis caused by stroke, end-stage neural degeneration, or neuromuscular diseases such as "amyotrophic lateral sclerosis" ("ALS"). People with LIS can use brain–computer interface (BCI) technology to help them communicate. The NIDCD-supported scientists significantly improved the performance of a BCI device by developing a program that combines data collected from electrical signals in the brain with data from tracking eye movement. This hybrid system improves the accuracy and speed at which users can type words using BCI technology. Future work will translate this technology from the lab into the clinic or home for individuals with LIS, potentially helping them communicate more easily and effectively with physicians, caretakers, and family.

Research in language and language disorders includes studies on characterization, genetic and brain causes, and diagnostic and treatment approaches relevant to communication across a person's life span.

Voice, Speech, and Language Disorders

- Language researchers supported by the NIDCD explore the genetic bases of child language disorders and characterize the linguistic and cognitive deficits in children and adults with language disorders. The NIDCD-supported studies have demonstrated that children with developmental speech and language problems are at considerable risk for learning disabilities and psychosocial problems that emerge during adolescence or adulthood.
- Researchers are developing effective diagnostic and intervention strategies for children with an autism spectrum disorder (ASD) or specific language impairment (SLI) and adults with aphasia. This research will further our understanding of the neural bases of language disorders.
- Research on the acquisition, characterization, and use of American sign language (ASL) is expanding knowledge of the language used by many individuals who are deaf.

Chapter 13 | Visual Processing Disorders

WHAT ARE VISUAL PROCESSING DISORDERS?
A visual processing disorder, also called a "perceptual disorder," is difficulty making sense of information received through the eyes. This is different from vision or sight loss or impairment. Individuals with visual processing disorders may have adequate eyesight, but their brains do not accept or interpret visible data appropriately. This defect can cause problems in many aspects of life, from identifying letters and symbols to differentiating objects around them and recalling what they have seen. Visual processing difficulties can influence self-esteem and socialization and impair learning.

CAUSES OF VISUAL PROCESSING DISORDERS
Although medical research has not determined the cause of visual processing abnormalities, evidence shows that traumatic brain injury (TBI) and preterm birth delivery may raise the risk of visual processing disorders. Some researchers believe that low birth weight may also play a significant role. Mild traumatic damage to the brain's visual areas could cause the disorder, but there is not enough data to confirm this.

SYMPTOMS OF VISUAL PROCESSING DISORDERS
Visual processing difficulties can be challenging to identify in children; however, the following symptoms are standard:
- Confusing words and mathematical symbols with similar appearances

"Visual Processing Disorders," © 2022 Infobase. Reviewed November 2022.

- Below-average reading and writing capabilities despite excellent spoken linguistic ability
- Frequently complaining of eye strain despite having normal eyesight
- Difficulties recalling sequences, numerals, or the spelling of words
- Inattention or difficulty paying attention to video presentations, video games, and movies
- Forgetful of letters, digits, or words
- Frequently bumping into objects
- Having crooked or badly spaced handwriting
- Having limited reading comprehension
- Having trouble telling time
- Having trouble writing or coloring within the lines
- Making mistakes when copying
- Poor spelling ability
- Skipping words or lines when reading
- Reversing letters or numbers when reading

DIAGNOSIS OF VISUAL PROCESSING DISORDERS

Researchers have identified many forms of visual processing disorders, each of which affects distinct abilities and poses specific difficulties. A child might have more than one condition at the same time, such as:
- **Visual discrimination**. The child has difficulty distinguishing between two similar-looking letters, shapes, patterns, or objects. They may confuse letters such as d and b, p and q, or h and n. There may also be difficulty distinguishing between triangular and square shapes.
- **Visual figure-ground discrimination**. A child with this disorder type cannot distinguish a shape or character from its background. It may be challenging to locate a specific piece of information on a page. A classic illustration of this disorder is an inability to complete a jigsaw puzzle.

Visual Processing Disorders

- **Visual sequencing**. The order and arrangement of images, words, or symbols are difficult to recognize for those with this disorder type. A child might misunderstand letters or struggle to hold their place on the page while reading and may miss lines or read the same line over and over.
- **Visual-spatial relationships**. Individuals with this condition have difficulty seeing objects in relation to space. They may have trouble determining how distant an object is from them and how far two things are from one another. Reading an analog clock or a map might also be difficult.
- **Visual closure**. Visual closure difficulties can occur in determining what an item is when only just pieces of it are visible. An example of this is when an individual may not recognize a familiar word if a letter is absent or identify a picture of a face if a part, such as a mouth, is missing.
- **Letter and symbol reversal**. People with this condition tend to reverse letters or numbers when reading or writing. They may also have difficulty with letter construction and misuse, or use interchangeably, similar-looking letters and digits.
- **Visual-motor processing**. Children with this condition have difficulty synchronizing the movement of body parts that rely on visual signals. They may look clumsy and uncoordinated or may bump into objects. They may also have trouble writing within lines or copying from a chalkboard.
- **Long- or short-term visual memory issues**. This makes it challenging to recall items shown to them shortly after they have been taken from view. A child's difficulty with memory games is evidence of this.

TREATMENT OF VISUAL PROCESSING DISORDERS

Although there is no treatment for visual processing impairments, there are a variety of interventions that can assist individuals in improving their abilities and adapting to the obstacles they confront. Educators can help children who have been diagnosed with visual processing difficulties by recognizing them and providing special education services, such as:

- **Individual informal support systems.** These systems include allowing the child to write answers on the same page as the questions, providing books with larger print, or having tests read aloud.
- **Individualized educational program (IEP).** This provides specific attention to the child that might include special services for developing and improving reading and writing abilities.
- **Response to intervention (RTI).** This program is used in some schools where all students are assessed to identify those who require special assistance.

It is generally understood that visual processing disorder cannot be cured, but patients can find some services to overcome their difficulties. Caregivers, including parents, play a vital role in assisting children with visual processing disorders to develop their abilities. They may write out schedules and instructions in large print, with each step numbered, or color-code important points. They might encourage the use of a ruler to guide the eyes during a reading session, provide thickly lined or dotted paper for writing, and provide a visual break whenever needed because long periods of visual input can be exhausting.

Above all, caregivers and educators aware of and monitoring the child's growth in skills and abilities can assist in determining whether modifications in classroom structure and resources are required. Implementing them appropriately will go a long way in effectively managing children with visual processing disorders.

References

Lynch, Matthew. "Visual Processing Disorder: What You Need to Know," The Edvocate, February 25, 2022.

Morin, Amanda. "Classroom Accommodations for Visual Processing Issues," Understood for All Inc., April 1, 2015.

Visual Processing Disorders

"Visual and Auditory Processing Disorders," LD OnLine, January 31, 2022.
"Visual Processing Disorder," White Swan Foundation, January 16, 2019.
"Visual Processing Disorders," MindWell Psychology, September 13, 2022.
"Visual Processing Disorders," Touch-type Read and Spell, May 11, 2017.
"What Is Visual Processing Disorder?" Advanced Vision Therapy, April 22, 2021.
"What Is Visual Processing Disorder?" Churchill Center & School, February 24, 2017.

Part 3 | Other Disorders That Make Learning Difficult

Chapter 14 | Attention Deficit Hyperactivity Disorder

WHAT IS ATTENTION DEFICIT HYPERACTIVITY DISORDER?
Attention deficit hyperactivity disorder (ADHD) is one of childhood's most common neurodevelopmental disorders. It is usually first diagnosed in childhood and often lasts into adulthood. Children with ADHD may have trouble paying attention, controlling impulsive behaviors (acting without thinking about the result), or being overly active.

TYPES OF ATTENTION DEFICIT HYPERACTIVITY DISORDER
The following are three different ways ADHD presents itself, depending on which types of symptoms are strongest in the individual:
- **Predominantly inattentive presentation**. It is hard for the individual to organize or finish a task, pay attention to details, or follow instructions or conversations. The person is easily distracted or forgets details of daily routines.
- **Predominantly hyperactive-impulsive presentation**. The person fidgets and talks a lot. It is hard for her or him to sit still for long (e.g., for a meal or while doing homework). Smaller children may run, jump, or climb constantly. The individual feels restless and

---

This chapter includes text excerpted from "Attention-Deficit/Hyperactivity Disorder (ADHD)," Centers for Disease Control and Prevention (CDC), August 9, 2022.

has trouble with impulsivity. Someone impulsive may interrupt others, grab things from people, or speak at inappropriate times. It is hard for the person to wait their turn or listen to directions. A person with impulsiveness may have more accidents and injuries than others.
- **Combined presentation**. Symptoms of the previous two types are equally present in the person. Because symptoms can change over time, the presentation may also change over time.

SIGNS AND SYMPTOMS OF ATTENTION DEFICIT HYPERACTIVITY DISORDER

It is normal for children to have trouble focusing and behaving at one time or another. However, children with ADHD do not just grow out of these behaviors. The symptoms continue, can be severe, and cause difficulty at school, at home, or with friends. A child with ADHD might:
- Daydream a lot.
- Forget or lose things a lot.
- Squirm or fidget.
- Talk too much.
- Make careless mistakes or take unnecessary risks.
- Have a hard time resisting temptation.
- Have trouble taking turns.
- Have difficulty getting along with others.

CAUSES OF ATTENTION DEFICIT HYPERACTIVITY DISORDER

Scientists are studying cause(s) and risk factors to find better ways to manage and reduce the chances of a person having ADHD. The cause(s) and risk factors for ADHD are unknown, but current research shows that genetics plays an important role. Some of the studies correlate genetic factors with ADHD.

In addition to genetics, scientists are studying other possible causes and risk factors, including:
- Brain injury
- Exposure to environmental risks (e.g., lead) during pregnancy or at a young age

Attention Deficit Hyperactivity Disorder

- Alcohol and tobacco use during pregnancy
- Premature delivery
- Low birth weight

Research does not support the popularly held views that ADHD is caused by eating too much sugar, watching too much television, parenting, or social and environmental factors such as poverty or family chaos. Of course, many things, including these, might worsen symptoms, especially in certain people. But the evidence is not strong enough to conclude that they are the main causes of ADHD.

DIAGNOSIS OF ATTENTION DEFICIT HYPERACTIVITY DISORDER

Deciding if a child has ADHD is a process with several steps. There is no single test to diagnose ADHD; many other problems, such as anxiety, depression, sleep problems, and certain learning disabilities, can have similar symptoms. One step involves having a medical exam, including hearing and vision tests, to rule out other problems with symptoms such as ADHD. Diagnosing ADHD usually includes a checklist for rating ADHD symptoms and taking a history of the child from parents, teachers, and sometimes the child.

TREATMENT FOR ATTENTION DEFICIT HYPERACTIVITY DISORDER

In most cases, ADHD is best treated with behavior therapy and medication. For preschool-aged children (4–5 years of age) with ADHD, behavior therapy, particularly training for parents, is recommended as the first line of treatment before medication is tried. What works best can depend on the child and family. Good treatment plans will include close monitoring, follow-ups, and changes, if needed, along the way.

MANAGING SYMPTOMS: STAYING HEALTHY

Being healthy is important for all children and can be especially important for children with ADHD. In addition to behavioral therapy and medication, having a healthy lifestyle can make it easier for

your child to deal with ADHD symptoms. Here are some healthy behaviors that may help:
- Developing healthy eating habits such as eating plenty of fruits, vegetables, and whole grains and choosing lean protein sources.
- Participating in daily physical activity oriented on age.
- Limiting the amount of daily screen time from TVs, computers, phones, and other electronics.
- Getting the recommended amount of sleep each night oriented on age.

ATTENTION DEFICIT HYPERACTIVITY DISORDER IN ADULTS

Attention deficit hyperactivity disorder can last into adulthood. Some adults have ADHD but have never been diagnosed. The symptoms can cause difficulty at work, at home, or in relationships. Symptoms may look different at older ages; for example, hyperactivity may appear as extreme restlessness. Symptoms can become more severe when the demands of adulthood increase.

OTHER CONCERNS AND CONDITIONS WITH ATTENTION DEFICIT HYPERACTIVITY DISORDER

Attention deficit hyperactivity disorder often occurs with other disorders. Many children with ADHD have other disorders as well as ADHD, such as behavior or conduct problems, learning disorders, anxiety, and depression.

Chapter 15 | Cerebral Palsy

WHAT IS CEREBRAL PALSY?
Cerebral palsy (CP) refers to a group of neurological disorders that appear in infancy or early childhood and permanently affect body movement and muscle coordination. CP is caused by damage to or abnormalities inside the developing brain that disrupt the brain's ability to control movement and maintain posture and balance. The term cerebral refers to the brain; palsy refers to the loss or impairment of motor function. CP affects the motor area of the brain's outer layer (called the "cerebral cortex"), the part of the brain that directs muscle movement.

In some cases, the cerebral motor cortex has not developed normally during fetal growth. In others, the damage results from injury to the brain either before, during, or after birth. In either case, the damage is not repairable, and the disabilities that result are permanent.

Children with CP exhibit a wide variety of symptoms, including:
- Lack of muscle coordination when performing voluntary movements (ataxia)
- Stiff or tight muscles and exaggerated reflexes (spasticity)
- Weakness in one or more arms or legs
- Walking on the toes, a crouched gait, or a "scissored" gait
- Variations in muscle tone, either too stiff or too floppy
- Excessive drooling or difficulties swallowing or speaking

This chapter includes text excerpted from "Cerebral Palsy: Hope through Research," National Institute of Neurological Disorders and Stroke (NINDS), July 25, 2022.

- Shaking (tremor) or random involuntary movements
- Delays in reaching motor skill milestones
- Difficulty with precise movements such as writing or buttoning a shirt

The symptoms of CP differ in type and severity from one person to the next and may even change in an individual over time. Symptoms vary greatly among individuals, depending on which brain parts have been injured. All people with cerebral palsy have problems with movement and posture. Some also have intellectual disabilities, seizures, abnormal physical sensations or perceptions, and other medical disorders. People with CP also may have impaired vision or hearing, language, and speech problems.

Cerebral palsy is the leading cause of childhood disabilities but does not always cause profound disabilities. While one child with severe CP might be unable to walk and need extensive, lifelong care, another child with mild CP might be only slightly awkward and require no special assistance. The disorder is not progressive, meaning it does not get worse over time. However, as the child ages, certain symptoms may become more or less evident.

A study by the Centers for Disease Control and Prevention (CDC) shows the average prevalence of cerebral palsy is 3.3 children per 1,000 live births.

There is no cure for cerebral palsy, but supportive treatments, medications, and surgery can help many individuals improve their motor skills and communication with the world.

WHAT ARE THE EARLY SIGNS?

The signs of cerebral palsy usually appear in the early months of life although specific diagnosis may be delayed until age two years or later. Infants with CP frequently have developmental delays, in which they cannot reach developmental milestones such as learning to roll over, sit, crawl, or walk. Some infants with CP have abnormal muscle tone. Decreased muscle tone (hypotonia) can make them appear relaxed, even floppy. Increased muscle tone (hypertonia) can make them seem stiff or rigid. In some cases, an early period of hypotonia will progress to hypertonia after the

Cerebral Palsy

first 2–3 months of life. Children with CP may also have unusual postures or favor one side of the body when they reach, crawl, or move. It is important to note that some children without CP also might have some of these signs. Some early warning signs:

- In a baby younger than six months of age:
  - Her or his head lags when you pick her or him up while she or he is lying on his back.
  - She or he feels stiff.
  - She or he feels floppy.
  - When you pick her or him up, her or his legs get stiff, and they cross or scissor.
- In a baby older than six months of age:
  - She or he does not roll over in either direction.
  - She or he cannot bring her or his hands together.
  - She or he has difficulty bringing her or his hands to her or his mouth.
  - She or he reaches out with only one hand while keeping the other fisted.
- In a baby older than 10 months of age:
  - She or he crawls in a lopsided manner, pushing off with one hand and leg while dragging the opposite hand and leg.
  - She or he cannot stand holding onto the support.

WHAT CAUSES CEREBRAL PALSY?

Cerebral palsy is caused by abnormal development of part of the brain or by damage to parts of the brain that control movement. This damage can occur before, during, or shortly after birth. Most children have congenital CP (i.e., they were born with it) although it may not be detected until months or years later. A few children have acquired cerebral palsy, meaning the disorder begins after birth. Some causes of acquired cerebral palsy include brain damage in the first few months or years of life, brain infections such as bacterial meningitis or viral encephalitis, problems with blood flow to the brain, or head injury from a motor vehicle accident, a fall, or child abuse.

In many cases, the cause of cerebral palsy is unknown. Possible causes include genetic abnormalities, congenital brain malformations, maternal infections or fevers, or fetal injury. The following types of brain damage may cause its characteristic symptoms:

- **Damage to the brain's white matter (periventricular leukomalacia, or PVL).** The brain's white matter is responsible for transmitting signals inside the brain and to the rest of the body. Damage from PVL looks like tiny holes in the white matter of an infant's brain. These gaps in brain tissue interfere with the normal transmission of signals. Researchers have identified a period of selective vulnerability in the developing fetal brain, a period of time between 26 and 34 weeks of gestation, in which periventricular white matter is particularly sensitive to insults and injury.
- **Abnormal development of the brain (cerebral dysgenesis).** Any interruption of the normal process of brain growth during fetal development can cause brain malformations that interfere with the transmission of brain signals. Mutations in the genes that control brain development during this early period can keep the brain from developing normally. Infections, fevers, trauma, or other conditions that cause unhealthy conditions in the womb also put an unborn baby's nervous system at risk.
- **Bleeding in the brain (intracranial hemorrhage).** Bleeding inside the brain from blocked or broken blood vessels is commonly caused by fetal stroke. Some babies suffer a stroke while still in the womb because of blood clots in the placenta that block blood flow in the brain. Other types of fetal stroke are caused by malformed or weak blood vessels in the brain or by blood-clotting abnormalities. Maternal high blood pressure (hypertension) is a common medical disorder during pregnancy and is more common in babies with fetal stroke. Maternal infection, especially pelvic inflammatory disease, has also been shown to increase the risk of fetal stroke.

- **Severe lack of oxygen in the brain**. Asphyxia, a lack of oxygen in the brain caused by an interruption in breathing or poor oxygen supply, is common for a brief period of time in babies due to the stress of labor and delivery. If the supply of oxygen is cut off or reduced for lengthy periods, an infant can develop a type of brain damage called "hypoxic-ischemic encephalopathy," which destroys tissue in the cerebral motor cortex and other brain areas. This damage can also be caused by severe maternal low blood pressure, rupture of the uterus, detachment of the placenta, problems involving the umbilical cord, or severe trauma to the head during labor and delivery.

WHAT ARE THE RISK FACTORS?

Some medical conditions or events during pregnancy and delivery may increase a baby's risk of being born with cerebral palsy. These risks include the following:

- **Low birth weight and premature birth**. Premature babies (born less than 37 weeks into pregnancy) and babies weighing less than five and a half pounds at birth have a much higher risk of developing cerebral palsy than full-term, heavier-weight babies. Tiny babies born at very early gestational ages are especially at risk.
- **Multiple births**. Twins, triplets, and other multiple births—even those born at term—are linked to an increased risk of cerebral palsy. The death of a baby's twin or triplet further increases the risk.
- **Infections during pregnancy**. Infections such as toxoplasmosis, rubella (German measles), cytomegalovirus, and herpes can infect the womb and placenta. Inflammation triggered by infection may then go on to damage the developing nervous system in an unborn baby. Maternal fever during pregnancy or delivery can also prevent this inflammatory response.
- **Blood type incompatibility between mother and child**. Rhesus (Rh) incompatibility is a condition

that develops when a mother's Rh blood type (either positive or negative) is different from the blood type of her baby. The mother's system does not tolerate the baby's different blood type, and her body will begin to make antibodies that will attack and kill her baby's blood cells, which can cause brain damage.
- **Exposure to toxic substances**. Mothers exposed to toxic substances during pregnancy, such as methyl mercury, are at a heightened risk of having a baby with CP.
- **Mothers with thyroid abnormalities, intellectual disability, excess protein in the urine, or seizures**. Mothers with these conditions are slightly more likely to have a child with CP.

There are also medical conditions during labor and delivery and immediately after delivery that act as warning signs for an increased risk of CP. However, most of these children will not develop CP. Warning signs include the following:
- **Breech presentation**. Babies with cerebral palsy are more likely to be in a breech position (feet first) instead of head first at the beginning of labor. Babies who are unusually floppy as fetuses are likelier to be born in the breech position.
- **Complicated labor and delivery**. A baby with vascular or respiratory problems during labor and delivery may already have suffered brain damage or abnormalities.
- **Small for gestational age**. Babies born smaller than normal for their gestational age are at risk for cerebral palsy because of factors that keep them from growing naturally in the womb.
- **Low Apgar score**. The Apgar score is a numbered rating that reflects a newborn's physical health. Doctors periodically score a baby's heart rate, breathing, muscle tone, reflexes, and skin color during the first minutes after birth. A low score 10–20 minutes after delivery is often considered an important sign of potential problems such as CP.

- **Jaundice**. More than 50 percent of newborns develop jaundice (yellowing of the skin or whites of the eyes) after birth when bilirubin, a substance normally found in bile, builds up faster than their livers can break it down and pass it from the body. Severe, untreated jaundice can kill brain cells and cause deafness and CP.
- **Seizures**. An infant with seizures faces a higher risk of being diagnosed later in childhood with CP.

HOW IS CEREBRAL PALSY DIAGNOSED?

Most children with CP are diagnosed during the first two years of life. But, if a child's symptoms are mild, it can be difficult for a doctor to make a reliable diagnosis before age four or five.

Doctors will order tests to evaluate the child's motor skills. During regular visits, the doctor will monitor the child's development, growth, muscle tone, age-appropriate motor control, hearing and vision, posture, and coordination, to rule out other disorders that could cause similar symptoms. Although symptoms may change over time, CP is not progressive. If a child continuously loses motor skills, the problem is more likely to be a condition other than CP—such as a genetic or muscle disease, metabolism disorder, or tumors in the nervous system. Lab tests can identify other conditions that may cause symptoms similar to those associated with CP.

Neuroimaging techniques that allow doctors to look into the brain (such as magnetic resonance imaging (MRI) scan) can detect abnormalities that indicate a potentially treatable movement disorder. Neuroimaging methods are as follows:
- **Cranial ultrasound** uses high-frequency sound waves to produce pictures of the brains of young babies. It is used for high-risk premature infants because it is the least intrusive of the imaging techniques. However, it is not as successful as computed tomography (CT) or magnetic resonance imaging (MRI) at capturing subtle changes in white matter—the type of brain tissue damaged in CP.

- **Computed tomography** uses x-rays to create images that show the structure of the brain and the areas of damage.
- **Magnetic resonance imaging** uses a computer, a magnetic field, and radio waves to create an anatomical picture of the brain's tissues and structures. MRI can show the location and type of damage and offers finer details than CT.

Another test, an electroencephalogram, uses a series of electrodes that are either taped or temporarily pasted to the scalp to detect electrical activity in the brain. Changes in the normal electrical pattern may help identify epilepsy.

Some metabolic disorders can masquerade as CP. Most childhood metabolic disorders have characteristic brain abnormalities or malformations that will show up on an MRI.

Other types of disorders can also be mistaken for CP or can cause specific types of CP. For example, coagulation disorders (which prevent blood from clotting or lead to excessive clotting) can cause prenatal or perinatal strokes that damage the brain and produce symptoms characteristic of CP, most commonly hemiparetic CP. Referrals to specialists such as a child neurologist, developmental pediatrician, ophthalmologist, or otologist aid in a more accurate diagnosis and help doctors develop a specific treatment plan.

WHAT ARE THE DIFFERENT FORMS OF CEREBRAL PALSY?

The specific forms of CP are determined by the extent, type, and location of a child's abnormalities. Doctors classify CP according to the type of movement disorder involved—spastic (stiff muscles), athetoid (writhing movements), or ataxic (poor balance and coordination)—plus any additional symptoms, such as weakness (paresis) or paralysis (plegia). For example, hemiparesis (hemi = half) indicates that only one side of the body is weakened. Quadriplegia (quad = four) means all four limbs are affected.

Cerebral Palsy

Spastic cerebral palsy is the most common type of disorder. People have stiff muscles and awkward movements. Forms of spastic cerebral palsy include the following:

- **Spastic hemiplegia/hemiparesis** typically affects the arm and hand on one side of the body but can also include the leg. Children with spastic hemiplegia generally walk later and tiptoe because of tight heel tendons. The arm and leg of the affected side are frequently shorter and thinner. Some children will develop an abnormal curvature of the spine (scoliosis). A child with spastic hemiplegia may also have seizures. The speech will be delayed and, at best, may be competent, but intelligence is usually normal.
- **Spastic diplegia/diparesis** involves muscle stiffness predominantly in the legs and less severely affects the arms and face although the hands may be clumsy. Tendon reflexes in the legs are hyperactive. The toes point up when the bottom of the foot is stimulated. Tightness in certain leg muscles makes the legs move like the arms of a scissor. Children may require a walker or leg braces. Intelligence and language skills are usually normal.
- **Spastic quadriplegia/quadriparesis** is the most severe form of cerebral palsy and is often associated with moderate-to-severe intellectual disability. It is caused by widespread damage to the brain or significant brain malformations. Children often have severe stiffness in their limbs but a floppy neck. They are rarely able to walk. Speaking and being understood is difficult. Seizures can be frequent and hard to control.

Dyskinetic cerebral palsy (including athetoid, choreoathetoid, and dystonic cerebral palsies) is characterized by slow and uncontrollable writhing or jerky movements of the hands, feet, arms, or legs. Hyperactivity in the muscles of the face and tongue makes some children grimace or drool. They find it difficult to sit straight or walk. Some children have problems hearing, controlling their breathing, and/or coordinating the muscle movements required for speaking. Intelligence is rarely affected in these forms of cerebral palsy.

Ataxic cerebral palsy affects balance and depth perception. Children with ataxic CP often have poor coordination and walk unsteadily with a wide-based gait. They have difficulty with quick or precise movements, such as writing or buttoning a shirt, or a hard time controlling voluntary movements, such as reaching for a book.

Mixed types of cerebral palsy refer to symptoms that do not correspond to any single type of CP but are a mix of types. For example, a child with mixed CP may have some muscles that are too tight and others that are too relaxed, creating a mix of stiffness and floppiness.

HOW IS CEREBRAL PALSY TREATED?

Cerebral palsy cannot be cured, but treatment often improves a child's capabilities. Many children go on to enjoy near-normal adult lives if their disabilities are properly managed. In general, the earlier treatment begins, the better chance children have of overcoming developmental disabilities or learning new ways to accomplish the tasks that challenge them.

There is no standard therapy that works for every individual with CP. Once the diagnosis is made and the type of CP is determined, a team of health-care professionals will work with a child and her or his parents to identify specific impairments and needs and then develop an appropriate plan to tackle the core disabilities that affect the child's quality of life.

Physical therapy is a cornerstone of CP treatment, usually in the first few years of life or soon after the diagnosis. Specific sets of exercises (such as resistive or strength training programs) and activities can maintain or improve muscle strength, balance, and motor skills and prevent contractures. Special braces (called "orthotic devices") may be used to improve mobility and stretch spastic muscles.

Cerebral Palsy

Occupational therapy focuses on optimizing upper body function, improving posture, and making the most of a child's mobility. Occupational therapists help individuals address new ways to meet everyday activities such as dressing, going to school, and participating in day-to-day activities.

Recreation therapy encourages participation in art and cultural programs, sports, and other events that help an individual expand physical and cognitive skills and abilities. Parents of children who participate in recreational therapies usually notice an improvement in their child's speech, self-esteem, and emotional well-being.

Speech and language therapy can improve a child's ability to speak more clearly; help with swallowing disorders; and learn new ways to communicate—using sign language and/or special communication devices such as a computer with a voice synthesizer or a special board covered with symbols of everyday objects and activities to which a child can point to indicate her or his wishes.

Treatments for problems with eating and drooling are often necessary when children with CP have difficulty eating and drinking because they have little control over the muscles that move their mouth, jaw, and tongue. They are also at risk for breathing food or fluid into the lungs, as well as for malnutrition, recurrent lung infections, and progressive lung disease.

Drug Treatments

Oral medications such as diazepam, baclofen, dantrolene sodium, and tizanidine are usually used as the first line of treatment to relax stiff, contracted, or overactive muscles. Some drugs have some risky side effects, such as drowsiness, changes in blood pressure, and risk of liver damage that require continuous monitoring. Oral medications are most appropriate for children who need only a mild reduction in muscle tone or who have widespread spasticity.

- **Botulinum toxin** (BT-A), injected locally, has become a standard treatment for overactive muscles in children with spastic movement disorders such as CP. BT-A relaxes contracted muscles by keeping nerve cells from over-activating muscle. The relaxing effect of a BT-A injection lasts approximately three months.

Undesirable side effects are mild and short-lived, consisting of pain upon injection and occasionally mild flu-like symptoms. BT-A injections are most effective when followed by a stretching program, including physical therapy and splinting. BT-A injections work best for children who have some control over their motor movements and have a limited number of muscles to treat, none of which is fixed or rigid.
- **Intrathecal baclofen therapy** uses an implantable pump to deliver baclofen, a muscle relaxant, into the fluid surrounding the spinal cord. Baclofen decreases the excitability of nerve cells in the spinal cord, which then reduces muscle spasticity throughout the body. The pump can be adjusted if muscle tone is worse at certain times of the day or night. The baclofen pump is most appropriate for individuals with chronic, severe stiffness, or uncontrolled muscle movement throughout the body.

Assistive Devices

Assistive devices such devices as computers, computer software, voice synthesizers, and picture books can greatly help some individuals with CP improve their communication skills. Other devices around the home or workplace make it easier for people with CP to adapt to activities of daily living.

Orthotic devices help compensate for muscle imbalance and increase independent mobility. Braces and splints use external force to correct muscle abnormalities and improve functions, such as sitting or walking. Other orthotics help stretch muscles or the position of a joint. Braces, wedges, special chairs, and other devices can help people sit more comfortably and make it easier to perform daily functions. Wheelchairs, rolling walkers, and powered scooters can help individuals who are not independently mobile. Vision aids include glasses, magnifiers, large print books, and computer typefaces. Some individuals with CP may need surgery to correct vision problems. Hearing aids and telephone amplifiers may help people hear more clearly.

CAN CEREBRAL PALSY BE PREVENTED?

Cerebral palsy related to genetic abnormalities cannot be prevented, but a few risk factors for congenital CP can be managed or avoided. For example, rubella, or German measles, is preventable if women are vaccinated against the disease before becoming pregnant. Rh incompatibilities can also be managed early in pregnancy. Acquired CP, often due to head injury, is often preventable using common safety tactics, such as using car seats for infants and toddlers.

Chapter 16 | Chromosomal Disorders

Chapter Contents
Section 16.1—What Are Chromosomal Disorders?.................. 139
Section 16.2—Down Syndrome 144
Section 16.3—47,XYY Syndrome... 148
Section 16.4—Fragile X Syndrome 150
Section 16.5—Klinefelter Syndrome.. 154
Section 16.6—Prader-Willi Syndrome 159
Section 16.7—Turner Syndrome 164
Section 16.8—Velocardiofacial Syndrome 168
Section 16.9—Williams Syndrome 171

Section 16.1 | **What Are Chromosomal Disorders?**

This section contains text excerpted from the following sources: Text beginning with the heading "What Are Chromosomes?" is excerpted from "Chromosome Abnormalities Fact Sheet," National Human Genome Research Institute (NHGRI), August 15, 2020; Text under the heading "Are Chromosomal Disorders Inherited?" is excerpted from "Are Chromosomal Disorders Inherited?" MedlinePlus, National Institutes of Health (NIH), April 19, 2021.

WHAT ARE CHROMOSOMES?

Chromosomes are the structures that hold genes. Genes are the individual instructions that tell our bodies how to develop and function; they govern physical and medical characteristics, such as hair color, blood type, and disease susceptibility.

Many chromosomes have two segments, called "arms," separated by a pinched region known as the "centromere." The shorter arm is called the "p" arm. The longer arm is called the "q" arm.

WHERE ARE THE CHROMOSOMES FOUND IN THE HUMAN BODY?

The human body is made up of individual units called "cells." Your body has many different cells, such as the skin, liver, and blood. In the center of most cells is a structure called the "nucleus." This is where chromosomes are located.

HOW MANY CHROMOSOMES DO HUMANS HAVE?

A human cell's typical number of chromosomes is 46: 23 pairs, holding an estimated 20,000–25,000 genes. One set of 23 chromosomes is inherited from the biological mother (from the egg), and the other is inherited from the biological father (from the sperm).

Of the 23 pairs of chromosomes, the first 22 pairs are called "autosomes." The final pair is called the "sex chromosomes." Sex chromosomes determine an individual's sex; females have two X chromosomes (XX), and males have an X and a Y chromosome (XY). The mother and father each contribute one set of 22 autosomes and one sex chromosome.

HOW DO SCIENTISTS STUDY CHROMOSOMES?

For a century, scientists studied chromosomes by looking at them under a microscope. For chromosomes to be seen this way, they need to be stained. Once stained, the chromosomes look like strings with light and dark "bands," and their picture can be taken. A picture, or chromosome map, of all 46 chromosomes is called a "karyotype." The karyotype can help identify abnormalities in the structure or the number of chromosomes.

To help identify chromosomes, the pairs numbered 1–22, with the 23rd pair labeled "X" and "Y." In addition, the bands that appear after staining are numbered; the higher the number, the farther that area is from the centromere.

In the past decade, newer techniques have allowed scientists and doctors to screen for chromosomal abnormalities without a microscope. These newer methods compare the patient's deoxyribonucleic acid (DNA) to a normal DNA sample. The comparison can find chromosomal abnormalities where the two samples differ.

One such method is called "noninvasive prenatal testing." This is a test to screen a pregnancy to determine whether a baby has an increased chance of having specific chromosome disorders. The test examines the baby's DNA in the mother's blood.

WHAT ARE CHROMOSOME ABNORMALITIES?

There are many types of chromosome abnormalities. However, they can be organized into two basic groups: numerical abnormalities and structural abnormalities.

- **Numerical abnormalities**. When an individual is missing one of the chromosomes from a pair, the condition is called "monosomy." The condition is called "trisomy" when an individual has more than two chromosomes instead of a pair. An example of a condition caused by numerical abnormalities is Down syndrome, marked by mental disability, learning difficulties, a characteristic facial appearance, and poor muscle tone (hypotonia) in infancy. An individual with

Chromosomal Disorders

Down syndrome has three copies of chromosome 21 rather than two; for that reason, the condition is also known as "trisomy 21." An example of monosomy, in which an individual lacks a chromosome, is Turner syndrome. In Turner syndrome, a female is born with only one sex chromosome, an X, and is usually shorter than average and unable to have children, among other difficulties.
- **Structural abnormalities**. A chromosome's structure can be altered in the following ways:
  - **Deletions**. A portion of the chromosome is missing or deleted.
  - **Duplications**. A portion of the chromosome is duplicated, resulting in extra genetic material.
  - **Translocations**. A portion of one chromosome is transferred to another chromosome. There are two main types of translocation. In a reciprocal translocation, segments from two different chromosomes have been exchanged. In a Robertsonian translocation, an entire chromosome has attached to another at the centromere.
  - **Inversions**. A portion of the chromosome has broken off, turned upside down, and reattached. As a result, the genetic material is inverted.
  - **Rings**. A portion of a chromosome has broken off and formed a circle or ring. This can happen with or without the loss of genetic material.

Most chromosome abnormalities occur as an accident in the egg or sperm. In these cases, the abnormality is present in every body cell. Some abnormalities happen after conception; some cells have the abnormality, and some do not.

Chromosome abnormalities can be inherited from a parent (such as a translocation) or be "de novo" (new to the individual). This is why chromosome studies are often performed on the parents when a child is found to have an abnormality.

HOW DO CHROMOSOME ABNORMALITIES HAPPEN?
Chromosome abnormalities usually occur when there is an error in cell division. There are two kinds of cell division: mitosis and meiosis.
- **Mitosis**. Mitosis results in two cells that are duplicates of the original cell. One cell with 46 chromosomes divides and becomes two cells with 46 chromosomes each. This kind of cell division occurs throughout the body, except in the reproductive organs. This is how most cells that make up our body are made and replaced.
- **Meiosis**. Meiosis results in cells with half the number of chromosomes 23 instead of the normal 46. This type of cell division occurs in the reproductive organs, resulting in the eggs and sperm.

In both processes, the correct number of chromosomes is supposed to end up in the resulting cells. However, errors in cell division can result in cells with too few or too many copies of a chromosome. Errors can also occur when the chromosomes are duplicated.

Other factors that can increase the risk of chromosome abnormalities are as follows:
- **Maternal age**. Women are born with all the eggs they will ever have. Some researchers believe that errors can crop up in the eggs' genetic material as they age. Older women are at higher risk of giving birth to babies with chromosome abnormalities than younger women. Because men produce new sperm throughout their lives, paternal age does not increase the risk of chromosome abnormalities.
- **Environment**. Although there is no conclusive evidence that specific environmental factors cause chromosome abnormalities, it is still possible that the environment may play a role in the occurrence of genetic errors.

Chromosomal Disorders

ARE CHROMOSOMAL DISORDERS INHERITED?

Although it is possible to inherit some types of chromosomal abnormalities, most chromosomal disorders (such as Down syndrome and Turner syndrome) are not passed from one generation to the next.

Changes in the number of chromosomes cause some chromosomal conditions. These changes are not inherited but occur as random events during the formation of reproductive cells (eggs and sperm). An error in cell division called "nondisjunction" results in reproductive cells with an abnormal number of chromosomes. For example, a reproductive cell may accidentally gain or lose one copy of a chromosome. If one of these atypical reproductive cells contributes to a child's genetic makeup, the child will have an extra or missing chromosome in each of the body's cells.

Changes in chromosome structure can also cause chromosomal disorders. Some changes in chromosome structure can be inherited, while others occur as random accidents during the formation of reproductive cells or in early fetal development. Because the inheritance of these changes can be complex, people concerned about this type of chromosomal abnormality may want to talk with a genetics professional.

Some cancer cells also change the number or structure of their chromosomes. Because these changes occur in somatic cells (cells other than eggs and sperm), they cannot be passed from one generation to the next.

Section 16.2 | Down Syndrome

> This section includes text excerpted from "Facts about Down Syndrome," Centers for Disease Control and Prevention (CDC), April 6, 2021.

WHAT IS DOWN SYNDROME?

Down syndrome is a condition in which a person has an extra chromosome. Chromosomes are small "packages" of genes in the body. They determine how a baby's body forms and functions as it grows during pregnancy and after birth. Typically, a baby is born with 46 chromosomes. Babies with Down syndrome have an extra copy of one of these chromosomes, chromosome 21. A medical term for having an extra copy of a chromosome is "trisomy." Down syndrome is also referred to as "Trisomy 21." This extra copy changes how the baby's body and brain develop, which can cause mental and physical challenges for the baby.

Even though people with Down syndrome might act and look similar, each person has different abilities. People with Down syndrome usually have an intelligence quotient (IQ)—a measure of intelligence in the mildly to moderately low range and are slower to speak than other children.

Some common physical features of Down syndrome are as follows:
- A flattened face, especially the bridge of the nose
- Almond-shaped eyes that slant up
- A short neck
- Small ears
- A tongue that tends to stick out of the mouth
- Tiny white spots on the iris (colored part) of the eye
- Small hands and feet
- A single line across the palm of the hand (palmar crease)
- Small pinky fingers that sometimes curve toward the thumb
- Poor muscle tone or loose joints
- Shorter in height as children and adults

Chromosomal Disorders

HOW MANY BABIES ARE BORN WITH DOWN SYNDROME?
Down syndrome remains the most common chromosomal condition diagnosed in the United States. Each year, about 6,000 babies born in the United States have Down syndrome. This means that Down syndrome occurs in about one in every 700 babies.

TYPES OF DOWN SYNDROME
There are three types of Down syndrome. People often cannot tell the difference between each type without looking at the chromosomes because the physical features and behaviors are similar.
- **Trisomy 21**. About 95 percent of people with Down syndrome have trisomy 21. With this type of Down syndrome, each cell in the body has three separate copies of chromosome 21 instead of the usual two copies.
- **Translocation Down syndrome**. This type accounts for a small percentage of people with Down syndrome (about 3%). This occurs when an extra part or a whole extra chromosome 21 is present but is attached or "translocated" to a different chromosome rather than being a separate chromosome 21.
- **Mosaic Down syndrome**. This type affects about two percent of people with Down syndrome. Mosaic means mixture or combination. For children with mosaic Down syndrome, some of their cells have three copies of chromosome 21, but others have the typical two copies of chromosome 21. Children with mosaic Down syndrome may have the same features as other children with Down syndrome. However, they may have fewer features of the condition due to some (or many) cells with a typical number of chromosomes.

CAUSES AND RISK FACTORS OF DOWN SYNDROME
- The extra chromosome 21 leads to the physical features and developmental challenges that can occur among

people with Down syndrome. Researchers know that an extra chromosome causes Down syndrome, but no one knows for sure why Down syndrome occurs or how many different factors play a role.
- One factor that increases the risk of having a baby with Down syndrome is the mother's age. Women who are 35 years or older when they become pregnant are more likely to have a pregnancy affected by Down syndrome than women who become pregnant at a younger age. However, most babies with Down syndrome are born to mothers less than 35 years old because there are many more births among younger women.

DIAGNOSIS OF DOWN SYNDROME

Two basic tests are available to detect Down syndrome during pregnancy: screening and diagnostic tests. A screening test can tell a woman and her health-care provider whether her pregnancy has a lower or higher chance of having Down syndrome. Screening tests do not provide an absolute diagnosis, but they are safer for the mother and the developing baby. Diagnostic tests can detect whether or not a baby will have Down syndrome, but they can be riskier for the mother and developing baby. Neither screening nor diagnostic tests can predict the full impact of Down syndrome on a baby; no one can predict this.

Screening Tests

Screening tests often include a combination of a blood test, which measures the number of various substances in the mother's blood (e.g., MS-AFP, triple screen, quad-screen), and an ultrasound, which creates a picture of the baby. During an ultrasound, one of the things the technician looks at is the fluid behind the baby's neck. Extra fluid in this region could indicate a genetic problem. These screening tests can help determine the baby's risk of Down syndrome. Rarely, screening tests can give an abnormal result even when there is nothing wrong with the baby. Sometimes, the test results are normal, and yet they miss a problem that does exist.

Chromosomal Disorders

Diagnostic Tests
Diagnostic tests are usually performed after a positive screening test to confirm a Down syndrome diagnosis. The following are the types of diagnostic tests:
- **Chorionic villus sampling (CVS)**. CVS examines material from the placenta.
- **Amniocentesis**. It examines the amniotic fluid (the fluid from the sac surrounding the baby).
- **Percutaneous umbilical blood sampling (PUBS)**. PUBS examines blood from the umbilical cord.

These tests look for chromosome changes that would indicate a Down syndrome diagnosis.

OTHER HEALTH PROBLEMS
Many people with Down syndrome have common facial features and no other major birth defects. However, some people with Down syndrome might have one or more major birth defects or other medical problems. Some of the more common health problems among children with Down syndrome are as follows:
- Hearing loss
- Obstructive sleep apnea (a condition where the person's breathing temporarily stops while asleep)
- Ear infections
- Eye diseases
- Heart defects present at birth

Health-care providers routinely monitor children with Down syndrome for these conditions.

TREATMENTS FOR DOWN SYNDROME
Down syndrome is a lifelong condition. Services early in life will often help babies and children with Down syndrome to improve their physical and intellectual abilities. Most of these services focus on helping children with Down syndrome develop to their full potential. These services include speech, occupational, and physical therapy,

typically offered through early intervention programs in each state. Children with Down syndrome may also need extra help or attention in school although many are included in regular classes.

Section 16.3 | 47,XYY Syndrome

This section includes text excerpted from "47,XYY Syndrome," MedlinePlus, National Institutes of Health (NIH), March 2, 2022.

WHAT IS 47,XYY SYNDROME?

47,XYY syndrome is characterized by an extra copy of the Y chromosome in each individual's cells. Although many people with this condition are taller than average, the chromosomal change sometimes causes no unusual physical features. Most individuals with 47,XYY syndrome have normal production of the male sex hormone testosterone and normal male sexual development, and they are usually able to father children.

47,XYY syndrome is associated with an increased risk of learning disabilities and delayed development of speech and language skills. Affected children can develop delayed motor skills (such as sitting and walking) or weak muscle tone (hypotonia). Other signs and symptoms of this condition include hand tremors or other involuntary movements (motor tics), seizures, and asthma. Individuals with 47,XYY syndrome have an increased risk of behavioral, social, and emotional difficulties compared with their unaffected peers. These problems include attention deficit hyperactivity disorder (ADHD), depression, anxiety, and autism spectrum disorder (ASD), a group of developmental conditions that affect communication and social interaction.

Physical features oriented to 47,XYY syndrome can include increased belly fat, a large head (macrocephaly), unusually large teeth (macrodontia), flat feet (pes planus), fifth fingers that curve inward (clinodactyly), widely spaced eyes (ocular hypertelorism), and abnormal side-to-side curvature of the spine (scoliosis). These characteristics vary widely among people with this condition.

Chromosomal Disorders

FREQUENCY OF 47,XYY SYNDROME
47,XYY syndrome occurs in about one in 1,000 newborns. Five to 10 children with 47,XYY syndrome are born in the United States daily. Many affected individuals are never diagnosed or not diagnosed until later in life.

CAUSES OF 47,XYY SYNDROME
People normally have 46 chromosomes in each cell. Two of the 46 chromosomes, known as "X" and "Y," are called "sex chromosomes" because they help determine whether a person will develop male or female sex characteristics. Females typically have two X chromosomes (46,XX), and males have one X chromosome and one Y chromosome (46,XY) in each cell.

47,XYY syndrome is caused by the presence of an extra copy of the Y chromosome in each of a male's cells. As a result of the extra Y chromosome, each cell has a total of 47 chromosomes instead of the usual 46. It is unclear why an extra copy of the Y chromosome is associated with tall stature, learning problems, and other features in some boys and men.

Some people with 47,XYY syndrome have an extra Y chromosome in only some of their cells. This phenomenon is called "46,XY/47" and "XYY mosaicism."

INHERITANCE OF 47,XYY SYNDROME
47,XYY syndrome is not inherited. The chromosomal change occurs as a random event during the formation of sperm cells. An error in cell division called "nondisjunction" can result in sperm cells with an extra copy of the Y chromosome. If one of these atypical reproductive cells contributes to a child's genetic makeup, the child will have an extra Y chromosome in each of the body's cells.

46, XY/47,XYY mosaicism is also not inherited. It occurs as a random event during cell division in early embryonic development. As a result, some of an affected person's cells have one X chromosome and one Y chromosome (46,XY), and others have one X chromosome and two Y chromosomes (47,XYY).

Section 16.4 | Fragile X Syndrome

This section includes text excerpted from "What Is Fragile X Syndrome?" Centers for Disease Control and Prevention (CDC), June 3, 2022.

WHAT IS FRAGILE X SYNDROME?

Fragile X syndrome (FXS) is a genetic disorder. FXS is caused by changes in a gene called "*Fragile X Messenger Ribonucleoprotein 1*" (*FMR1*). *FMR1* usually makes an *FMR1* protein (FMRP) needed for brain development. People who have FXS do not make this protein. Those with fragile X-associated disorders have changes in the *FMR1* gene but usually still make some of the protein.

Fragile X syndrome affects both males and females. However, females often have milder symptoms than males. The exact number of people with FXS is unknown, but a review of research studies estimated that about one in 7,000 males and about one in 11,000 females had been diagnosed with FXS.

HOW IS FRAGILE X SYNDROME INHERITED?

Understanding how FXS is inherited helps know about the changes in the *FMR1* gene that cause FXS and other fragile X-associated disorders. There is a place in the *FMR1* gene where the DNA pattern of the chemical letters, cytosine-guanine-guanine (CGG), is repeated repeatedly. People have different numbers of these CGG repeats, but most have less than 45 repeats. People with FXS nearly always have more than 200 repeats, many more than normal. Having more than 200 repeats causes the *FMR1* gene to "turn off" so that it cannot make FMRP (the protein made by the *FMR1* gene). When a person's *FMR1* gene has more than 200 repeats, so it cannot make FMRP; the person has FXS.

Each person is in one of the four groups shown below, oriented on the number of CGG repeats in the person's *FMR1* gene. The number of CGG repeats that a person has can be determined by a blood test ordered by a health-care provider or genetic counselor. People with different numbers of CGG repeats have different risks of developing fragile X-associated disorders and having children with FXS.

Chromosomal Disorders

A female has two copies of the *FMR1* gene, one on her two X chromosomes. The number of CGG repeats on each copy of the *FMR1* gene is usually different. For example, a female might have 30 CGG repeats on one copy of her *FMR1* gene but 70 CGG repeats on her other. The group where the female is in normal, intermediate, premutation, or full mutation is oriented on her *FMR1* gene copy with the greatest number of CGG repeats. A male has only one copy of the *FMR1* gene on his only X chromosome, so the group in which a male is in is oriented on the number of CGG repeats in that one copy.

Normal: 5–44 Repeats
Most males have about 5–44 repeats of the chemical letters, CGG, in their *FMR1* gene, and most females also have 5–44 repeats in each of their *FMR1* genes. This is considered a normal number of repeats. People with a normal number of repeats do not have FXS and do not pass a higher chance of having FXS to their children.

Intermediate: 45–54 Repeats
People who have an intermediate number of repeats (45–54) do not have FXS and are not at risk of having children with FXS. However, they may have a slightly higher chance of having some symptoms related to other fragile X-associated disorders and may pass the slightly higher chance of having these disorders to their children.

Premutation: 55–200 Repeats
People who have 55–200 repeats are said to have a "premutation" in the *FMR1* gene. They do not have FXS, but they might have, or may later develop, other fragile X-associated disorders. In addition, people with a premutation can have children with a premutation or full mutation (FXS). However, the chances of having a child with a premutation or a full mutation are different for women with a premutation than they are for men with a premutation, as described below:
- The number of repeats in the egg cells of a woman with a premutation can increase from the premutation range

(55–200 repeats) to the full mutation range (more than 200 repeats). Therefore, a woman with a premutation can pass on a full mutation. The more CGG repeats a woman with a premutation has, the more likely her child will inherit an *FMR1* gene with a full mutation and, therefore, have FXS. With each pregnancy, a woman with a premutation in one of her *FMR1* genes has a 50 percent chance of passing on either the premutation or a full mutation to her child (daughters or sons) and a 50 percent chance of not passing on either the premutation or the full mutation.
- A man with a premutation will pass on his premutation to his daughters but not his sons. A man with a premutation will not pass on a full mutation to any of his children.

Full Mutation: More Than 200 Repeats
People with a full mutation (more than 200 repeats) have FXS.
- With each pregnancy, women have a 50 percent chance of passing fragile X on to their child (sons or daughters).

SIGNS AND SYMPTOMS OF FRAGILE X SYNDROME
Signs that a child might have FXS include the following:
- **Developmental delays** (not sitting, walking, or talking at the same time as other children the same age)
- **Learning disabilities** (trouble learning new skills)
- **Social and behavior problems** (such as not making eye contact, anxiety, trouble paying attention, hand flapping, acting and speaking without thinking, and being very active)

Males with FXS usually have some degree of intellectual disability ranging from mild to severe. Females with FXS can have normal intelligence or some degree of intellectual disability. Autism spectrum disorder (ASD) also occurs more frequently in people with FXS.

TESTING/DIAGNOSIS OF FRAGILE X SYNDROME

Fragile X syndrome can be diagnosed by testing a person's deoxyribonucleic acid (DNA) from a blood test. A doctor or genetic counselor can order the test. Testing can also be done to find changes in the *FMR1* gene that can lead to fragile X-associated disorders.

A diagnosis of FXS can be helpful to the family because it can provide a reason for a child's intellectual disabilities and behavioral problems. This allows the family and other caregivers to learn more about the disorder and manage care so the child can reach her or his full potential. However, the results of DNA tests can affect other family members and raise many issues. So anyone considering FXS testing should consider having genetic counseling before getting tested.

TREATMENTS FOR FRAGILE X SYNDROME

There is no cure for FXS. However, treatment services can help people learn important skills. Services can include therapy to learn to talk, walk, and interact with others. In addition, medicine can be used to help control some issues, such as behavior problems. To develop the best treatment plan, people with FXS, parents, and health-care providers should work closely with one another and with everyone involved in treatment and support—which may include teachers, childcare providers, coaches, therapists, and other family members. Taking advantage of all the resources available will help guide success.

EARLY INTERVENTION SERVICES

Early intervention services help children from birth to three years (36 months) old learn important skills. These services may improve a child's development. Even if the child has not been diagnosed with FXS, they may be eligible for services. These services are provided through an early intervention system in each state. Through this system, you can ask for an evaluation. In addition, treatment for particular symptoms, such as speech therapy for language delays, often does not need to wait for a formal diagnosis. While early intervention is extremely important, treatment services at any age can be helpful.

WHAT TO DO IF YOU THINK YOUR CHILD MIGHT HAVE FRAGILE X SYNDROME

Local public school systems can provide services and support for children three years of age and older. Children can access some services even if they do not attend public school. When parents are concerned about a child's development, it can be very challenging to figure out the right steps. States have created parent centers. These centers help families learn how and where to have their children evaluated and how to find services.

Section 16.5 | Klinefelter Syndrome

This section contains text excerpted from the following sources: Text beginning with the heading "What Is Klinefelter Syndrome?" is excerpted from "Klinefelter Syndrome," MedlinePlus, National Institutes of Health (NIH), April 1, 2019; Text beginning with the heading "What Are the Symptoms of Klinefelter Syndrome?" is excerpted from "About Klinefelter Syndrome," National Human Genome Research Institute (NHGRI), May 19, 2019.

WHAT IS KLINEFELTER SYNDROME?

Klinefelter syndrome is a chromosomal condition in boys and men that can affect physical and intellectual development. Most commonly, affected individuals are taller than average and are unable to father biological children (infertile); however, the signs and symptoms of Klinefelter syndrome vary among boys and men with this condition. In some cases, the features of the condition are so mild that the condition is not diagnosed until puberty or adulthood, and researchers believe that up to 75 percent of affected men and boys are never diagnosed.

Boys and men with Klinefelter syndrome typically have small testes that produce a reduced amount of testosterone (primary testicular insufficiency). Testosterone is the hormone that directs male sexual development before birth and during puberty. Without treatment, testosterone shortage can lead to delayed or incomplete puberty, breast enlargement (gynecomastia), decreased muscle mass, decreased bone density, and reduced facial and body hair. As a result of the small testes and decreased hormone production,

Chromosomal Disorders

affected males are infertile but may benefit from assisted reproductive technologies. Some affected individuals also have differences in their genitalia, including undescended testes (cryptorchidism), the opening of the urethra on the underside of the penis (hypospadias), or an unusually small penis (micropenis).

Other physical changes associated with Klinefelter syndrome are usually subtle. Older children and adults with the condition tend to be somewhat taller than their peers. Other differences can include abnormal fusion of certain bones in the forearm (radioulnar synostosis), curved pinky fingers (fifth finger clinodactyly), and flat feet (pes planus).

Children with Klinefelter syndrome may have low muscle tone (hypotonia) and problems with coordination that may delay the development of motor skills, such as sitting, standing, and walking. Affected boys often have learning disabilities, resulting in mild delays in speech and language development and problems with reading. Boys and men with Klinefelter syndrome tend to have better receptive language skills (the ability to understand speech) than expressive language skills (vocabulary and speech production). They may have difficulty communicating and expressing themselves.

Individuals with Klinefelter syndrome tend to have anxiety, depression, impaired social skills, behavioral problems such as emotional immaturity and impulsivity, attention deficit hyperactivity disorder (ADHD), and limited problem-solving skills (executive functioning). About 10 percent of boys and men with Klinefelter syndrome have autism spectrum disorder (ASD).

Nearly half of all men with Klinefelter syndrome develop metabolic syndrome, a group of conditions that include type 2 diabetes, high blood pressure (hypertension), increased belly fat, and high levels of fats (lipids) such as cholesterol and triglycerides in the blood. Compared with unaffected men, adults with Klinefelter syndrome also have an increased risk of developing involuntary trembling (tremors), breast cancer (if gynecomastia develops), thinning and weakening of the bones (osteoporosis), and autoimmune disorders such as systemic lupus erythematosus and rheumatoid arthritis.

FREQUENCY OF KLINEFELTER SYNDROME
Klinefelter syndrome affects about one in 650 newborn boys. It is among the most common sex chromosome disorders, which are conditions caused by changes in the number of sex chromosomes (X and Y chromosomes).

CAUSES OF KLINEFELTER SYNDROME
Klinefelter syndrome is a sex chromosome disorder in boys and men that results from the presence of an extra X chromosome in cells. People typically have 46 chromosomes in each cell, two of which are the sex chromosomes. Females have two X chromosomes (46,XX), and males have one X chromosome and one Y chromosome (46,XY). Most often, boys and men with Klinefelter syndrome have the usual X and Y chromosomes, plus one extra X chromosome, for a total of 47 (47,XXY).

Boys and men with Klinefelter syndrome have an extra copy of multiple genes on the X chromosome. The activity of these extra genes may disrupt many aspects of development, including sexual development before birth and at puberty, and are responsible for the common signs and symptoms of Klinefelter syndrome. Researchers are working to determine which genes contribute to the specific developmental and physical differences that can occur with Klinefelter syndrome.

Some people with features of Klinefelter syndrome have an extra X chromosome in only some of their cells; other cells typically have one X chromosome and one Y chromosome. (Rarely, other cells may have additional chromosome abnormalities.) These individuals describe the condition as mosaic Klinefelter syndrome (46,XY/47,XXY). It is thought that less than 10 percent of individuals with Klinefelter syndrome have the mosaic form. Boys and men with mosaic Klinefelter syndrome may have milder signs and symptoms than those with the extra X chromosome in all of their cells, depending on what proportion of cells have the additional chromosome.

Several conditions resulting from more than one extra sex chromosome in each cell are sometimes described as variants of Klinefelter syndrome. These conditions include 48,XXXY syndrome,

Chromosomal Disorders

48,XXYY syndrome, and 49,XXXXY syndrome. Like Klinefelter syndrome, these conditions affect male sexual development and can be associated with learning disabilities and speech and language development problems. However, the features of these disorders tend to be more severe than those of Klinefelter syndrome and affect more parts of the body. As doctors and researchers have learned more about the differences between these sex chromosome disorders, they have started considering them separate conditions.

INHERITANCE OF KLINEFELTER SYNDROME

Klinefelter syndrome is not inherited; an extra X chromosome is added during the formation of reproductive cells (eggs or sperm) in an affected person's parents. During cell division, an error called "nondisjunction" prevents X chromosomes from being distributed normally among reproductive cells as they form. Typically, as cells divide, each egg cell gets a single X chromosome, and each sperm cell gets either an X or Y chromosome. However, because of nondisjunction, an egg or sperm cell can also end up with an extra copy of the X chromosome.

If an egg cell with an extra X chromosome (XX) is fertilized by a sperm cell with one Y chromosome, the resulting child will have Klinefelter syndrome. Similarly, if a sperm cell with both an X chromosome and a Y chromosome (XY) fertilizes an egg cell with a single X chromosome, the resulting child will have Klinefelter syndrome.

Mosaic Klinefelter syndrome (46,XY/47,XXY) is also not inherited. It occurs as a random error during cell division early in fetal development. As a result, some of the body's cells have the usual one X chromosome and one Y chromosome (46,XY), and others have an extra copy of the X chromosome (47,XXY).

WHAT ARE THE SYMPTOMS OF KLINEFELTER SYNDROME?

Males with Klinefelter syndrome may have the following symptoms:
- Small
- Firm testes
- A small penis

- Sparse pubic, armpit, and facial hair
- Enlarged breasts (called "gynecomastia")
- Tall stature
- Abnormal body proportions (long legs, short trunk)

School-age children may be diagnosed if referred to a doctor to evaluate learning disabilities. The diagnosis may also be considered in the adolescent male when puberty is not progressing as expected. Adult males may come to the doctor because of infertility.

Klinefelter syndrome is associated with an increased risk for breast cancer, a rare tumor called "extragonadal germ cell tumor," "lung disease," "varicose veins," and "osteoporosis." Men who have Klinefelter syndrome also have an increased risk for autoimmune disorders such as lupus, rheumatoid arthritis, and Sjogren's syndrome.

HOW IS KLINEFELTER SYNDROME DIAGNOSED?

A chromosomal analysis (karyotype) is used to confirm the diagnosis. In this procedure, a small blood sample is drawn. White blood cells are then separated from the sample, mixed with tissue culture medium, incubated, and checked for chromosomal abnormalities, such as an extra X chromosome.

The chromosome analysis looks at several cells, usually at least 20, which allows for diagnosing genetic conditions in both the full and mosaic states. In some cases, low-level mosaicism may be missed. However, if mosaicism is suspected (oriented on hormone levels, sperm counts, or physical characteristics), additional cells can be analyzed from within the same blood draw.

HOW IS KLINEFELTER SYNDROME TREATED?

Testosterone therapy increases strength, promotes muscular development, grows body hair, improves mood and self-esteem, and increases energy and concentration.

Most men who have Klinefelter syndrome are not able to father children. However, some men with an extra X chromosome have fathered healthy offspring, sometimes with the help of infertility specialists.

Chromosomal Disorders

Most men with Klinefelter syndrome can expect a normal and productive life. Early diagnosis, in conjunction with educational interventions, medical management, and strong social support, will optimize each individual's potential in adulthood.

Section 16.6 | Prader-Willi Syndrome

This section contains text excerpted from the following sources: Text beginning with the heading "What Is Prader-Willi Syndrome?" is excerpted from "Prader–Willi Syndrome," MedlinePlus, National Institutes of Health (NIH), May 13, 2022; Text under the heading "What Are the Treatments for Prader-Willi Syndrome?" is excerpted from "What Are the Treatments for Prader-Willi Syndrome (PWS)?" Eunice Kennedy Shriver National Institute of Child Health and Human Development (NICHD), December 29, 2021.

WHAT IS PRADER-WILLI SYNDROME?

Prader-Willi syndrome (PWS) is a complex genetic condition affecting many body parts. This condition is characterized by weak muscle tone (hypotonia), feeding difficulties, poor growth, and delayed development in infancy. In childhood, affected individuals develop extreme hunger, leading to chronic overeating (hyperphagia) and obesity. Some people with PWS, particularly those with obesity, also develop type 2 diabetes (the most common form of diabetes).

People with PWS typically have mild-to-moderate intellectual impairment and learning disabilities. Behavioral problems include temper outbursts, stubbornness, and compulsive behavior, such as picking at the skin. Sleep abnormalities can also occur. Additional features of this condition include distinctive facial features such as a narrow forehead, almond-shaped eyes, a triangular mouth; short stature; and small hands and feet. Some people with PWS have unusually fair skin and light-colored hair. Both affected males and affected females have underdeveloped genitals. Puberty is delayed or incomplete, and most affected individuals cannot have children (infertile).

FREQUENCY OF PRADER-WILLI SYNDROME

Prader-Willi syndrome affects an estimated one in 10,000–30,000 people worldwide.

CAUSES OF PRADER-WILLI SYNDROME

Prader-Willi syndrome is caused by the loss of function of genes in a particular region of chromosome 15. People normally inherit one copy of this chromosome from each parent. Some genes are turned on (active) only on the copy inherited from a person's father (the paternal copy). This parent-specific gene activity results from a process called "genomic imprinting."

Most PWS (about 70%) occurs when each cell's segment of the paternal chromosome 15 is deleted. People with this chromosomal change are missing certain critical genes in this region because the genes on the paternal copy have been deleted, and the genes on the maternal copy are turned off (inactive). In another 25 percent of cases, a person with PWS has two copies of chromosome 15 inherited from her or his mother (maternal copies) instead of one from each parent. This situation is called "maternal uniparental disomy." Rarely, PWS can also be caused by a chromosomal rearrangement called a "translocation" or by a genetic alteration or other change that abnormally turns off (inactivates) genes on the paternal chromosome 15.

It appears likely that the characteristic features of PWS result from the loss of function of several genes on chromosome 15. Among these are genes that provide instructions for making molecules called "*small nucleolar ribonucleic acid*" (*snoRNAs*). These molecules have a variety of functions, including helping to regulate other types of RNA molecules. (RNA molecules are essential in producing proteins and other cell activities.) Studies suggest that the loss of a particular group of *snoRNA* genes, known as the "SNORD116 cluster," may play a major role in causing the signs and symptoms of PWS. However, it is unknown how a missing SNORD116 cluster could contribute to intellectual disability, behavioral problems, and the physical features of the disorder.

In some people with PWS, the loss of a gene called "*oculocutaneous albinism II*" (*OCA2*) is associated with unusually fair skin and light-colored hair. The *OCA2* gene is located on the segment of chromosome 15 that is often deleted in people with this disorder. However, loss of the *OCA2* gene does not cause the other signs and symptoms of PWS. The protein produced from this gene helps determine the coloring (pigmentation) of the skin, hair, and eyes.

Chromosomal Disorders

Researchers are studying other genes on chromosome 15 that may also be oriented to this condition's major signs and symptoms.

INHERITANCE OF PRADER-WILLI SYNDROME

Most PWS cases are not inherited, particularly caused by a deletion in the paternal chromosome 15 or by maternal uniparental disomy. These genetic changes occur as random events during the formation of reproductive cells (eggs and sperm) or early embryonic development. Affected people typically have no history of the disorder in their family.

Rarely, a genetic change responsible for PWS can be inherited. For example, it is possible for a genetic change that abnormally turns off genes on the paternal chromosome 15 to be passed from one generation to the next.

WHAT ARE THE TREATMENTS FOR PRADER-WILLI SYNDROME?

Parents can enroll infants with PWS in early intervention programs. However, even if a PWS diagnosis is delayed, treatments are valuable at any age.

The types of treatment depend on the individual's symptoms. The health-care provider may recommend the following:

- **Use of special nipples or tubes for feeding difficulties**. Difficulty in sucking is one of the most common symptoms of newborns with Prader-Willi syndrome. Special nipples or tubes are used for several months to feed newborns and infants who are unable to suck properly to make sure that the infant is fed adequately and grows. To ensure that the child is growing properly, the health-care provider will monitor height, weight, and body mass index (BMI) monthly during infancy.
- **Strict supervision of daily food intake**. Once overeating starts between ages two and four years, supervision will help minimize food hoarding and stealing and prevent rapid weight gain and severe obesity. Parents should lock refrigerators and all cabinets containing food. No medications have proven beneficial in reducing food-seeking behavior. A

well-balanced, low-calorie diet and regular exercise are essential and must be maintained for the rest of the individual's life. People with PWS rarely need more than 1,000–1,200 calories per day. Height, weight, and BMI should be monitored every six months during the first 10 years of life after infancy and once a year after age 10 for the rest of the person's life to make sure she or he is maintaining a healthy weight. Ongoing consultation with a dietitian to guarantee adequate vitamin and mineral intake, including calcium and vitamin D, might be needed.

- **Growth hormone (GH) therapy.** GH therapy has been demonstrated to increase height, lean body mass, and mobility; decrease fat mass; and improve movement and flexibility in individuals with PWS from infancy through adulthood. When given early in life, it also may prevent or reduce behavioral difficulties. Additionally, GH therapy can help improve speech, improve abstract reasoning, and often allow information to be processed more quickly. It also has been shown to improve sleep quality and resting energy expenditure. GH therapy usually is started during infancy or at diagnosis with PWS. This therapy often continues during adulthood at 20–25 percent of the recommended dose for children.
- **Treatment of eye problems by a pediatric ophthalmologist.** Many infants have trouble getting their eyes to focus together. These infants should be referred to a pediatric ophthalmologist who has expertise in working with infants with disabilities.
- **Treatment of curvature of the spine by an orthopedist.** An orthopedist should evaluate and treat, if necessary, the curvature of the spine (scoliosis). Treatment will be the same as that for people with scoliosis who do not have PWS.
- **Sleep studies and treatment.** Sleep disorders are common with PWS. Treating a sleep disorder can help improve the quality of sleep. The same treatments that

health-care providers use with the general population can apply to individuals with PWS.
- **Physical therapy**. Muscle weakness is a serious problem among individuals with PWS. For children younger than age three, physical therapy may increase muscular strength and help such children achieve developmental milestones. For older children, daily exercise will help build lean body mass.
- **Behavioral therapy**. People with PWS have difficulty controlling their emotions. Using behavioral therapy can help. Stubbornness, anger, and obsessive-compulsive behavior, including an obsession with food, should be handled with behavioral management programs using firm limit-setting strategies. Structure and routines are also advised.
- **Medications**. Medications, especially serotonin reuptake inhibitors (SRIs), may reduce obsessive-compulsive symptoms. SRIs also may help manage psychosis.
- **Early interventions/special needs programs**. Individuals with PWS have varying degrees of intellectual difficulty and learning disabilities. Early intervention programs, including speech therapy for delays in acquiring language and for difficulties with pronunciation, should begin as early as possible and continue throughout childhood. Special education is almost always necessary for school-age children. Groups that offer training in social skills may also prove beneficial. An individual aide is often useful in helping PWS children focus on schoolwork.
- **Sex hormone treatments and/or corrective surgery**. These treatments are used to treat small genitals (penis, scrotum, clitoris).
- **Replacement of sex hormones**. Replacement of sex hormones during puberty may result in the development of adequate secondary sex characteristics (e.g., breasts, pubic hair, a deeper voice).

- **Placement in group homes during adulthood.** Group homes offer the necessary structure and supervision for adults with PWS, helping them avoid compulsive eating, severe obesity, and other health problems.

Section 16.7 | Turner Syndrome

This section includes text excerpted from documents published by two public domain sources. The text under the headings marked 1 is excerpted from "About Turner Syndrome," National Human Genome Research Institute (NHGRI), September 24, 2013. Reviewed October 2022; Text under the headings marked 2 are excerpted from "Turner Syndrome," MedlinePlus, National Institutes of Health (NIH), October 1, 2017. Reviewed October 2022.

WHAT IS TURNER SYNDROME?[1]

Turner syndrome (TS) is a chromosomal condition that alters development in females. Women with this condition tend to be shorter than average and are usually unable to conceive a child (infertile) because of an absence of ovarian function. Other features of this condition that can vary among women with TS include extra skin on the neck (webbed neck), puffiness or swelling (lymphedema) of the hands and feet, skeletal abnormalities, heart defects, and kidney problems. The TS is a chromosomal condition oriented to the X chromosome.

Researchers have not yet determined which genes on the X chromosome are responsible for most signs and symptoms of TS. They have, however, identified one gene called the *"short-stature homeobox"* (*SHOX*) gene that is important for bone development and growth. Missing one copy of this gene likely causes short stature and skeletal abnormalities in women with TS.

WHAT ARE THE SYMPTOMS OF TURNER SYNDROME?[1]

Girls who have TS are shorter than average. They often have a normal height for the first three years of life but then have a slow growth rate. At puberty, they do not have the usual growth spurt.

Nonfunctioning ovaries are another symptom of TS. Normally, a girl's ovaries begin to produce sex hormones (estrogen and

Chromosomal Disorders

progesterone) at puberty. This does not happen in most girls who have TS. They do not start their periods or develop breasts without hormone treatment at puberty.

Even though many women who have Turner have nonfunctioning ovaries and are infertile, their vaginas and womb are totally normal.

Girls with TS may have frequent middle ear infections in early childhood. Recurrent infections can lead to hearing loss in some cases. Girls with TS are usually of normal intelligence with good verbal and reading skills. Some girls, however, have problems with math, memory skills, and fine-finger movements.

Additional symptoms of TS include the following:
- An especially wide neck (webbed neck) and a low or indistinct hairline
- A broad chest and widely spaced nipples
- Arms that turn out slightly at the elbow
- A heart murmur that is sometimes associated with narrowing of the aorta (blood vessels exiting the heart)
- A tendency to develop high blood pressure (so this should be checked regularly)
- Minor eye problems that are corrected by glasses
- Scoliosis (spine deformity) that occurs in 10 percent of adolescent girls with TS
- The thyroid gland that becomes underactive in about 10 percent of women with TS (regular blood tests are necessary to detect it early and, if necessary, treat it with thyroid replacement)
- Older or overweight women with TS that are slightly more at risk of developing diabetes
- Osteoporosis that can develop because of a lack of estrogen, but this can largely be prevented by hormone replacement therapy

CAUSES OF TURNER SYNDROME[2]

Turner syndrome is oriented to the X chromosome, one of the two sex chromosomes. People typically have two sex chromosomes in each cell: females have two X chromosomes, while males have one X chromosome and one Y chromosome. TS results when one normal X chromosome is present in a female's cells and the other sex chromosome is missing or structurally altered. The missing genetic material affects development before and after birth.

About half of individuals with TS have monosomy X, which means each cell in the individual's body has only one copy of the X chromosome instead of the usual two sex chromosomes. TS can also occur if one of the sex chromosomes is partially missing or rearranged rather than completely absent. Some women with TS have a chromosomal change in only some of their cells, known as "mosaicism." Women with TS caused by X chromosome mosaicism have mosaic TS.

IS TURNER SYNDROME INHERITED?[1]

Turner syndrome is not usually inherited in families. TS occurs when one of the two X chromosomes normally found in women is missing or incomplete. Although the exact cause of TS is unknown, it appears to occur due to a random error during the formation of either the eggs or sperm.

Humans have 46 chromosomes containing all of a person's genes and DNA. Two of these chromosomes, the sex chromosomes, determine a person's gender. Both of the sex chromosomes in females are called "X chromosomes" (written as XX). Males have an X chromosome and a Y chromosome (written as XY). The two sex chromosomes help a person develop fertility and the sexual characteristics of their gender.

In TS, the girl does not have the usual pair of two complete X chromosomes. The most common scenario is that the girl has only one X chromosome in her cells. Some girls with TS have two X chromosomes, but one of the X chromosomes is incomplete. In another scenario, the girl has some cells with two X chromosomes in her body, but other cells have only one. This is called "mosaicism."

FREQUENCY OF TURNER SYNDROME[2]

Turner syndrome occurs in about one in 2,500 newborns worldwide, but it is much more common among pregnancies that do not survive to term (miscarriages and stillbirths).

HOW IS TURNER SYNDROME DIAGNOSED?[1]

A diagnosis of TS may be suspected when several typical physical features are observed, such as a webbed neck, a broad chest, and widely spaced nipples. Sometimes, the diagnosis is made at birth because of heart problems, an unusually wide neck, or swelling of the hands and feet.

The two main clinical features of TS are short stature and the lack of development of the ovaries.

Many girls are diagnosed in early childhood when a slow growth rate and other features are identified. Diagnosis sometimes takes place later when puberty does not occur. TS may be suspected in pregnancy during an ultrasound test. This can be confirmed by prenatal testing—chorionic villous sampling or amniocentesis—to obtain cells from the unborn baby for chromosomal analysis. If a diagnosis is confirmed prenatally, the baby may be under the care of a specialist pediatrician immediately after birth.

A blood test confirms the diagnosis, called a "karyotype." This is used to analyze the chromosomal composition of the female.

WHAT IS THE TREATMENT FOR TURNER SYNDROME?[1]

During childhood and adolescence, girls may be under the care of a pediatric endocrinologist or a specialist in childhood conditions of hormones and metabolism. Growth hormone injections are beneficial in some individuals with TS. Injections often begin in early childhood and may increase final adult height by a few inches.

Estrogen replacement therapy is usually started at normal puberty, around 12 years, to start breast development. Estrogen and progesterone are given a little later to begin a monthly "period," which is necessary to keep the womb healthy. Estrogen is also given to prevent osteoporosis. Babies born with a heart murmur or narrowing of the aorta may need surgery to correct the problem. A heart expert (cardiologist) will assess and follow up on any treatment necessary.

Girls who have TS are more likely to get middle ear infections. Repeated infections may lead to hearing loss and should be evaluated by the pediatrician. An ear, nose, and throat specialist (ENT) may be involved in caring for this health issue.

High blood pressure is quite common in women who have TS. In some cases, the elevated blood pressure is due to a narrowing of the aorta or a kidney abnormality. However, most of the time, no specific cause for the elevation is identified. If necessary, blood pressure should be checked routinely and treated with medication. Women with TS have a slightly higher risk of having an underactive thyroid or developing diabetes. This should also be monitored and treated if necessary during routine health maintenance visits.

Regular health checks are very important. Special clinics for the care of girls and women with TS are available in some areas, with access to various specialists. Early preventive care and treatment are very important. Almost all women are infertile, but pregnancy with donor embryos may be possible. Appropriate medical treatment and support allow a woman with TS to lead a normal, healthy, and happy life.

Section 16.8 | Velocardiofacial Syndrome

This section includes text excerpted from "About Velocardiofacial Syndrome," National Human Genome Research Institute (NHGRI), June 29, 2017. Reviewed October 2022.

WHAT IS VELOCARDIOFACIAL SYNDROME?

Velocardiofacial syndrome (VCFS) is a genetic condition that is sometimes hereditary. The VCFS is characterized by a combination of medical problems that vary from child to child. These medical problems include cleft palate, or an opening in the roof of the mouth, and other differences in the palate; heart defects; problems fighting infection; low calcium levels; differences in the way the kidneys are formed or work; a characteristic facial appearance; learning problems; and speech and feeding problems.

The term "velocardiofacial" comes from the Latin words "velum" meaning palate, "cardia" meaning heart, and "facies" having to do with the face. Not all of these identifying features are found in each child born with VCFS. The most common features are palatal differences (~75%), heart defects (75%), problems fighting infection

Chromosomal Disorders

(77%), low calcium levels (50%), differences in the kidney (35%), characteristic facial appearance (numbers vary depending on the individual's ethnic and racial background), learning problems (~90%), speech problem (~75%), and feeding problems (35%).

Two genes—*catechol-O-methyltransferase* (*COMT*) and *T-Box Transcription Factor 1* (*TBX1*)—are associated with VCFS. However, not all of the genes that cause VCFS have been identified. Most children with this syndrome are missing a small part of chromosome 22. Chromosomes are threadlike structures found in every cell of the body. Each chromosome contains hundreds of genes. A human cell normally contains 46 chromosomes (23 from each parent). The location or address of the missing segment in individuals with VCFS is 22q11.2.

The velocardiofacial syndrome is also called the "22q11.2 deletion syndrome." It also has other clinical names such as DiGeorge syndrome, conotruncal anomaly face syndrome (CTAF), autosomal dominant Opitz G/BBB syndrome, or Cayler cardiofacial syndrome. As a result of this deletion, about 30 genes are generally absent from this chromosome. VCFS affects about one in 4,000 newborns. VCFS may affect more individuals because some people with the 22q11.2 deletion may not be diagnosed as they have very few signs and symptoms.

WHAT ARE THE SYMPTOMS OF VELOCARDIOFACIAL SYNDROME?

Despite the involvement of a very specific portion of chromosome 22, there is great variation in the symptoms of this syndrome. At least 30 different symptoms have been associated with the 22q11 deletion. Most of these symptoms are not present in all individuals who have VCFS.

Symptoms include cleft palate, usually of the soft palate (the roof of the mouth nearest the throat, which is behind the bony palate), heart problems, asymmetrical faces (elongated face, almond-shaped eyes, wide nose, small ears), eye problems, feeding problems that include food coming through the nose (nasal regurgitation) because of the palatal differences, middle-ear infections (otitis media), low calcium due to hypoparathyroidism (low levels of the parathyroid hormone that can result in seizures), immune system problems that make it difficult for the body to fight infections, differences in the way the kidneys are formed or how they work, weak muscles, differences in the spine such as curvature of the spine (scoliosis) or bony abnormalities in the neck or upper back, and tapered fingers. Children are born with these features.

Children who have VCFS also often have learning difficulties and developmental delays. About 65 percent of individuals with the 22q11.2 deletion have a nonverbal learning disability. When tested, their verbal intelligence quotient (IQ) scores are greater than 10 points higher than their performance IQ scores. This combination of test scores brings down the full-scale IQ scores, but they would not represent the abilities of the individual accurately. As a result of this type of learning disability, students will have relative strengths in reading and rote memorization but will struggle with math and abstract reasoning. These individuals may also have communication and social interaction problems, such as autism. As adults, these individuals have an increased risk of developing mental illnesses such as depression, anxiety, and schizophrenia.

IS VELOCARDIOFACIAL SYNDROME INHERITED?

Velocardiofacial syndrome is due to a 22q11.2 deletion. Most often, neither parent has the deletion, so it is new in the child (93%) and the chance for the couple to have another child with VCFS is quite low (close to zero). However, once the deletion is present in a person, she or he has a 50 percent chance of having children who also have the deletion. The 22q11 deletion happens as an accident when the egg or sperm is formed early in fetal development.

In less than 10 percent of cases, a person with VCFS inherits the deletion in chromosome 22 from a parent. When VCFS is inherited in families, this means that other family members may be affected as well.

Since some people with the 22q11.2 deletion are very mildly affected, it is suggested that all parents of children with the deletion have tested. Furthermore, some people with the deletion have no symptoms but have the deletion in some of their cells but not all. This is called "mosaicism." Even others have the deletion only in their egg or sperm cells but not in their blood cells. It is

Chromosomal Disorders

recommended that all parents of a child with a 22q11.2 deletion seek genetic counseling before or during a subsequent pregnancy to learn more about their chances of having another child with VCFS.

WHAT IS THE TREATMENT FOR VELOCARDIOFACIAL SYNDROME?

Treatment is oriented on the type of symptoms that are present. For example, newborns treat heart defects as they would normally be via surgical interventions. Individuals with low calcium levels are given calcium supplements and frequent vitamin D to help them absorb the calcium. Palate problems are treated by a team of specialists called a "cleft palate" or "craniofacial team" and again often require surgical interventions and intensive speech therapy. Infections are generally treated aggressively with antibiotics in infants and children with immune problems.

Early intervention and speech therapies are started when possible at one year of age to assess and treat developmental delays.

Section 16.9 | Williams Syndrome

This section includes text excerpted from "Williams Syndrome," MedlinePlus, National Institutes of Health (NIH), May 31, 2022.

WHAT IS WILLIAMS SYNDROME?

Williams syndrome (WS) is a developmental disorder that affects many parts of the body. This condition is characterized by mild-to-moderate intellectual disability or learning problems, unique personality characteristics, distinctive facial features, and heart and blood vessel (cardiovascular) problems.

People with WS typically struggle with visual-spatial tasks such as drawing and assembling puzzles. Still, they tend to do well on tasks that involve spoken language, music, and learning by repetition (rote memorization). Affected individuals have outgoing, engaging personalities and tend to take an extreme interest in other people. Attention deficit disorder (ADD), problems with anxiety, and phobias are common among people with this disorder.

Young children with WS have distinctive facial features, including a broad forehead, puffiness around the eyes, a flat bridge of the nose, full cheeks, and a small chin. Many affected people have dental problems, such as teeth that are small, widely spaced, crooked, or missing. Older children and adults typically have longer faces with wide mouths and full lips.

The cardiovascular disease called "supravalvular aortic stenosis" (SVAS) occurs frequently in WS patients. SVAS is a narrowing of the large blood vessel (the aorta) that carries blood from the heart to the rest of the body. If this condition is not treated, the aortic narrowing can lead to shortness of breath, chest pain, and heart failure. Narrowing of other vessels, including the artery from the heart to the lungs (pulmonary stenosis) and the arteries that supply blood to the heart (coronary artery stenosis), can also occur. Other heart and blood vessel problems, including high blood pressure (hypertension) and stiff blood vessels, have also been reported in people with WS. Individuals with WS have an increased risk of complications with anesthesia.

Additional signs and symptoms of WS include abnormalities of connective tissue (tissue that supports the body's joints and organs), such as joint problems and soft, loose skin. Affected people may also have increased calcium levels in the blood (hypercalcemia) in infancy, developmental delays, problems with coordination, and short stature. Medical problems involving vision or hearing, including sensitivity to sound (hyperacusis), are frequently associated with WS. In addition, problems with the digestive tract and the urinary system are also possible. Obesity or diabetes can develop in adulthood.

FREQUENCY OF WILLIAMS SYNDROME

Williams syndrome affects an estimated one in 7,500–18,000 people.

CAUSES OF WILLIAMS SYNDROME

Williams syndrome is caused by the loss (deletion) of genetic material from a specific region of chromosome 7. The deleted region includes 25–27 genes, and researchers believe that a loss of several of these genes contributes to the characteristic features of this disorder.

Elastin (*ELN*), *General transcription factor II-I* (*GTF2I*), *General transcription factor II-I repeat domain-containing protein 1* (*GTF2IRD1*), and *LIM Domain Kinase 1* (*LIMK1*) are among the genes that are typically deleted in people with WS. Researchers have found that loss of the *ELN* gene is associated with connective tissue abnormalities and cardiovascular disease (specifically supravalvular aortic stenosis) found in many people with this disease. Studies suggest that deletion of *GTF2I*, *GTF2IRD1*, *LIMK1*, and perhaps other genes may help explain the characteristic difficulties with visual-spatial tasks, unique behavioral characteristics, and other cognitive difficulties seen in people with WS. Loss of the *GTF2IRD1* gene may also contribute to the distinctive facial features often associated with this condition.

Researchers believe that the presence or absence of the *neutrophil cytosolic factor 1* (*NCF1*) gene on chromosome 7 impacts the risk of developing hypertension in people with WS. When the *NCF1* gene is included in the part of the deleted chromosome, affected individuals are less likely to develop hypertension. Therefore, the loss of this gene appears to be a protective factor. People with WS whose *NCF1* gene is not deleted have a higher risk of developing hypertension.

Several other genes are commonly part of the deletion on chromosome 7. Loss of some of these genes appears to be involved in particular signs and symptoms of the condition, and their relationship to the condition is under investigation. However, it is unknown what role, if any, the loss of many of these other genes plays in WS.

INHERITANCE OF WILLIAMS SYNDROME

Most cases of WS are not inherited. The chromosomal alteration usually occurs as a random event during the formation of reproductive cells (eggs or sperm) in a parent of an affected individual. These cases occur in people with no history of the disorder in their family. However, the risk of having a child with WS is increased if an unaffected parent has a chromosomal change called an "inversion" in the region of chromosome 7 associated with WS.

The WS is considered an autosomal dominant condition because one copy of the altered chromosome 7 in each cell is sufficient to cause the disorder. In a small percentage of cases, people with WS inherit the chromosomal deletion from a parent with the condition.

Chapter 17 | Epilepsy-Aphasia Spectrum

WHAT IS AN EPILEPSY-APHASIA SPECTRUM?

An epilepsy-aphasia spectrum is a group of conditions that have overlapping signs and symptoms. A key feature of these conditions is the impairment of language skills (aphasia). Language problems can affect speaking, reading, and writing. Another feature of epilepsy-aphasia spectrum disorders is certain patterns of abnormal electrical activity in the brain, which are detected by a test called an "electroencephalogram" (EEG). Many people with conditions in this spectrum develop recurrent seizures (epilepsy), and some have mild-to-severe intellectual disabilities. The conditions in the epilepsy-aphasia spectrum, which all begin in childhood, include Landau-Kleffner syndrome (LKS), epileptic encephalopathy with continuous spike-and-wave during sleep syndrome (ECSWS), autosomal dominant rolandic epilepsy with speech dyspraxia (ADRESD), intermediate epilepsy-aphasia disorder (IEAD), atypical childhood epilepsy with centrotemporal spikes (ACECTS), and childhood epilepsy with centrotemporal spikes (CECTS).

LKS and ECSWS are at the severe end of the spectrum. Both usually feature a characteristic abnormal pattern of electrical activity in the brain called "continuous spike" and "waves" during slow-wave sleep (CSWS). This pattern occurs while the affected child is sleeping, specifically during deep (slow-wave) sleep.

Most children with LKS develop normally in early childhood although some speak later than their peers. However, affected

---

This chapter includes text excerpted from "Epilepsy-Aphasia Spectrum," MedlinePlus, National Institutes of Health (NIH), November 1, 2016. Reviewed November 2022.

children lose language skills beginning around age five. This loss typically begins with verbal agnosia, which is the inability to understand speech. As LKS develops, the ability to express speech is also impaired. Approximately 70 percent of children with LKS have seizures, typically of a type described as focal (or partial), because the seizure activity occurs in specific regions of the brain rather than affecting the entire brain.

About half of children with ECSWS develop normally in early childhood, while others have delayed development of speech and motor skills. Although children with ECSWS typically lose a range of previously acquired skills, including those involved in language, movement, learning, or behavior, not everyone with ECSWS has aphasia. Seizures occur in approximately 80 percent of children with ECSWS and can include a variety of types, such as atypical absence seizures, which involve short periods of staring blankly; hemiclonic seizures, which cause rhythmic jerking of one side of the body; or generalized tonic-clonic seizures, which cause stiffening and rhythmic jerking of the entire body.

CECTS is at the mild end of the epilepsy-aphasia spectrum. Affected children have rolandic seizures; these seizures are triggered by abnormal activity in an area of the brain called the "rolandic region," which is part of the cerebrum. The seizures, which usually occur during sleep, cause twitching, numbness, or tingling of the face or tongue, often causing drooling and impairing speech. In most people with CECTS, the seizures disappear by the end of adolescence. Most affected individuals develop normally although some have difficulty coordinating the movements of the mouth and tongue needed for clear speech (dyspraxia) or impairment of language skills.

The other conditions in the epilepsy-aphasia spectrum are less common and fall in the middle of the spectrum. Children with IEAD usually have delayed development or regression of language skills. Some have seizures, and most have abnormal electrical activity in their brains during sleep although it is not prominent enough to be classified as CSWS. ACECTS features seizures and developmental regression that can affect movement, language, and attention. Children with ACECTS have abnormal electrical activity in the brain that is sometimes classified as CSWS. ADRESD is characterized by focal seizures, speech difficulties due to dyspraxia, and learning disability.

FREQUENCY OF EPILEPSY-APHASIA SPECTRUM
The prevalence of the epilepsy-aphasia spectrum is unknown. Most of the conditions in the spectrum are rare; however, CECTS is one of the most common forms of epilepsy in children, accounting for 8–25 percent of cases. It is estimated to occur in one in 5,000 children younger than 16.

CAUSES OF EPILEPSY-APHASIA SPECTRUM
Variants (also known as "mutations") in the *GRIN2A* gene can cause conditions in the epilepsy-aphasia spectrum. These variants are more common in the more severe conditions; they are found in up to 20 percent of people with LKS or ECSWS and about five percent of people with CECTS. In affected people without a *GRIN2A* gene variant, the cause of the condition is unknown. Some affected individuals have a brain abnormality that may contribute to the condition. Researchers suspect that changes in other, unidentified genes may also be associated with epilepsy-aphasia spectrum disorders.

The *GRIN2A* gene provides instructions for making the GluN2A protein, which is one component (subunit) of a subset of N-methyl-D-aspartate (NMDA) receptors. NMDA receptors transmit signals that turn on nerve cells (neurons) in the brain. Signaling through these receptors is involved in normal brain development, changes in the brain in response to experience (synaptic plasticity), learning, and memory. The GluN2A subunit determines where in the brain the receptor is located and how it functions. Receptors containing this subunit are found in regions of the brain involved in speech and language, among other regions. These receptors also appear to play a role in brain signaling during slow-wave sleep.

Variants in the *GRIN2A* gene lead to altered NMDA receptor signaling in the brain. As a result, neurons may be abnormally turned on, which can cause seizures and other abnormal brain activity and may lead to the death of the neurons. Changes in *GluN2A* appear to particularly affect signaling in regions of the brain involved in speech and language and disrupt brain activity during slow-wave sleep, leading to several of the signs and symptoms of this group of conditions.

It is not clear why some people with a *GRIN2A* gene variant have a relatively mild condition and others have more severe signs and symptoms, even within the same family. Variations in other genes and environmental factors may also play a role in the development of the condition.

INHERITANCE OF EPILEPSY-APHASIA SPECTRUM

Conditions in the epilepsy-aphasia spectrum that are caused by *GRIN2A* gene variants are inherited in an autosomal dominant pattern, which means one copy of the altered gene in each cell is sufficient to cause the disorder. Individuals with an epilepsy-aphasia spectrum disorder may have family members with a condition in the epilepsy-aphasia spectrum or a related disorder such as isolated seizures or speech and language problems.

In some cases, an affected person inherits the variant from one affected parent. Other cases result from new variants in the gene and occur in people with no history of the disorder in their family.

Chapter 18 | Fetal Alcohol Spectrum Disorders

Chapter Contents
Section 18.1—Alcohol Use and Pregnancy................................ 181
Section 18.2—Facts about Fetal Alcohol Spectrum
              Disorders 184

Section 18.1 | Alcohol Use and Pregnancy

This section contains text excerpted from "Fetal Alcohol Spectrum Disorders (FASDs)," Centers for Disease Control and Prevention (CDC), December 14, 2021.

ALCOHOL USE DURING PREGNANCY

There is no known safe amount of alcohol use during pregnancy or while trying to get pregnant. There is also no safe time for alcohol use during pregnancy. All types of alcohol are equally harmful, including all wines and beer. Fetal alcohol spectrum disorders (FASDs) are preventable if a baby is not exposed to alcohol before birth.

WHY IS ALCOHOL DANGEROUS?

Alcohol in the mother's blood passes to the baby through the umbilical cord. Alcohol use during pregnancy can cause miscarriage, stillbirth, and a range of lifelong physical, behavioral, and intellectual disabilities. These disabilities are known as "FASDs." Children with FASDs might have the following characteristics and behaviors:

- Abnormal facial features, such as a smooth ridge between the nose and upper lip (this ridge is called the "philtrum")
- Small head size
- Shorter-than-average height
- Low body weight
- Poor coordination
- Hyperactive behavior
- Difficulty with attention
- Poor memory
- Difficulty in school (especially with math)
- Learning disabilities
- Speech and language delays
- Intellectual disability or low intelligence quotient (IQ)
- Poor reasoning and judgment skills
- Sleep and sucking problems as a baby

- Vision or hearing problems
- Problems with the heart, kidney, or bones

HOW MUCH ALCOHOL IS DANGEROUS?

There is no known safe amount of alcohol use during pregnancy.

WHEN IS ALCOHOL DANGEROUS?

There is no safe time for alcohol use during pregnancy. Alcohol can cause problems for the baby throughout pregnancy, including before a woman knows she is pregnant. Alcohol use in the first three months of pregnancy can cause the baby to have abnormal facial features. Growth and central nervous system problems (e.g., low birth weight, behavioral problems) can occur from alcohol use anytime during pregnancy. The baby's brain develops throughout pregnancy and can be affected by exposure to alcohol at any time. It is never too late to stop alcohol use during pregnancy. Stopping alcohol use will improve the baby's health and well-being.

ALCOHOL AND PREGNANCY: QUESTIONS AND ANSWERS

Q: You just found out you are pregnant. You have stopped drinking now, but you were drinking in the first few weeks of your pregnancy before you knew you were pregnant. What should you do now?

A: Most importantly, after learning of your pregnancy, you have completely stopped alcohol use. It is never too late to stop alcohol use during pregnancy. Because brain growth occurs throughout pregnancy, stopping alcohol use will improve the baby's health and well-being. If you used any amount of alcohol while you were pregnant, talk with your child's health-care provider as soon as possible and share your concerns. Make sure you get regular prenatal checkups.

Q: Is it okay to drink a little or at certain times during pregnancy?

A: There is no known safe amount of alcohol use during your pregnancy or when you are trying to get pregnant. There is also no safe time for alcohol use during pregnancy. Alcohol can cause

Fetal Alcohol Spectrum Disorders

problems for your baby throughout pregnancy, including before you know you are pregnant. FASDs are preventable if a baby is not exposed to alcohol before birth.

Q: You drank wine during your last pregnancy, and your baby turned out fine. Why should you not drink again during this pregnancy?

A: Every pregnancy is different. Alcohol use during pregnancy might affect one baby more than another. You could have one child who is born healthy and another child who is born with problems.

Q: If you drank when you were pregnant, does that mean your baby will have FASD?

A: If you used any amount of alcohol while you were pregnant, talk with your child's health-care provider as soon as possible and share your concerns. You may not know right away if your child has been affected. FASDs include a range of physical and intellectual disabilities that are not always easy to identify when a child is a newborn. Some of these effects may not be known until your child is in school. There is no cure for FASDs. However, identifying and intervening with children with these conditions as early as possible can help them reach their full potential.

Q: If a woman has an FASD but does not drink during pregnancy, can her child have FASD? Is FASD hereditary?

A: FASDs are not genetic or hereditary. If a baby is exposed to alcohol during pregnancy, the baby can be born with FASD. But, if a woman has an FASD, her own child cannot have an FASD unless she uses alcohol during pregnancy.

Q: Can a father's drinking cause harm to the baby?

A: How alcohol affects the male sperm is currently being studied. Whatever the effects are found to be, they are not FASDs. These disorders are caused specifically when a baby is exposed to alcohol during pregnancy. However, the father's role is important. He can help the woman avoid alcohol use during pregnancy. He can encourage her to abstain from alcohol by avoiding social situations that involve drinking. He can also help her by avoiding alcohol himself.

Section 18.2 | Facts about Fetal Alcohol Spectrum Disorders

This section includes text excerpted from "Basics about FASDs," Centers for Disease Control and Prevention (CDC), January 11, 2022.

WHAT ARE FETAL ALCOHOL SPECTRUM DISORDERS?

Fetal alcohol spectrum disorders (FASDs) are a group of conditions that can occur in a person who was exposed to alcohol before birth. These effects can include physical problems and problems with behavior and learning. Often, a person with an FASD has a mix of these problems.

SIGNS AND SYMPTOMS OF FETAL ALCOHOL SPECTRUM DISORDERS

Fetal alcohol spectrum disorders refer to a collection of diagnoses that represent the range of effects that can happen to a person exposed to alcohol before birth. These conditions can affect each person differently and range from mild to severe. A person with an FASD might have the following:

- Low body weight
- Poor coordination
- Hyperactive behavior
- Difficulty with attention
- Poor memory
- Difficulty in school (especially with math)
- Learning disabilities
- Speech and language delays
- Intellectual disability or low intelligence quotient (IQ)
- Poor reasoning and judgment skills
- Sleep and sucking problems as a baby
- Vision or hearing problems
- Problems with the heart, kidneys, or bones
- Shorter-than-average height
- Small head size
- Abnormal facial features, such as a smooth ridge between the nose and upper lip (this ridge is called the "philtrum")

Fetal Alcohol Spectrum Disorders

CAUSES AND PREVENTIONS OF FETAL ALCOHOL SPECTRUM DISORDERS

Fetal alcohol spectrum disorders can occur when a person is exposed to alcohol before birth. Alcohol in the mother's blood passes to the baby through the umbilical cord.

There is no known safe amount of alcohol during pregnancy or when trying to get pregnant. There is also no safe time to drink during pregnancy. Alcohol can cause problems for a developing baby throughout pregnancy, including before a woman knows she is pregnant. All types of alcohol are equally harmful, including all wines and beer.

To prevent FASDs, a woman should avoid alcohol if she is pregnant or might be pregnant. This is because a woman could get pregnant and not know for up to 4–6 weeks.

It is never too late to stop alcohol use during pregnancy. Because brain growth occurs throughout pregnancy, stopping alcohol use will improve the baby's health and well-being. FASDs are preventable if a baby is not exposed to alcohol before birth.

DIAGNOSES OF FETAL ALCOHOL SPECTRUM DISORDERS

Different FASD diagnoses are oriented on particular symptoms and include:

- **Fetal alcohol syndrome (FAS).** FAS represents the most involved end of the FASD spectrum. People with FAS have a central nervous system (CNS) problems, abnormal facial features, and growth problems. People with FAS can have learning, memory, attention span, communication, vision, or hearing problems. They might have a mix of these problems. People with FAS often have trouble in school and getting along with others.
- **Alcohol-related neurodevelopmental disorder (ARND).** People with ARND might have intellectual disabilities and problems with behavior and learning. They might do poorly in school and have difficulties with math, memory, attention, judgment, and poor impulse control.

- **Alcohol-related birth defects (ARBD).** People with ARBD might have problems with the heart, kidneys, bones, or hearing. They might have a mix of these.
- **Neurobehavioral disorder associated with prenatal alcohol exposure (ND-PAE).** ND-PAE was first included as a recognized condition in the *Diagnostic and Statistical Manual 5* (DSM 5) of the American Psychiatric Association (APA) in 2013. A child or youth with ND-PAE will have problems in the following three areas:
  - Thinking and memory, where the child may have trouble planning or may forget material she or he has already learned.
  - Behavior problems, such as severe tantrums, mood issues (e.g., irritability), and difficulty shifting attention from one task to another.
  - The trouble with day-to-day living can include problems with bathing, dressing for the weather, and playing with other children. In addition, to be diagnosed with ND-PAE, the mother of the child must have consumed more than minimal levels of alcohol before the child's birth, which APA defines as more than 13 alcoholic drinks per month of pregnancy (i.e., any 30-day period of pregnancy) or more than two alcoholic drinks in one sitting.

Areas Evaluated for Fetal Alcohol Spectrum Disorders Diagnoses

The term FASDs is not meant for use as a clinical diagnosis. Diagnosing FASDs can be hard because there is no medical test for these conditions, like a blood test. And other disorders, such as attention deficit hyperactivity disorder (ADHD) and Williams syndrome, have some symptoms like FAS. To diagnose FASDs, doctors look for:
- Prenatal alcohol exposure although confirmation is not required to make a diagnosis
- Central nervous system problems (e.g., small head size, problems with attention and hyperactivity, poor coordination)

Fetal Alcohol Spectrum Disorders

- Lower-than-average height, weight, or both
- Abnormal facial features (e.g., the smooth ridge between the nose and upper lip)

TREATMENT OF FETAL ALCOHOL SPECTRUM DISORDERS

Fetal alcohol spectrum disorders last a lifetime. There is no cure for FASDs, but research shows that early intervention treatment services can improve a child's development. There are many treatment options, including medication to help with some symptoms, behavior and education therapy, parent training, and other alternative approaches. No one treatment is right for every child. Good treatment plans will include close monitoring, follow-ups, and changes as needed along the way.

Also, "protective factors" can help reduce the effects of FASDs and help people with these conditions reach their full potential. Protective factors include:

- Diagnosis before six years of age
- Loving, nurturing, and stable home environment during the school years
- Absence of violence
- Involvement in special education and social services

Chapter 19 | Gerstmann Syndrome

WHAT IS GERSTMANN SYNDROME?

Gerstmann syndrome is a cognitive impairment resulting from damage to a specific area of the brain—the left parietal lobe in the angular gyrus region. It may occur after a stroke or in association with damage to the parietal lobe. It is characterized by four primary symptoms: a writing disability (agraphia or dysgraphia), a lack of understanding of the rules for calculation or arithmetic (acalculia or dyscalculia), an inability to distinguish right from left, and an inability to identify fingers (finger agnosia). The disorder should not be confused with Gerstmann-Sträussler-Scheinker disease, transmissible spongiform encephalopathy.

In addition to exhibiting the above symptoms, many adults also experience aphasia (difficulty expressing oneself when speaking, understanding speech, or reading and writing).

There are few reports of the syndrome, sometimes called "developmental Gerstmann syndrome," in children. The cause is not known. Most cases are identified when children reach school age, a time when they are challenged with writing and math exercises. Generally, children with the disorder exhibit poor handwriting and spelling skills and difficulty with math functions, including adding, subtracting, multiplying, and dividing. An inability to differentiate right from left and discriminate among individual fingers may also be apparent. In addition to the four primary symptoms, many children also suffer from constructional apraxia, an inability

---

This chapter includes text excerpted from "Gerstmann's Syndrome," National Institute of Neurological Disorders and Stroke (NINDS), July 25, 2022.

to copy simple drawings. Frequently, there is also an impairment in reading. The disorder may affect children with high intellectual functioning and those with brain damage.

TREATMENT OF GERSTMANN SYNDROME

There is no cure for Gerstmann syndrome. Treatment is symptomatic and supportive. Occupational and speech therapies may help diminish dysgraphia and apraxia. In addition, calculators and word processors may help school children cope with the disorder's symptoms.

PROGNOSIS OF GERSTMANN SYNDROME

In adults, many of the symptoms diminish over time. Although it has been suggested that in children, symptoms may diminish over time, it appears that most children probably do not overcome their deficits but learn to adjust to them.

Chapter 20 | Hearing Disabilities

Chapter Contents
Section 20.1—Hearing Loss in Children 193
Section 20.2—Hearing Loss Treatment and
　　　　　　　Intervention Services 196

Section 20.1 | Hearing Loss in Children

This section includes text excerpted from "Hearing Loss in Children," Centers for Disease Control and Prevention (CDC), July 19, 2022.

Hearing loss can affect a child's ability to develop communication, language, and social skills. The earlier children with hearing loss get services, the more likely they will reach their full potential. If you are a parent and you suspect your child has hearing loss, trust your instincts and speak with your child's doctor. Do not wait!

WHAT IS HEARING LOSS?

Hearing loss can happen when any part of the ear is not working in the usual way. This includes the outer ear, middle ear, inner ear, hearing (acoustic) nerve, and auditory system.

SIGNS AND SYMPTOMS OF HEARING LOSS

The signs and symptoms of hearing loss are different for each child. If you think your child might have hearing loss, ask the child's doctor for a hearing screening as soon as possible. Do not wait!

Even if a child has passed a hearing screening, it is important to look for the following signs.

Signs in Babies

- Does not startle at loud noises.
- Does not turn to the source of a sound after six months.
- Does not say single words, such as "dada" or "mama," by one year of age.
- Turns head when she or he sees you but not if you only call out her or his name. This sometimes is mistaken for not paying attention or ignoring but could result from partial or complete hearing loss.
- Seems to hear some sounds but not others.

Signs in Children
- Speech is delayed.
- Speech is not clear.
- Does not follow directions. This sometimes is mistaken for not paying attention or ignoring but could result from partial or complete hearing loss.
- Often says, "Huh?"
- Turns the TV volume up too high.

Babies and children should reach milestones in how they play, learn, communicate, and act. A delay in these milestones could signify hearing loss or other developmental problems.

CAUSES AND RISK FACTORS OF HEARING LOSS
Hearing loss can happen at any time during life—from before birth to adulthood. Here are some of the things that can increase the chance that a child will have hearing loss:
- **A genetic cause**. About one out of two cases of hearing loss in babies is due to genetic causes. Some babies with a genetic cause for their hearing loss might have family members who also have hearing loss. About one out of three babies with genetic hearing loss have a "syndrome." This means they have other conditions besides hearing loss, such as Down syndrome or Usher syndrome.
- **Maternal infections during pregnancy, complications after birth, and head trauma**. One in four cases of hearing loss in babies is due to maternal infections during pregnancy, complications after birth, and head trauma. For example, the child:
  - Was exposed to infection before birth.
  - Spent five days or more in a hospital neonatal intensive care unit (NICU) or had complications while in the NICU.
  - Needed a special procedure such as a blood transfusion to treat bad jaundice.
  - Has head, face, or ears shaped or formed in a different way than usual.

Hearing Disabilities

- Has a condition such as a neurological disorder that may be associated with hearing loss.
- Had an infection around the brain and spinal cord called "meningitis."
- Received a bad injury to the head that required a hospital stay.

SCREENING AND DIAGNOSIS

Hearing screening can tell if a child might have hearing loss. Hearing screening is easy and is not painful. Babies are often asleep while being screened. It takes a very short time—usually only a few minutes.

Babies

All babies should have a hearing screening no later than one month after birth. Most babies have their hearing screened while still in the hospital. If a baby does not pass a hearing screening, it is very important to get a full hearing test as soon as possible but no later than three months after birth.

Children

Children should have their hearing tested before they enter school or any time there is a concern about the child's hearing. Children who do not pass the hearing screening need a full hearing test as soon as possible.

TREATMENTS AND INTERVENTION SERVICES FOR HEARING LOSS

No single treatment or intervention is the answer for every person or family. Good treatment plans will include close monitoring, follow-ups, and any changes needed along the way. There are many communication options for children with hearing loss and their families. Some of these options include:

- Learning other ways to communicate, such as sign language
- Technology to help with communication, such as hearing aids and cochlear implants

- Medicine and surgery to correct some types of hearing loss
- Family support services

PREVENTION OF HEARING LOSS

The following are tips for parents to help prevent hearing loss in their children:
- Have a healthy pregnancy.
- Make sure your child gets all the regular childhood vaccines.
- Keep your child away from high noise levels, such as very loud toys.

Section 20.2 | Hearing Loss Treatment and Intervention Services

This section includes text excerpted from "Hearing Loss Treatment and Intervention Services," Centers for Disease Control and Prevention (CDC), July 18, 2022.

No single treatment or intervention is the answer for every child or family. Good intervention plans will include close monitoring, follow-ups, and any changes needed along the way. There are many different options for children with hearing loss and their families.

Some of the treatment and intervention options include:
- Working with a professional (or team) who can help a child and family learn to communicate.
- Getting a hearing device, such as a hearing aid.
- Joining support groups.
- Taking advantage of other resources available to children with hearing loss and their families.

EARLY INTERVENTION AND SPECIAL EDUCATION
Early Intervention (0–3 Years)

Hearing loss can affect a child's ability to develop speech, language, and social skills. The earlier a child who is deaf or hard of hearing starts getting services, the more likely the child's speech, language, and social skills will reach their full potential.

Early intervention program services help young children with hearing loss learn the language and other important skills. Research shows that early intervention services can greatly improve a child's development.

Babies with hearing loss should receive intervention services as soon as possible but no later than six months.

Many services are available through the Individuals with Disabilities Education Improvement Act 2004 (IDEA 2004). Services for children from birth through 36 months of age are called "early intervention" or "Part C services." Even if your child has not been diagnosed with hearing loss, she or he may be eligible for early intervention treatment services. The IDEA 2004 says that children under three years (36 months) at risk of developmental delays may be eligible for services. These services are provided through an early intervention system in your state. Through this system, you can ask for an evaluation.

Special Education (3–22 Years)
Special education is instruction specifically designed to address the educational and related developmental needs of older children with disabilities or those experiencing developmental delays. Services for these children are provided through the public school system. These services are available through the IDEA 2004, Part B.

Early Hearing Detection and Intervention Program
Every state has an early hearing detection and intervention (EHDI) program. EHDI works to identify infants and children with hearing loss. EHDI also promotes timely follow-up testing and services or interventions for any family whose child has a hearing loss. If your child has a hearing loss or if you have any concerns about your child's hearing, contact your local EHDI program coordinator to find available services in your state.

TECHNOLOGY

Many people who are deaf or hard of hearing have some hearing. The amount of hearing a deaf or hard-of-hearing person has is called "residual hearing." Technology does not "cure" hearing loss but may help a child with hearing loss to make the most of their residual hearing. For those parents who choose to have their child use technology, there are many options, including:
- Hearing aids
- Cochlear or brainstem implants
- Bone-anchored hearing aids
- Other assistive devices

Hearing Aids

Hearing aids make sounds louder. They can be worn by people of any age, including infants. Babies with hearing loss may understand sounds better using hearing aids. This may allow them to learn speech skills at a young age.

There are many styles of hearing aids. They can help with many types of hearing loss. A young child is usually fitted with behind-the-ear style hearing aids because they are better suited to growing ears.

Cochlear and Auditory Brainstem Implants

A cochlear implant may help many children with severe-to-profound hearing loss—even when very young. It gives the child a way to hear when a hearing aid is not enough. Unlike a hearing aid, cochlear implants do not make sounds louder. A cochlear implant sends sound signals directly to the hearing nerve.

Persons with severe-to-profound hearing loss due to an absent or very small hearing nerve or severely abnormal inner ear (cochlea) may not benefit from a hearing aid or cochlear implant. Instead, an auditory brainstem implant may provide some hearing. An auditory brainstem implant directly stimulates the hearing pathways in the brainstem, bypassing the inner ear and hearing nerve.

Both cochlear and brainstem implants have two main parts. The parts are placed inside the inner ear, the cochlea, or base of

Hearing Disabilities

the brain; the brainstem during surgery; and the parts outside the ear that send sounds to the parts inside the ear.

Bone-Anchored Hearing Aids

This type of hearing aid can be considered when a child has conductive, mixed, or unilateral hearing loss and is specifically suitable for children who cannot otherwise wear "in-the-ear" or "behind-the-ear" hearing aids.

Other Assistive Devices

Besides hearing aids, other devices help people with hearing loss. The following are some examples of other assistive devices:

- **Frequency modulation (FM) system**. An FM system is a device that helps people with hearing loss hear in background noise. FM stands for frequency modulation. It is the same type of signal used for radios. FM systems send sound from a microphone used by someone speaking to a person wearing the receiver. This system is sometimes used with hearing aids. An extra piece is attached to the hearing aid that works with the FM system.
- **Captioning**. Many television programs, videos, and digital versatile discs (DVDs) are captioned. Television sets made after 1993 are made to show the captioning. You do not have to buy anything special. Captions show the conversation spoken on a program's soundtrack at the bottom of the television screen.
- **Other devices**. There are many other devices available for children with hearing loss. Some of these are as follows:
  - Text messaging
  - Telephone amplifiers
  - Flashing and vibrating alarms
  - Audio loop systems
  - Infrared listening devices
  - Portable sound amplifiers
  - Text telephone or teletypewriter (TTY)

MEDICAL AND SURGICAL

Medications or surgery may also help make the most of a person's hearing. This is especially true for conductive hearing loss or one that involves a part of the outer or middle ear that is not working in the usual way.

A chronic ear infection can cause one type of conductive hearing loss. A chronic ear infection is a buildup of fluid behind the eardrum in the middle ear space. Most ear infections are managed with medication or careful monitoring. Infections that do not go away with medication can be treated with a simple surgery involving putting a tiny tube into the eardrum to drain the fluid.

Another type of conductive hearing loss is caused by the outer or middle ear not forming correctly while the baby is growing in the mother's womb. The outer and middle ears need to work together for sound to be sent correctly to the inner ear. If any of these parts did not form correctly, there might be hearing loss in that ear. This problem may be improved and perhaps even corrected with surgery. An ear, nose, and throat doctor (otolaryngologist) is the health-care professional who usually takes care of this problem.

Placing a cochlear implant, auditory brainstem implant, or bone-anchored hearing aid will also require surgery.

LEARNING LANGUAGE

Without extra help, children with hearing loss have problems learning the language. These children can then be at risk for other delays. Families who have children with hearing loss often need to change their communication habits or learn special skills (such as sign language) to help their children learn the language. These skills can be used with hearing aids, cochlear or auditory brainstem implants, and other devices that help children hear.

FAMILY SUPPORT SERVICES

For many parents, their child's hearing loss is unexpected. Parents sometimes need time and support to adapt to the child's hearing loss.

Hearing Disabilities

Parents of children with recently identified hearing loss can seek different support. Support is anything that helps a family and may include advice, information, having the chance to get to know other parents that have a child with hearing loss, locating a deaf mentor, finding childcare or transportation, giving parents time for personal relaxation, or just being a supportive listener.

Chapter 21 | Pervasive Developmental Disorders

Chapter Contents
Section 21.1—What Are Pervasive Developmental
 Disorders? 205
Section 21.2—Asperger Syndrome 206
Section 21.3—Autism Spectrum Disorder 208
Section 21.4—Rett Syndrome 209

Section 21.1 | What Are Pervasive Developmental Disorders?

This section includes text excerpted from "Pervasive Developmental Disorders," National Institute of Neurological Disorders and Stroke (NINDS), July 25, 2022.

DEFINITION OF PERVASIVE DEVELOPMENTAL DISORDERS

The diagnostic category of pervasive developmental disorder (PDD) is characterized by delays in socialization and communication skills development. Parents may note symptoms as early as infancy although the typical age of onset is before three years. Symptoms may include problems with using and understanding language; difficulty relating to people, objects, and events; unusual play with toys and other objects; difficulty with changes in routine or familiar surroundings; and repetitive body movements or behavior patterns.

Autism (a developmental brain disorder characterized by impaired social interaction and communication skills and a limited range of activities and interests) is the most characteristic and best-studied PDD. Other types of PDD include Asperger syndrome, childhood disintegrative disorder, and Rett syndrome. Children with PDD vary widely in abilities, intelligence, and behaviors. Some children do not speak at all; others speak in limited phrases or conversations; and some have relatively normal language development. Repetitive play skills and limited social skills are generally evident. Unusual responses to sensory information, such as loud noises and lights, are also common.

TREATMENT OF PERVASIVE DEVELOPMENTAL DISORDERS

There is no known cure for PDD. Medications address specific behavioral problems; therapy for children with PDD should be specialized according to need. Some children with PDD benefit from specialized classrooms in which the class size is small and instruction is given on a one-to-one basis. Others function well in standard special education or regular classes with additional support.

PROGNOSIS OF PERVASIVE DEVELOPMENTAL DISORDERS

Early intervention, including appropriate and specialized educational programs and support services, is critical in improving the outcome of individuals with PDD. PDD is not fatal and does not affect normal life expectancy.

Section 21.2 | Asperger Syndrome

This section includes text excerpted from "Asperger Syndrome," National Institute of Neurological Disorders and Stroke (NINDS), July 25, 2022.

WHAT IS ASPERGER SYNDROME?

Asperger syndrome (AS) is a developmental disorder. It is an autism spectrum disorder (ASD), one of a distinct group of neurological conditions characterized by a greater or lesser degree of impairment in language and communication skills, as well as repetitive or restrictive patterns of thought and behavior. Other ASDs include classic autism, Rett syndrome, childhood disintegrative disorder, and pervasive developmental disorder not otherwise specified (usually referred to as "PDD-NOS"). Unlike children with autism, children with AS retain their early language skills.

The most distinguishing symptom of AS is a child's obsessive interest in a single object or topic to the exclusion of any other. Children with AS want to know everything about their topic of interest, and their conversations with others will be about little else. Their expertise, high level of vocabulary, and formal speech patterns make them seem like little professors. Other characteristics of AS include repetitive routines or rituals, peculiarities in speech and language, socially and emotionally inappropriate behavior and the inability to interact successfully with peers, problems with nonverbal communication, and clumsy and uncoordinated motor movements.

Children with AS are isolated because of their poor social skills and narrow interests. They may approach other people but make normal conversation impossible by inappropriate or eccentric

Pervasive Developmental Disorders

behavior or by wanting only to talk about their singular interest. Children with AS usually have a history of developmental delays in motor skills, such as pedaling a bike, catching a ball, or climbing outdoor play equipment. They are often awkward and poorly coordinated, with a walk that can appear stilted or bouncy.

TREATMENT FOR ASPERGER SYNDROME
The ideal treatment for AS coordinates therapies that address the three core symptoms of the disorder:
- Poor communication skills
- Obsessive or repetitive routines
- Physical clumsiness

There is no single best treatment package for all children with AS, but most professionals agree that the earlier the intervention, the better.

An effective treatment program builds on the child's interests, offers a predictable schedule, teaches tasks as simple steps, actively engages the child's attention in highly structured activities, and provides regular behavior reinforcement. It may include social skills training, cognitive-behavioral therapy (CBT), medication for coexisting conditions, and other measures.

PROGNOSIS OF ASPERGER SYNDROME
With effective treatment, children with AS can learn to cope with their disabilities but may still find social situations and personal relationships challenging. Many adults with AS can work successfully in mainstream jobs although they may continue to need encouragement and moral support to maintain an independent life.

Section 21.3 | Autism Spectrum Disorder

This section includes text excerpted from "What Is Autism Spectrum Disorder," Centers for Disease Control and Prevention (CDC), March 31, 2022.

WHAT IS AUTISM SPECTRUM DISORDER?

Autism spectrum disorder (ASD) is a developmental disability caused by differences in the brain. Some people with ASD have a known difference, such as a genetic condition. Other causes are not yet known. Scientists believe multiple causes of ASD act together to change the most common ways people develop. There is still much to learn about these causes and how they impact people with ASD.

People with ASD may behave, communicate, interact, and learn in ways that are different from most others. Often, nothing about how they look sets them apart from other people. The abilities of people with ASD can vary significantly. For example, some people with ASD may have advanced conversation skills, whereas others may be nonverbal. Some people with ASD need a lot of help daily; others can work and live with a little to no support.

ASD begins before the age of three years and can last throughout a person's life although symptoms may improve over time. Some children show ASD symptoms within the first 12 months of life. In others, symptoms may not show up until 24 months of age or later. Some children with ASD gain new skills and meet developmental milestones until around 18–24 months of age, and then they stop gaining new skills or lose the skills they once had.

As children with ASD become adolescents and young adults, they may have difficulties developing and maintaining friendships, communicating with peers and adults, or understanding what behaviors are expected in school or on the job. They may come to the attention of health-care providers because they also have conditions such as anxiety, depression, or attention deficit hyperactivity disorder (ADHD), which occur more often in people with ASD than those without ASD.

SIGNS AND SYMPTOMS OF AUTISM SPECTRUM DISORDER

People with ASD often have problems with social communication and interaction and restricted or repetitive behaviors or interests.

People with ASD may also have different ways of learning, moving, or paying attention. It is important to note that some people without ASD might also have these symptoms. For people with ASD, these characteristics can make life very challenging.

SCREENING AND DIAGNOSIS OF AUTISM SPECTRUM DISORDER

Diagnosing ASD can be difficult since there is no medical test to diagnose the disorder, such as a blood test. Doctors look at the child's behavior and development to make a diagnosis. ASD can sometimes be detected at 18 months of age or younger. By age two, a diagnosis by an experienced professional can be considered reliable. However, many children do not receive a final diagnosis until they are much older. Some people are not diagnosed until they are adolescents or adults. This delay means that people with ASD might not get the early help they need.

TREATMENT AND INTERVENTION SERVICES FOR AUTISM SPECTRUM DISORDER

Current treatments for ASD seek to reduce symptoms that interfere with daily functioning and quality of life. ASD affects each person differently, meaning that people with ASD have unique strengths and challenges and different treatment needs. Treatment plans usually involve multiple professionals and are catered to the individual.

Section 21.4 | Rett Syndrome

This section includes text excerpted from "Rett Syndrome," MedlinePlus, National Institutes of Health (NIH), October 1, 2018. Reviewed November 2022.

WHAT IS RETT SYNDROME?

Rett syndrome is a brain disorder that occurs almost exclusively in girls. The most common form of the condition is known as "classic Rett syndrome." After birth, girls with classic Rett syndrome have 6–18 months of apparently normal development before developing severe problems with language and communication, learning, coordination, and other brain functions. Early in childhood, affected girls lose purposeful use of their hands and begin making repeated hand wringing, washing, or clapping motions. They tend to grow more slowly than other children, and about three-quarters have a small head size (microcephaly). Other signs and symptoms that can develop include breathing abnormalities, spitting or drooling, unusual eye movements such as intense staring or excessive blinking, cold hands and feet, irritability, sleep disturbances, seizures, and abnormal side-to-side curvature of the spine (scoliosis). Researchers have described several variants or atypical forms of Rett syndrome, which can be milder or more severe than the classic form.

Rett syndrome is part of a spectrum of disorders with the same genetic cause. Other disorders on the spectrum include PPM-X syndrome, MECP2 duplication syndrome, and MECP2-related severe neonatal encephalopathy. These other conditions can affect males.

FREQUENCY OF RETT SYNDROME

This condition affects an estimated one in 9,000–10,000 females.

CAUSES OF RETT SYNDROME

Mutations in a gene called "*MECP2*" underlie almost all cases of classic Rett syndrome and some variant forms of the condition. This gene provides instructions for making a protein (MeCP2) that is critical for normal brain function. Although the exact function of the MeCP2 protein is unclear, it is likely involved in maintaining connections (synapses) between nerve cells (neurons). It may also be necessary for the normal function of other types of brain cells.

The MeCP2 protein is thought to help regulate the activity of genes in the brain. This protein may also control the production of different versions of certain proteins in brain cells. Mutations in the *MECP2* gene alter the MeCP2 protein or result in the production of less protein, which appears to disrupt the normal function of neurons and other cells in the brain. Specifically, studies suggest that changes in the MeCP2 protein may reduce the activity of certain

Pervasive Developmental Disorders

neurons and impair their ability to communicate with one another. It is unclear how these changes lead to the specific features of Rett syndrome.

Several conditions with signs and symptoms overlapping those of Rett syndrome have been found to result from mutations in other genes. These conditions, including FOXG1 syndrome and CDKL5 deficiency disorder, were previously thought to be variant forms of Rett syndrome. However, doctors and researchers have identified some important differences between the conditions, so they are now usually considered to be separate disorders.

INHERITANCE OF RETT SYNDROME

In more than 99 percent of people with Rett syndrome, there is no history of the disorder in their family. Many of these cases result from new mutations in the *MECP2* gene.

A few families with more than one affected family member have been described. These cases helped researchers determine that classic Rett syndrome and variants caused by *MECP2* gene mutations have an X-linked dominant pattern of inheritance. A condition is considered X-linked if the mutated gene that causes the disorder is located on the X chromosome, one of the two sex chromosomes. The inheritance is dominant if one copy of the altered gene in each cell is sufficient to cause the condition.

Males with mutations in the *MECP2* gene often die in infancy. However, a small number of males with a genetic change involving *MECP2* have developed signs and symptoms similar to those of Rett syndrome, including intellectual disability, seizures, and movement problems. In males, this condition is described as *MECP2-related severe neonatal encephalopathy*. The signs and symptoms in some males with a *MECP2* gene mutation are on the milder end of the spectrum.

Chapter 22 | Tourette Syndrome

Chapter Contents
Section 22.1—Tourette Syndrome: Basics 215
Section 22.2—Co-occurring Conditions of Tourette
　　　　　　　Syndrome 217

Section 22.1 | Tourette Syndrome: Basics

This section includes text excerpted from "What Is Tourette Syndrome?" Centers for Disease Control and Prevention (CDC), May 17, 2022.

WHAT IS TOURETTE SYNDROME?

Tourette syndrome (TS) is a condition of the nervous system. TS causes people to have "tics." Tics are sudden twitches, movements, or sounds that people repeatedly make. People who have tics cannot stop their bodies from doing these things. For example, a person might keep blinking over and over. Or a person might make a grunting sound unwillingly.

Having tics is a little bit like having hiccups. Even though you might not want to hiccup, your body does it anyway. Sometimes, people can stop themselves from doing a certain tic for a while, but it is hard. Eventually, the person has to do the tic.

TYPES OF TICS

There are two types of tics:
- **Motor tics**. These tics are movements of the body. Examples of motor tics include blinking, shrugging the shoulders, or jerking an arm.
- **Vocal tics**. These tics are sounds that a person makes with her or his voice. Examples of vocal tics include humming, clearing the throat, or yelling a word or phrase.

Tics can be:
- **Simple tics**. These tics involve just a few parts of the body. Examples of simple tics include squinting the eyes or sniffing.
- **Complex tics**. These tics usually involve several different body parts and can have a pattern. An example of a complex tic is bobbing the head while jerking an arm and jumping up.

SYMPTOMS OF TOURETTE SYNDROME
The main symptoms of TS are tics. Symptoms usually begin when a child is 5–10 years of age. The first symptoms are often motor tics in the head and neck area. Tics usually are worse during times that are stressful or exciting. They tend to improve when a person is calm or focused on an activity.

The types of tics and how often a person has tics change significantly over time. Even though the symptoms might appear, disappear, and reappear, these conditions are considered chronic.

In most cases, tics decrease during adolescence and early adulthood and sometimes disappear entirely. However, many people with TS experience tics into adulthood; sometimes, tics can worsen during adulthood.

Although the media often portray people with TS as involuntarily shouting out swear words (called "coprolalia") or constantly repeating the words of other people (called "echolalia"), these symptoms are rare. They are not required for a diagnosis of TS.

CAUSES AND RISK FACTORS OF TOURETTE SYNDROME
Doctors and scientists do not know the exact cause of TS. Research suggests that it is an inherited genetic condition. It means it is passed on from parent to child through genes.

DIAGNOSIS OF TOURETTE SYNDROME
No single test, such as a blood test, can diagnose TS. Health professionals look at the person's symptoms to diagnose TS and other tic disorders. The tic disorders differ in terms of the type of tic present (motor, vocal, or a combination of both) and how long the symptoms have lasted. TS can be diagnosed if a person has both motor and vocal tics and has had tic symptoms for at least a year.

TREATMENT FOR TOURETTE SYNDROME
Although there is no cure for TS, treatments are available to help manage the tics. Many people with TS have tics that do not get in the way of their daily life and, therefore, do not need any treatment.

Tourette Syndrome

However, medication and behavioral treatments are available if tics cause pain or injury; interfere with school, work, or social life; or cause stress.

Section 22.2 | Co-occurring Conditions of Tourette Syndrome

This section includes text excerpted from "What Is Tourette Syndrome?" Centers for Disease Control and Prevention (CDC), May 17, 2022.

Tourette syndrome (TS) often occurs with other related conditions (co-occurring conditions). These conditions include attention deficit hyperactivity disorder (ADHD), obsessive-compulsive disorder (OCD), and other behavioral or conduct problems. People with TS and related conditions can be at higher risk for learning, behavioral, and social problems.

The symptoms of other disorders can complicate the diagnosis and treatment of TS and create extra challenges for people with TS and their families, educators, and health professionals. Most children diagnosed with TS also have other mental health, behavioral, or developmental condition. Conditions that commonly occur with TS include:

- Anxiety or depression
- ADHD
- Autism spectrum disorder (ASD)
- Behavioral problems, such as oppositional defiant disorder (ODD) or conduct disorder (CD)
- Developmental delays or intellectual disabilities
- Learning disorders
- Obsessive-compulsive behaviors
- Speech or language disorders

Because co-occurring conditions are so common among people with TS, it is important for doctors to assess every child with TS for other conditions and problems.

ATTENTION DEFICIT HYPERACTIVITY DISORDER
Attention deficit hyperactivity disorder is a common co-occurring condition among children with TS. Children with ADHD have trouble paying attention and controlling impulsive behaviors. They might act without thinking about what the result will be, and in some cases, they are also overly active. It is normal for children to have trouble focusing and behaving at one time or another. However, for children with ADHD, symptoms can continue, can be severe, and cause difficulty at school, at home, or with friends.

OBSESSIVE-COMPULSIVE BEHAVIORS
People with obsessive-compulsive behaviors have unwanted thoughts (obsessions) that they feel a need to respond to (compulsions). Examples of obsessive-compulsive behaviors are having to think about, say, or do something over and over. More than a third of people with TS have OCD. Sometimes, it is difficult to tell the difference between complex tics that a child with TS may have and obsessive-compulsive behaviors.

BEHAVIOR OR CONDUCT PROBLEMS
Oppositional Defiant Disorder
Children with ODD show negative, defiant, and hostile behaviors toward adults or authority figures. ODD usually starts before a child is eight years of age but no later than early adolescence. Children with ODD might show symptoms most often with people they know well, such as family members or a regular care provider. The behavior problems associated with ODD are more severe or persistent than what might be expected for the child's age and result in major problems in school, at home, or with peers.

Examples of ODD behaviors include:
- Losing one's temper a lot.
- Arguing with adults or refusing to comply with adults' rules or requests.
- Getting angry or being resentful or vindictive often.
- Annoying others on purpose or easily becoming annoyed with others.

- Blaming other people often for one's own mistakes or misbehavior.

Conduct Disorder

Children with conduct disorder (CD) act aggressively toward others and break the rules, laws, and social norms. They might have more injuries and difficulty with friends. In addition, the symptoms of CD happen in more than one area in the child's life (e.g., at home, in the community, and at school).

Behavior problems can be highly disruptive for the child and others in the child's life. It is important to get a diagnosis and treatment plan from a mental health professional as soon as possible. Effective treatments for disruptive behaviors include behavior therapy training for parents.

Rage

Some people with TS have anger that is out of control or episodes of "rage." Rage that happens repeatedly and is disproportionate to the situation that triggers it may be diagnosed as a mood disorder, such as intermittent explosive disorder. Symptoms might include extreme verbal or physical aggression. Examples of verbal aggression include extreme yelling, screaming, and cursing. Examples of physical aggression include extreme shoving, kicking, hitting, biting, and throwing objects. Rage symptoms are more likely to occur among those with other behavioral disorders such as ADHD, ODD, or CD.

Among people with TS, symptoms of rage are more likely to occur at home than outside the home. Treatment can include behavior therapy, learning how to relax, and social skills training. Some of these methods will help individuals and families better understand what can cause the symptoms of rage, how to avoid encouraging these behaviors, and how to use appropriate discipline for these behaviors. In addition, treating other behavioral disorders that the person might have, such as ADHD, ODD, or CD, can help to reduce symptoms of rage.

ANXIETY
There are many different types of anxiety disorders with many different causes and symptoms. These include generalized anxiety disorder, OCD, panic disorder, posttraumatic stress disorder, separation anxiety, and different types of phobias. Separation anxiety is most common among young children. These children feel very worried when they are apart from their parents.

DEPRESSION
Everyone feels worried, anxious, sad, or stressed from time to time. However, if these feelings do not go away and they interfere with daily life (e.g., keeping a child home from school or other activities or keeping an adult from working or attending social activities), a person might have depression. Having either a depressed mood or a loss of interest or pleasure for at least two weeks might mean that someone has depression. Children and teens with depression might be irritable instead of sad.

To be diagnosed with depression, other symptoms also must be present, such as:
- Changes in eating habits or weight gain or loss
- Changes in sleep habits
- Changes in activity level (others notice increased activity or that the person has slowed down)
- Less energy
- Feelings of worthlessness or guilt
- Difficulty thinking, concentrating, or making decisions
- Repeated thoughts of death
- Thoughts or plans about suicide or a suicide attempt

Depression can be treated with counseling and medication.

OTHER HEALTH CONCERNS
Children with TS can also have other health conditions that require care. Among the more common health conditions that can occur with TS are:
- Asthma
- Hearing loss or vision problems

- Bone, joint, or muscle problems
- Brain injury or concussion

A study by the Centers for Disease Control and Prevention (CDC) showed that the rates of asthma and hearing or vision problems were similar to children without TS, but bone, joint, or muscle problems, as well as brain injury or concussion, were higher for children with TS. Children with TS were also less likely to receive effective coordination of care or have a medical home, which means a primary care setting where a team of providers provides healthcare and preventive services.

EDUCATIONAL CONCERNS

As a group, people with TS have levels of intelligence similar to those of people without TS. However, people with TS might be more likely to have learning differences, a learning disability, or a developmental delay that affects their ability to learn.

Many people with TS have problems with writing, organizing, and paying attention. People with TS might have problems processing what they hear or see. This can affect the person's ability to learn by listening to or watching a teacher. Or the person might have problems with their other senses (such as how things feel, smell, taste, and move) that affect learning and behavior. Children with TS might have trouble with social skills that affect their ability to interact with others.

As a result of these challenges, children with TS might need extra help in school. Many times, these concerns can be addressed with accommodations and behavioral interventions (e.g., help with social skills).

Accommodations can include things such as providing a different testing location or extra testing time, providing tips on how to be more organized, giving the child less homework, or letting the child use a computer to take notes in class. Children also might need behavioral interventions and therapy, or they may need to learn strategies to help with stress, paying attention, or other symptoms.

Chapter 23 | Traumatic Brain Injury

WHAT IS TRAUMATIC BRAIN INJURY?

Traumatic brain injury (TBI) is an injury to the brain from trauma or force, such as a bump or blow to the head or an object, such as a bullet entering the skull. TBI can cause problems with brain function. Some TBIs result in mild, temporary problems. A more severe TBI can lead to serious physical, mental, and emotional symptoms, coma, and even death. People or children who have already experienced a brain injury or brain disease are at higher risk for developing TBI. TBI includes (but is not limited to) several types of injury to the brain:

- **Skull fracture**. Skull fracture occurs when the skull cracks. Pieces of broken bone from the skull may cut into the brain and injure it, or an object such as a bullet may pierce the skull and enter the brain.
- **Contusion**. A contusion is a brain bruise where swollen brain tissue combines with blood released from broken blood vessels to increase pressure on the brain. A contusion can occur from the brain shaking back and forth against the skull, such as from a car crash, sports injury, or shaken baby syndrome.
- **Intracranial hematoma**. This injury occurs when a major blood vessel in or around the brain is damaged

---

This chapter includes text excerpted from "Traumatic Brain Injury (TBI)," *Eunice Kennedy Shriver* National Institute of Child Health and Human Development (NICHD), November 24, 2020.

and begins bleeding. The pooling of blood puts pressure on the brain.

A concussion is among the most common forms of TBI. It can happen when the head or body is moved back and forth quickly, such as during a car crash, sports injury, or a head blow. Concussions are often called "mild TBIs" because they are not life-threatening. However, they can still cause serious problems, especially if the person has experienced a concussion.

People may also experience nontraumatic brain injuries that result from a problem, such as a stroke, infection, or broken blood vessel, inside the brain or skull. A nontraumatic brain injury may have some of the same symptoms as someone with a TBI. Both traumatic and nontraumatic brain injuries can have serious, long-term effects on a person's ability to think and function.

TBI can happen to anyone, but some people are more likely to experience a TBI than others. For example, according to the Centers for Disease Control and Prevention (CDC), young children, teenagers, and adults aged 65 or older are at higher risk for TBI. The CDC statistics also show that males are at higher risk than females in most age groups.

WHAT ARE COMMON TRAUMATIC BRAIN INJURY SYMPTOMS?

Traumatic brain injury symptoms vary depending on the following:
- The type of injury
- How severe the injury is
- What area of the brain is injured

TBIs can both be local (the exact place on the brain where the injury occurred) and include the surrounding tissues, which can also be affected by the damage to the initial site. This means some symptoms appear immediately, while others may appear several days or weeks later and evolve over time. A person with TBI may or may not lose consciousness. Loss of consciousness, sometimes called a "blackout," does not necessarily mean the TBI is severe, especially if the blackout lasts only a short time.

Traumatic Brain Injury

Symptoms of Mild Traumatic Brain Injury
A person with a mild TBI may experience any of the following:
- Headache
- Confusion
- Lightheadedness
- Dizziness
- Blurred vision
- Ringing in the ears, also known as "tinnitus"
- Tiredness or sleepiness
- A bad taste in the mouth
- A change in sleep habits
- Behavior or mood changes
- The trouble with memory, concentration, attention, or thinking
- Loss of consciousness lasting a few seconds to minutes
- Sensitivity to light or sound
- Nausea or vomiting

Symptoms of Moderate or Severe Traumatic Brain Injury
A person with moderate or severe TBI may have some of the symptoms listed for mild TBI. In addition, the person may experience any of the following:
- Headache that gets worse or will not go away
- Loss of vision in one or both eyes
- Repeated vomiting or continued nausea
- Slurred speech
- Convulsions or seizures
- An inability to wake up from sleep
- Enlargement of the pupil (dark center) of one or both eyes
- Numbness or tingling of arms or legs
- Uncoordinated or "clumsy" movements
- Increased confusion, restlessness, or agitation
- Loss of consciousness lasting a few minutes to hours

A person who suffers a blow to the head or other injury that may cause a TBI should seek medical attention, even if none of the symptoms listed are present. Sometimes, symptoms do not appear until well after the injury.

WHAT CAUSES TRAUMATIC BRAIN INJURY?

A TBI is caused by an external force that injures the brain. It can occur when a person's head is hit, bumped, or jolted. It can also occur when an object, such as a bullet, pierces the skull or when the body is shaken or hit hard enough to cause the brain to slam into the skull.

Among the leading causes of TBI are falls, motor vehicle crashes and traffic-related accidents, being struck by or against an object, and assaults.

Many TBIs, especially in young people, happen while people are playing sports or doing recreational activities. Some activities that lead to emergency department visits for TBI are bicycling, football, playground activities, basketball, and soccer. The leading causes of TBI in the military are gunshots, fragments from an explosion, blasts, falls, motor vehicle crashes, and assaults.

HOW DO HEALTH-CARE PROVIDERS DIAGNOSE TRAUMATIC BRAIN INJURY?

Health-care providers use different tests and measures to diagnose TBI. Multiple measures are often used to diagnose TBI and map treatment and recovery paths. Some of these tests are described in the following sections. In addition to "neuro-checks"—a series of quick questions and tasks that help health-care providers assess how well a TBI patient's brain and body are working—some in-depth tests help reveal levels of injury or damage in TBI patients.

Imaging Tests

Health-care providers who suspect TBI usually take images of a person's brain. These imaging tests can include the following:
- **Computerized tomography (CT).** A CT or "computerized axial tomography" ("CAT") scan takes

Traumatic Brain Injury

x-rays from many angles to create a complete picture of the brain. It can quickly show whether the brain is bleeding, is bruised, or has other damage.
- **Magnetic resonance imaging (MRI)**. MRI uses magnets and radio waves to produce more detailed images than CT scans. An MRI likely would not be used as part of an initial TBI assessment because it takes too long to complete. It may be used in follow-up examinations, though.

Glasgow Coma Scale

The Glasgow Coma Scale (GCS) gives health-care providers a way to measure a person's functioning in three key areas:
- **Ability to speak**, such as whether the person speaks normally, speaks in a way that does not make sense, or cannot speak at all
- **Ability to open eyes**, including whether the person opens her or his eyes only when asked
- **Ability to move**, ranging from moving one's arms easily and on purpose to not moving even in response to pain

A health-care provider rates a person's responses in these categories and calculates a total score. A score of 13 or higher indicates a mild TBI; nine through 12 indicates a moderate TBI; and eight or below indicates a severe TBI. Doctors can also use the GCS to monitor a patient's recovery progress.

Measurements for Level of Traumatic Brain Injury

Health-care providers sometimes rank TBI by the person's level of consciousness, memory loss, and GCS score (refer to Table 23.1).

Other Tests

Other tests for TBI may include:
- **Speech and language tests**. These tests determine how well the patient can speak and use language, including

Table 23.1. Measurements for Level of Traumatic Brain Injury

Mild TBI	Moderate TBI	Severe TBI
Did not lose consciousness or was unconscious for less than 30 minutes.	Unconsciousness lasted for more than 30 minutes and up to 24 hours.	Unconsciousness lasted for more than 24 hours.
Memory loss lasted less than 24 hours.	Memory loss lasted anywhere from 24 hours to 7 days.	Memory loss lasted more than seven days.
GCS was 13–15.	GCS was 9–12.	GCS was eight or lower.

how well the muscles needed to form words work and how well the patient can read and write.
- **Social communication skills tests and role-playing scenarios.** These determine whether a person's behavior or actions have been affected.
- **Tests of swallowing abilities.** These tests are to ensure the patient can swallow safely and receive enough nutrition.
- **Tests of breathing abilities and lung function.** These tests are to determine whether breathing assistance or extra oxygen is needed.
- **Cognition tests or questions.** These are to see how the patient's thinking, reasoning, problem-solving, understanding, and remembering abilities.
- **Neuropsychological assessments.** These assessments are to learn more about the patient's brain and social functions, including the ability to control one's behavior and actions.

Blood Tests

Blood tests to diagnose TBI are an emerging area of research. In 2018, the U.S. Food and Drug Administration (FDA) approved a blood test that detects two proteins, ubiquitin c-terminal hydrolase L1 (UCH-L1) and glial fibrillary acidic protein (GFAP), released by the brain into the bloodstream when a mild concussion occurs.

Traumatic Brain Injury

The test can help identify individuals whose injury is unlikely to appear on a CT scan, eliminating the need for an unhelpful test. The blood test may also provide a way to quickly diagnose military personnel for a mild concussion.

Researchers at the National Institute of Nursing Research (NINR) and the National Institute of Child Health and Human Development (NICHD) found that testing for the blood protein tau could help identify athletes who need more recovery before safely returning to play after a sports-related concussion.

WHAT ARE THE TREATMENTS FOR TRAUMATIC BRAIN INJURY?

Various treatments can help a person recover from TBI and sometimes reduce or eliminate certain physical, emotional, and cognitive problems associated with TBI. The treatment specifics, including the type, setting, and length, depend on the injury's severity and the area of the injured brain.

Treatment for Mild Traumatic Brain Injury

Mild TBI, sometimes called a "concussion," may not require specific treatment other than rest. However, following a health-care provider's instructions for complete rest and slowly returning to normal activities after a mild TBI is very important. If a person returns to normal activities too soon and starts experiencing TBI symptoms, the healing process may take much longer. Certain activities, such as working on a computer and concentrating hard, can tire the brain even though they are not physically demanding. A person with a concussion might need to reduce these activities or take frequent breaks to let the brain rest.

In addition, alcohol and other drugs can slow recovery and increase the chances of reinjury. Reinjury during recovery can slow healing and increase the chances of long-term problems, including permanent brain damage and even death.

Emergency Treatment for Traumatic Brain Injury

Emergency care generally focuses on stabilizing and keeping the patient alive, ensuring the brain gets enough oxygen, controlling blood and brain pressure, and preventing further injury to the head or neck. Once the patient is stable, other types of care for TBI can begin.

Sometimes, surgery is needed as part of emergency care to reduce damage to the brain. Surgery may include:
- **Removing blood clots or pools.** Bleeding in the brain or between the brain and skull can lead to large areas of clotted blood, sometimes called "hematomas." These clotted or pooling blood pressure areas on the brain can damage brain tissues.
- **Repairing skull fractures.** Setting severe skull fractures or removing pieces of the skull or other debris from the brain area can help start the healing process of the skull and surrounding tissues.
- **Relieving pressure inside the skull (called "intracranial pressure" or "ICP").** Increased pressure from swelling, blood, and other things in the skull damage the brain. A TBI patient's ICP is monitored during emergency care. Sometimes, making a hole in the skull or adding a shunt or drain is needed to relieve pressure inside the skull and allow excess fluid to drain.

Medications

Medications can help treat symptoms of TBI and lower the risk of some associated conditions. Some medications are useful immediately after a TBI, while others treat symptoms and problems related to recovery from TBI sometime after the initial injury. These medications may include the following:
- **Antianxiety medication** to lessen feelings of nervousness and fear
- **Anticoagulants** to prevent blood clots and improve blood flow
- **Anticonvulsants** to prevent seizures
- **Antidepressants** to treat symptoms of depression and mood instability, which are also called "mood swings"
- **Diuretics** to help remove fluid that can increase pressure inside the brain

Traumatic Brain Injury

- **Muscle relaxants** to reduce muscle spasms and relax constricted muscles
- **Stimulants** to increase alertness and attention

Researchers continue to explore medications that may aid recovery from TBI.

Rehabilitation Therapies

Therapies can help people with TBI recover functions, relearn skills, and find new ways to do things that take their new health status into account. Rehabilitation can include several different kinds of therapy for physical, emotional, and cognitive difficulties and various activities, such as daily self-care, driving, and interacting with others. Depending on the injury, these treatments may be needed only briefly after the injury, occasionally throughout a person's life, or on an ongoing basis.

Therapy usually begins in the hospital and can continue in several places, including rehabilitation hospitals, skilled nursing facilities, homes, schools, and outpatient programs. Rehabilitation generally involves several health-care specialists, the person's family, and someone who manages the team. They often work together to design a treatment program to meet a person's specific needs and improve their abilities to function at home and in the community.

Rehabilitation therapy may include the following:
- **Physical therapy**. To build physical strength, balance, and flexibility and help restore energy levels.
- **Occupational therapy**. To learn or relearn how to perform daily tasks, such as getting dressed, cooking, and bathing.
- **Speech therapy**. To improve the ability to form words, speak aloud, and use other communication skills that can include instruction on how to use special communication devices and treatment of trouble swallowing, called "dysphagia."
- **Psychological counseling**. To learn coping skills, work on interpersonal relationships, and improve general emotional well-being that can include medication and

other ways to address chemical imbalances that may result from TBI.
- **Vocational counseling.** To help a patient return to work and community living by finding appropriate work opportunities and ways to deal with workplace challenges.
- **Cognitive therapy.** To improve memory, attention, perception, learning, planning, and judgment.

WHAT ARE THE POSSIBLE EFFECTS OF TRAUMATIC BRAIN INJURY?

Traumatic brain injury can have various effects depending on the type of injury, the severity of the injury, and what part of the brain is injured. According to the CDC, these health effects can sometimes remain long-term or even permanent.

Immediate Problems

Sometimes, a person will have medical complications after the injury. People with more severe TBI are more likely to have complications. Some complications of TBI include seizures, nerve damage, blood clots, narrowing of blood vessels, stroke, coma, and infections in the brain.

The likelihood of many of these problems decreases as more time passes and the person's condition stabilizes. However, some problems, such as seizures, may continue even after a person's condition is stable.

Longer-Term Effects

Traumatic brain injury may cause problems with various brain functions, and some of these problems do not appear until days or months after the injury. Some problems may be temporary, while others may persist throughout a person's life after the injury. Possible longer-term effects of TBI include problems with:
- **Cognition**, such as difficulty learning, remembering, making decisions, and reasoning

Traumatic Brain Injury

- **Senses**, such as double vision, a bitter taste in the mouth or loss of the sense of taste, ringing in the ears, and tingling or pain
- **Communication**, such as trouble talking, reading, writing, and explaining feelings or thoughts
- **Behavior**, including difficulty with social situations, relationships, self-control, and aggression
- **Emotions**, including depression, anxiety, mood swings, and irritability

Chapter 24 | Visual Impairment in Children

Vision is one of our five senses. Being able to see gives us tremendous access to learning about the world around us—people's faces and the subtleties of expression, what different things look like and how big they are, and the physical environments where we live and move, including approaching hazards.

When a child has a visual impairment, it is caused for immediate attention. It is because so much learning typically occurs visually. When vision loss goes undetected, children are delayed in developing a wide range of skills. While they can do virtually all the activities and tasks that sighted children take for granted, children who are visually impaired often need to learn to do them in a different way or using different tools or materials. Central to their learning will be touching, listening, smelling, tasting, moving, and using whatever vision they have. The assistance of parents, family members, friends, caregivers, and educators can be indispensable in that process. More will be said about this in a moment.

TYPES OF VISUAL IMPAIRMENTS

Not all visual impairments are the same although the umbrella term "visual impairment" may be used to describe generally the consequence of an eye condition or disorder.

The eye has different parts that work together to create our ability to see. When a part of the eye does not work right or communicate well with the brain, vision is impaired.

This chapter includes text excerpted from "Visual Impairment, Including Blindness," Center for Parent Information & Resources (CPIR), U.S. Department of Education (ED), April 1, 2017. Reviewed November 2022.

To understand the particular visual impairment a child has, it is helpful to understand the anatomy of the eye and the functions of its different parts.

Most of us are familiar with visual impairments such as nearsightedness and farsightedness. Less familiar visual impairments include:

- **Strabismus**, where the eyes look in different directions and do not focus simultaneously on a single point
- **Congenital cataracts**, where the lens of the eye is cloudy
- **Retinopathy of prematurity**, which may occur in premature babies when the light-sensitive retina has not developed sufficiently before birth
- **Retinitis pigmentosa**, a rare inherited disease that slowly destroys the retina
- **Coloboma**, where a portion of the structure of the eye is missing
- **Optic nerve hypoplasia**, which is caused by underdeveloped fibers in the optic nerve and which affects depth perception, sensitivity to light, and acuity of vision
- **Cortical visual impairment** (CVI), which is caused by damage to the part of the brain related to vision, not to the eyes themselves

Because there are many different causes of visual impairment, the degree of impairment a child experiences can range from mild to severe (up to, and including, blindness). The degree of impairment will depend on the following:

- The particular eye condition a child has
- What aspect of the visual system is affected (e.g., ability to detect light, shape, or color; ability to see things at a distance, up close, or peripherally)
- How much correction is possible through glasses, contacts, medicine, or surgery

Visual Impairment in Children

The term "blindness" does not necessarily mean that a child cannot see anything at all. A child who is considered legally blind may very well be able to see the light, shapes, colors, and objects (albeit indistinctly). Having such residual vision can be a valuable asset for the child in learning, movement, and life.

SIGNS OF A VISUAL IMPAIRMENT

It is very important to diagnose and address visual impairment in children as soon as possible. Some vision screening may occur at birth, especially if the baby is born prematurely or there is a family history of vision problems, but baby wellness visits as early as six months should also include basic vision screening to ensure that a little one's eyes are developing and functioning as might be expected.

Common signs that a child may have a visual impairment include the following:

- Eyes that do not move together when following an object or a face
- Crossed eyes, eyes that turn out or in, eyes that flutter from side to side or up and down, or eyes that do not seem to focus
- Eyes that bulge, dance, or bounce in rapid rhythmic movements
- Pupils that are unequal in size or that appear white instead of black
- Repeated shutting or covering of one eye
- An unusual degree of clumsiness, such as frequent bumping into things or knocking things over
- Frequent squinting, blinking, eye rubbing, or face crunching, especially when there is no bright light present
- Sitting too close to the TV or holding toys and books too close to the face
- Avoiding tasks and activities that require good vision

If any of these symptoms are present, parents will want to have their child's eyes professionally examined. Early detection and treatment are very important to the child's development.

HOW COMMON ARE VISUAL IMPAIRMENTS?

Very common, especially as we grow older. But there are many causes of visual impairments that have nothing to do with the aging process, and children certainly can be—and are—affected. In the United States, there are approximate:
- 455,462 children with vision difficulty (the term "vision difficulty" refers only to children who have serious difficulty seeing even when wearing glasses and those who are blind)
- 42,000 children with severe vision impairment (unable to see words and letters in ordinary newsprint)
- 61,739 children in educational settings who are legally blind

Each year states must report to the U.S. Department of Education (ED) how many children with visual impairments received special education and related services in schools under the Individuals with Disabilities Education Act (IDEA), the nation's special education law. Data for the school year 2015–2016 indicate that the following numbers of children were served in the United States and its outlying areas:
- 2,799 children (aged 3–5) with visual impairment
- 24,944 children (aged 6–21) with visual impairment

UNDERSTANDING HOW CHILDREN WITH VISUAL IMPAIRMENTS LEARN

Children with visual impairments can certainly learn and do learn well, but they lack the easy access to visual learning that sighted children have. The enormous amount of learning that takes place via vision must now be achieved using other senses and methods.

Hands are a primary information-gathering tool for children with visual impairments. So are the senses of smell, touch, taste,

Visual Impairment in Children

and hearing. Until the child holds the "thing" to be learned and explores its dimensions—let us say, a stuffed animal, a dog, a salt shaker, or a CD player—she or he cannot grasp its details. That is why sensory learning is so powerful for children with visual impairment and why they need to have as many opportunities as possible to experience objects directly and sensorially.

THE HELP AVAILABLE UNDER THE INDIVIDUALS WITH DISABILITIES EDUCATION ACT

If you suspect (or know) that your child has a visual impairment, you will be pleased to know there is a lot of help available under the IDEA—beginning with a free evaluation of your child. IDEA requires that all children suspected of having a disability be evaluated without cost to their parents to determine if they do have a disability and, because of the disability, need special services under IDEA. Those special services are as follows:

- **Early intervention**. A system of services to support infants and toddlers with disabilities (before their third birthday) and their families.
- **Special education and related services**. Services that are available through the public school system for school-aged children, including preschoolers (aged 3–21).

Visual impairment, including blindness, is one of the disabilities specifically mentioned and defined in IDEA. If a child meets the definition of visual impairment in IDEA as well as the state's criteria (if any), then she or he is eligible to receive early intervention services or special education and related services under IDEA (depending on her or his age).

- **To identify the early intervention program in your neighborhood**. Ask your child's pediatrician for a referral. You can also call the local hospital's maternity ward or pediatric ward and ask for the contact information of the local early intervention program.
- **Accessing special education and related services**. If your child is between 3 and 21 years of age, it is

recommended that you get in touch with your local public school system. Calling the public school in your neighborhood is an excellent place to start. The school should be able to tell you the next steps to having your child evaluated free of charge. If found eligible, your child can begin receiving services specially designed to address her or his educational needs and other needs associated with the disability.
- **Developing a written plan of services**. In both cases—in early intervention for a baby or toddler with a visual impairment and in special education for a school-aged child, parents work together with program professionals to develop a plan of services the child will receive based on her or his needs. In early intervention, that plan is called the "Individualized Family Service Plan" (IFSP). In special education, the plan is called the "individualized education program" (IEP). Parents are part of the team that develops their child's IFSP or IEP.

HOW INDIVIDUALS WITH DISABILITIES EDUCATION ACT DEFINES VISUAL IMPAIRMENT

The IDEA provides the nation with definitions of many disabilities that can make children eligible for special education and related services in schools. Visual impairment is one such disability the law defines—as visual impairment including blindness, which means an impairment in vision that, even with correction, adversely affects a child's educational performance. The term includes both partial sight and blindness.

WORKING WITH THE MEDICAL COMMUNITY

If you have a child with a visual impairment, you will probably find yourself dealing with a variety of eye care professionals who become involved in diagnosing and addressing your child's specific disability or eye condition. Wondering who these professionals might be, what qualifications they should have, and what kind of expertise they can bring to your child's care?

Visual Impairment in Children

FamilyConnect is an excellent source of this information. FamilyConnect is an online multimedia community created by the American Foundation for the Blind (AFB) and the National Association for Parents of Children with Visual Impairments (NAPVI).

ADAPTING THE ENVIRONMENT
Making adaptations to the environment where a child with visual impairment lives, works, or plays makes evident sense, but it may be difficult for families, day-care providers, or school personnel to decide what kinds of adaptations are necessary to ensure the child's safety while also encouraging her or his ability to do things independently.

EDUCATIONAL CONSIDERATIONS
Children with visual impairments need to learn the same subjects and academic skills as their sighted peers although they will probably do so in adapted ways. They must also learn an expanded set of skills that are distinctly vision-related, including learning how to:
- Move about safely and independently, which is known as "orientation and mobility" (O&M).
- Use assistive technologies designed for children with visual impairments.
- Use what residual vision they have effectively and efficiently.
- Read and write in Braille, if determined appropriate by the IEP team of the child after a thorough evaluation.

These are just some of the skills that need to be discussed by the student's IEP team and included in the IEP if the team decides that is appropriate. Each of the above skill areas—and more—can be addressed under the umbrella of special education and related services for a child with a visual impairment.

TIPS FOR TEACHERS
- Learn as much as you can about the student's specific visual impairment. What aspects of vision are affected,

and how does that affect the student's ability to move about the classroom, see the board, or read a textbook? Parents (and the student!) can be an excellent source of this information.
- Learn about the many instructional and classroom accommodations that truly help students with visual impairments learn. Strongly support the student by making sure that needed accommodations are provided for classwork, homework, and testing. These will help the student learn successfully.
- If you are not part of the student's IEP team, ask for a copy of her or his IEP. The student's educational goals will be listed there, as well as the services and classroom accommodations she or he is to receive.
- Consult with others (e.g., special educators, the O&M specialist) who can help you identify strategies for teaching and supporting this student, ways to adapt the curriculum, and how to address the student's IEP goals in your classroom.
- Find out if your state or school district has materials or resources available to help educators address the learning needs of children with visual impairments. It is amazing how many do!
- Communicate with the student's parents. Regularly share information about how the student is doing at school and at home.

TIPS FOR PARENTS
- Learn as much as you can about your child's specific visual impairment. The more you know, the more you can help yourself and your child.
- Understand that your child is receiving small bits of information at a time, not all at once through vision. Help your child explore new things with her or his senses and build up a concept of the "whole." For example, your child might need to be shown a banana, help you peel it, feel the banana without its skin, have a bite of it, and then help

you mash it in her or his bowl to understand the qualities of bananas and that bananas can be eaten in different ways.
- Encourage curiosity and explore new things and places often with your child. Give lots of opportunities to touch and investigate objects, ask questions, and hear explanations of what something is, where it comes from, and so on.
- Learn how to adapt your home, given the range and degree of your child's visual impairment. Help your son or daughter explore the house and learn to navigate it safely.
- Encourage your child's independence by letting her or him do things rather than you doing them. Teach how to do a chore by using hands-on guidance and give lots of practice opportunities with feedback. Now, your child knows the skill, too.
- Work with the early interventionists or school staff (depending on your child's age) to build a solid individualized plan of services and supports that address your child's unique developmental and educational needs.
- Talk to other parents of children who have visual impairments similar to that of your child. They can be a great source of support and insight into the challenges and joys of raising a child with vision problems.
- Keep in touch with the professionals working with your child. Offer support. Demonstrate any assistive technology your child uses and provide any information teachers will need. Find out how you can augment your child's learning at home.

Chapter 25 | Emotional Disturbance

WHAT IS EMOTIONAL DISTURBANCE?

Emotional disturbance means a condition exhibiting one or more of the following characteristics over a long period of time and to a marked degree that adversely affects a child's educational performance:

- An inability to learn that cannot be explained by intellectual, sensory, or health factors
- An inability to build or maintain satisfactory interpersonal relationships with peers and teachers
- Inappropriate types of behavior or feelings under normal circumstances
- A general pervasive mood of unhappiness or depression
- A tendency to develop physical symptoms or fears associated with personal or school problems

Emotional disturbance includes schizophrenia. The term does not apply to socially maladjusted children unless it is determined that they have an emotional disturbance.

This chapter contains text excerpted from the following sources: Text under the heading "What Is Emotional Disturbance?" is excerpted from "Sec. 300.8 (C) (4)," U.S. Department of Education (ED), May 2, 2017. Reviewed November 2022; Text under the heading "Warning Signs and Risk Factors for Emotional Distress" is excerpted from "Warning Signs and Risk Factors for Emotional Distress," Substance Abuse and Mental Health Services Administration (SAMHSA), May 16, 2022; Text under the heading "Children Identified with Emotional Disturbance" is excerpted from "OSEP Fast Facts: Children Identified with Emotional Disturbance," U.S. Department of Education (ED), May 6, 2020.

WARNING SIGNS AND RISK FACTORS FOR EMOTIONAL DISTRESS

It is common to feel stress symptoms before or after a crisis. Natural and human-caused disasters can devastate people's lives because they sometimes cause physical injury, damage to property, or the loss of a home or place of employment. Anyone who sees or experiences this can be affected in some way. Most stress symptoms are temporary and will resolve on their own in a fairly short amount of time. However, for some people, particularly children and teens, these symptoms may last for weeks or months and influence their relationships with families and friends. Common warning signs of emotional distress include:

- Eating or sleeping too much or too little.
- Pulling away from people and things.
- Having low or no energy.
- Having unexplained aches and pains, such as constant stomachaches or headaches.
- Feeling helpless or hopeless.
- Excessive smoking, drinking, or using drugs, including prescription medications.
- Worrying a lot of the time; feeling guilty but not sure why.
- Thinking of hurting or killing yourself or someone else.
- Having difficulty readjusting to home or work life.

For those who have lived through a natural or human-caused disaster, the event's anniversary may renew feelings of fear, anxiety, and sadness. Certain sounds, such as sirens, can also trigger emotional distress. These and other environmental sensations can take people back to the disaster or cause them to fear it will happen again. These "trigger events" can happen at any time.

Warning Signs and Risk Factors for Children and Teens

Children are often the most vulnerable of those impacted during and after a disaster. According to the National Child Traumatic Stress Network, a growing body of research has established that children as young as infancy may be affected by events that threaten their safety or the safety of their parents or caregivers.

Emotional Disturbance

Disasters are unfamiliar events not easily understood by children, who can find them emotionally confusing and frightening. During the turmoil, they may be left with someone unfamiliar to them and provided with limited information. Some warning signs of distress in children aged 6–11 include:
- Withdrawing from playgroups and friends.
- Competing more for the attention of parents and teachers.
- Being unwilling to leave home.
- Being less interested in schoolwork.
- Becoming aggressive.
- Having added conflict with peers or parents.
- Having difficulty concentrating.

For teens, the impact of disasters varies depending on how much of a disruption the disaster causes their family or community. Teens aged 12–18 are likely to have physical complaints when under stress or be less interested in schoolwork, chores, or other responsibilities.

Although some teens may compete vigorously for attention from parents and teachers after a disaster, they also may:
- Become withdrawn.
- Resist authority.
- Become disruptive or aggressive at home or in the classroom.
- Experiment with high-risk behaviors such as underage drinking or prescription drug misuse and abuse.

Children and teens most at risk for emotional distress include those who:
- Survived a previous disaster.
- Experienced temporary living arrangements, loss of personal property, and parental unemployment in a disaster.
- Lost a loved one or friend involved in a disaster.

Most young people need additional time to experience their world as a secure place and receive some emotional support to recover from their distress. The reactions of children and teens to a disaster are strongly influenced by how parents, relatives, teachers, and caregivers respond to the event. They often turn to these individuals for comfort and help. Teachers and other mentors play an especially important role after a disaster or other crisis by reinforcing normal routines to the extent possible, especially if new routines have to be established.

Warning Signs and Risk Factors for Adults

Adults impacted by disasters face the difficult challenge of balancing roles as first responders, survivors, and caregivers. They are often overwhelmed by the sheer magnitude of responsibility and immediate crisis response and recovery tasks. They must also take the time to address their physical and emotional needs and those of their family members and community. Warnings of signs of stress in adults may include the following:

- Crying spells or bursts of anger
- Difficulty eating
- Losing interest in daily activities
- Increasing physical distress symptoms such as headaches or stomach pains
- Fatigue
- Feeling guilty, helpless, or hopeless
- Avoiding family and friends

Adults most at risk of experiencing severe emotional stress and posttraumatic stress disorder include those with a history of:

- Exposure to other traumas, including severe accidents, abuse, assault, combat, or rescue work
- Chronic medical illness or psychological disorders
- Chronic poverty, homelessness, or discrimination
- Recent or subsequent major life stressors or emotional strain, such as single parenting

Adults most at risk for emotional stress include:

- Those who survived a previous disaster
- Those who lost a loved one or friend involved in a disaster

Emotional Disturbance

- Those who lack economic stability and/or knowledge of the English language
- Older adults that may lack mobility or independence

As with children and teens, adults also need time to return to normal routines. It is important that people try to accept whatever reactions they have related to the disaster. Take every day one at a time and focus on taking care of your own disaster-related needs and those of your family.

CHILDREN IDENTIFIED WITH EMOTIONAL DISTURBANCE

A child or youth, who was evaluated by the Individuals with Disabilities Education Act (IDEA) Sections 300.304 through 300.311 as having an emotional disturbance, is eligible for special education and related services under the IDEA, Part B, and, by reason thereof, needs special education and related services.

Percentage of Students with Disabilities Identified with Emotional Disturbance, Statewise

The states with the largest percentages of students with disabilities identified with emotional disturbance are Minnesota (13.41%) and Vermont (17.36%). The states with the smallest percentages of students with disabilities identified with emotional disturbance are Utah, Arkansas, Louisiana, Tennessee, Alabama, South Carolina, West Virginia, and North Carolina (1–3%).

In 2018–2019, the percentage of students with disabilities identified with emotional disturbance was 5.45 percent. States reported a range from 1.65 to 17.36 percent of students with disabilities identified with emotional disturbance.

Number of Students with Disabilities, Aged 6–21, by English Language Proficiency

The number of students with disabilities (refer to Figure 25.1) aged 6–21, by English language proficiency, served under IDEA, Part B, in the United States, outlying areas, and freely associated states: the school year 2018–2019. The discrepancy between English

Learning Disabilities Sourcebook, Seventh Edition

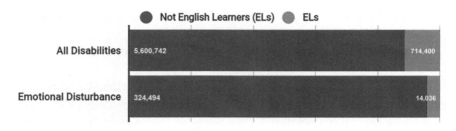

Figure 25.1. Number of Students with Disabilities by English Language Proficiency

learners (EL) defined as having emotional disturbance (95.85% EL and 4.15% not EL) and all pupils with disabilities (88.69% EL and 11.31% not EL) may be seen in this stacked bar chart.

Percentage of Students with Disabilities Identified with Emotional Disturbance, Aged 6–21

The percentage of students with disabilities (refer to Figure 25.2) identified with emotional disturbance, aged 6–21, served under IDEA, Part B, in the United States, outlying areas, and freely associated states: between the school years 2008–2009 and 2018–2019. It demonstrates the percentage of students with disabilities identified with emotional disturbance over a 10-year period.

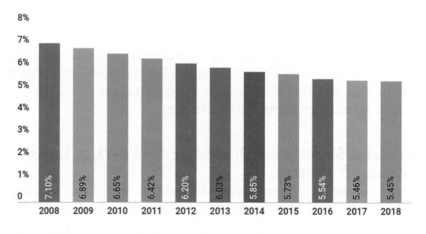

Figure 25.2. Percentage of Students with Disabilities Identified with Emotional Disturbance

Emotional Disturbance

The percentage of students with disabilities identified with emotional disturbance decreased from 7.1 percent in 2008–2009 to 5.45 percent in 2018–2019. Data from 2008 to 2011 include the United States and outlying areas; data from 2012 to 2018 include the United States, outlying areas, and freely associated states.

Percentage of Students with Disabilities Exiting School, Aged 14–21, by Basis of Exit

The percentage of students with disabilities exiting school, aged 14–21, by basis of exit, served under IDEA, Part B, in the United States, outlying areas, and freely associated states: the school year 2017–2018. It compares the percentage of all students with disabilities exiting school to students identified with emotional disturbance: graduated with a regular high school diploma of 73 and 60 percent, dropped out at 16 and 32 percent, and received a certificate of 10 and six percent, respectively (refer to Figure 25.3).

In the school year 2017–2018, students identified with emotional disturbance, aged 14–21, exiting school were more likely to drop out and less likely to graduate than all students with disabilities. Percentages do not equal 100 percent due to not including the counts of children who died, graduated with an alternate diploma, or reached maximum age.

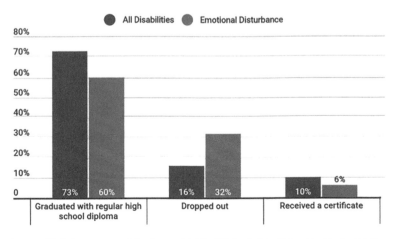

Figure 25.3. Percentage of Students with Disabilities Exiting School by Basis of Exit

Percentage of Students with Disabilities, Aged 6–21, by Educational Environment

The percentage of students with disabilities (refer to Figure 25.4), aged 6–21, by the educational environment, served under IDEA, Part B, in the United States, outlying areas, and freely associated states: the school year 2018–2019.

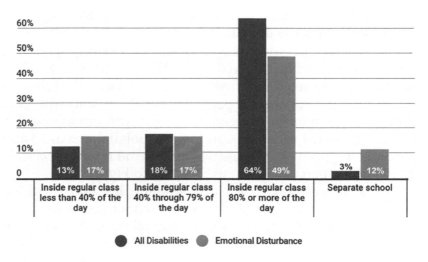

Figure 25.4. Percentage of Students with Disabilities by Educational Environment

In the school year 2018–2019, students identified with emotional disturbance were more likely to be served in a separate school than all students with disabilities. Percentages do not equal 100 percent due to not including the counts of children who receive services in a residential facility, home/hospital, or correctional facility or are parentally placed in private schools.

Number of Students with Disabilities, Aged 6–21, by Race and Ethnicity

The number of students with disabilities, aged 6–21, by race and ethnicity, served under IDEA, Part B, in the United States, outlying areas, and freely associated states: the school year 2018–2019. It also compares the number of all students with disabilities (American Indian or Alaska Native 85,534, Asian157,284, Black or African

Emotional Disturbance

American 1,129,554, Hispanic/Latinx 1,716,195, Native Hawaiian or other Pacific Islanders 23,384, two or more races 251,413, and White 2,951,864) to students identified with emotional disturbance (American Indian or Alaska Native 4,645, Asian 3,635, Black or African American 80,600, Hispanic/Latinx 63,105, Native Hawaiian or other Pacific Islanders 875, two or more races 19,025, and White 172,545) by race and ethnicity (refer to Figure 25.5).

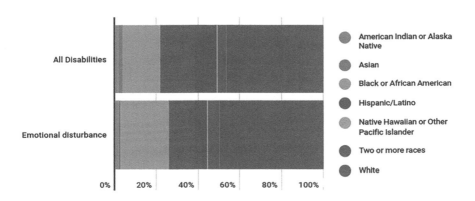

Figure 25.5. Percentage of Students with Disabilities by Race and Ethnicity

In the school year 2018–2019, when compared to all students with disabilities, Black or African American students were more likely to be identified with emotional disturbance than others, and Hispanic/Latinx students were less likely to be identified with emotional disturbance than others.

In the school year 2016–2017, Black or African American and Hispanic/Latinx students were less likely to be identified with autism, while White and Asian students with disabilities were more likely to be identified with autism when compared to all students with disabilities.

Total Disciplinary Removals per Child or Student with a Disability, Aged 3–21, by Disability Type

The total disciplinary removals per child or student with a disability (refer to Figure 25.6), aged 3–21, by disability type, served

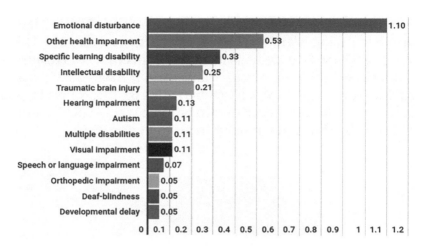

Figure 25.6. Total Disciplinary Removals per Child or Student with a Disability

under IDEA, Part B, in the United States, outlying areas, and freely associated states: the school year 2017–2018. It demonstrates the total disciplinary removers per child or student with a disability by disability type. Students identified with emotional disturbance have the most removals by change at 1.1 removals per child, followed by other health impairments at 0.53, specific learning disability at 0.33, intellectual disability at 0.25, traumatic brain injury at 0.21, hearing impairment at 0.13, autism at 0.11, multiple disabilities at 0.11, visual impairment at 0.11, speech or language impairment at 0.07, orthopedic impairment at 0.05, deaf-blindness at 0.05, and developmental delay at 0.05.

Children and students reported in these categories may be subject to multiple disciplinary removals. Children and students reported in these categories may be subject to multiple disciplinary removals. Data for Maine, Minnesota, Montana, Vermont, Wyoming, and Wisconsin were excluded, and data for the Virgin Islands and Vermont were unavailable.

A disciplinary removal is defined as any instance in which a child with a disability is removed from her/his educational placement for disciplinary purposes, including in-school suspension, out-of-school suspension, expulsion, removal by school personnel to an interim alternative educational setting for drug or weapon

Emotional Disturbance

offenses or serious bodily injury, and removal by hearing officer for likely injury to the child or others.

Percentage of Students with Disabilities, Aged 6–21, by Gender

The percentage of students with disabilities, aged 6–21, by gender, served under IDEA, Part B, in the United States, outlying areas, and freely associated states: the school year 2018–2019. It demonstrates the difference between the percentage of all male (66%) and female (34%) students with disabilities. It demonstrates the difference between the percentage of males (72%) and females (28%) identified with emotional disturbance (refer to Figure 25.7). Males were more likely to be identified with emotional disturbance than females compared to all students with disabilities.

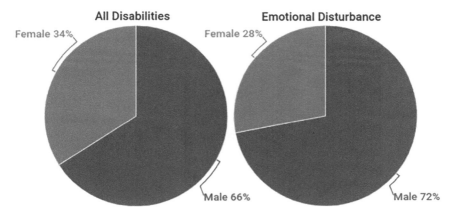

Figure 25.7. Percentage of Students with Disabilities by Gender

Part 4 | Learning Disabilities Interventions and Educational Process

Chapter 26 | Decoding Learning Disabilities Interventions

Children with learning disabilities face significant academic and emotional challenges as they struggle to master these skills. Learning disabilities are caused by differences in brain function that affect how a person's brain processes information. They do not indicate a person's intelligence; people with learning disabilities are just as bright as others. While learning disabilities can last a person's lifetime, they may be lessened with the right educational support.

Dr. Brett Miller, Ph.D., the program director of the Reading, Writing, and Related Learning Disabilities Program at the National Institute of Child Health and Human Development (NICHD), oversees the NICHD-funded research portfolio focused on learning disabilities. The program aims to understand how children learn to read, write, and do math; why some children struggle to acquire these skills; and what can be done to help them.

TEACHING CHILDREN WITH LEARNING DISABILITIES
An Example of NICHD-Funded Research on Learning Disabilities

The NICHD has resulted from a study on the investment in the Learning Disabilities Research Centers (LDRC). This study picked up kids at the end of fifth grade who were more than one year

---

This chapter includes text excerpted from "Decoding Learning Disabilities," *Eunice Kennedy Shriver* National Institute of Child Health and Human Development (NICHD), December 30, 2017. Reviewed November 2022.

behind in their reading level. They were given explicit, systematic, and direct instruction in reading for one, two, or three years. The children were directly and explicitly taught the component reading skills—including the rules of phonics—building their reading skills from the ground up. They were also given plenty of opportunities to practice their reading and enhance their understanding of the text more generally.

Children who made good progress within the first year transitioned to less intensive interventions. Those who continued to struggle got the second year of even more intensive intervention: smaller group instruction and more direct and explicit instruction. And those who continued to have difficulty went into the third year of intervention, which was even more intensive than the first two years.

The NICHD found that children with three years of intensive intervention show robust growth in reading comprehension and word-level reading. And so this is a success story.

The flip side is that while NICHD shows these gains, they could not reduce the gap between the reading levels of these children and their peers. Their peers also continued to develop their reading skills, so the gap remained.

Does This Study Have Implications for Teaching Children with Learning Disabilities?

This and other studies suggest that children with learning disabilities need direct, explicit, and systematic instruction, whether you are talking about reading or mathematics.

These children will likely need more time to build their skills and receive instruction in smaller groups so that they get more focused attention—it can be a small group, or it can one-on-one—depending upon the needs of the child and how significant their learning challenges are.

The NICHD knows that their most efficient and effective interventions are for our youngest learners. Starting young helps reduce the impact the disability has on their broader academic development.

Decoding Learning Disabilities Interventions

When Should These Interventions Begin?
The NICHD knows the risk factors when kids roll into kindergarten. For instance, if a parent has a learning disability, they know the children are at increased risk for a learning disability.

If NICHD knows a child has a higher risk of having reading difficulties going into preschool or kindergarten, they can monitor them to see how they perform and give them very explicit, direct, and systematic instruction early on. Fortunately, this type of instruction benefits those who struggle and those who do not, so it is effective for all kids.

So It Could Be Given within the Context of the Entire Class?
Exactly, and that is the hope and intent.

THE SCIENCE OF LEARNING DISABILITIES
What Do Brain Imaging Studies Tell Us?
Reading requires coordinated activity drawing on several different parts of the brain.

Brain imaging studies give us a window into understanding reading and reading disabilities. For the kids who develop typically with reading compared to those who do not, NICHD sees more focal activation in areas on the brain's left hemisphere and activation of parts of the left hemisphere that relate to improved word reading.

Kids who struggle with reading show more dispersed activation in the left hemisphere. But, if they successfully respond to reading intervention, they show a brain activation pattern that looks much more like individuals who do not struggle to read.

This is a remarkable example of what NICHD calls "neuroplasticity"; that is, you give an intervention in the classroom, and when the intervention is successful, you see changes in the structure and function of the brain.

Are There Genes Associated with Learning Disabilities?
Learning disabilities are complex conditions, and no single gene causes a learning disability or a reading disability. At this point, you

have identified about nine dyslexia susceptibility genes. If you have one of these genes, it does not mean that you will have dyslexia; you are at higher risk for dyslexia. This is one piece of information that could help us ascertain who would be at risk for problems.

Are There New Technologies to Help People with Learning Disabilities?

There are several resources now that individuals with learning disabilities have available to them to help support their learning. For example, there is software that reads the book to you. There are efforts to have more books recorded. Recorded books benefit from reading that sounds more natural and with appropriate intonation, as opposed to the reading software. But it is not practical to record every book, so reading will still be a necessary skill.

For individuals who have problems with writing, there are tools to help structure sentences and organize paragraphs and longer papers.

TIPS FOR PARENTS TO HELP THEIR CHILDREN

If you are a parent of a younger child, you can create a language-rich environment by talking with and reading with your child. This can help your child understand language structure—where to pause and allow someone else to talk—and improve her or his vocabulary.

You should read books to your child daily, giving them the story, vocabulary, background, and an understanding of how text is structured, how reading flows from left to right, and how the pages are turned. You can ask children questions to encourage them to think about what you have been reading and what is coming next in the story.

You can point out numbers in your environment for children with a math disability (dyscalculia). You can incorporate opportunities to learn about numbers when you are going to the grocery store or doing everyday tasks. For example, when you see three apples, you can count them. You are taking advantage of these opportunities to immerse your child in language and mathematical reasoning–rich environments.

Decoding Learning Disabilities Interventions

For children in school, create a positive environment where you celebrate successes and work with the challenges. It is important for parents to be role models who read and are engaged in their own lifelong learning. You can show children the calculations or measurements you are doing, like how you do the bills or measure the length of objects with a tape measure. You can have writing activities such as diaries, blogs, or other activities that are engaging and fun for your children.

Chapter 27 | Early Intervention Strategies

Chapter Contents
Section 27.1—Early Intervention: An Overview 267
Section 27.2—Parent Notification and Consent in Early
 Intervention 269
Section 27.3—Writing the Individualized Family Service
 Plan for Your Child 274
Section 27.4—Providing Early Intervention Services
 in Natural Environments 278
Section 27.5—Response to Intervention 283

Section 27.1 | Early Intervention: An Overview

This section contains text excerpted from the following sources: Text beginning with the heading "What Is Early Intervention?" is excerpted from "What Is Early Intervention?" Centers for Disease Control and Prevention (CDC), August 9, 2022; Text under the heading "Prevention and Early Intervention" is excerpted from "Prevention and Early Intervention," Youth.gov, July 9, 2022.

WHAT IS EARLY INTERVENTION?

- Early intervention is the term used to describe the services and supports that are available to babies and young children with developmental delays and disabilities and their families.
- It may include speech therapy, physical therapy, and other types of services based on the needs of the child and family.
- It can have a significant impact on a child's ability to learn new skills and overcome challenges and can increase success in school and life.
- Programs are available in every state and territory. These publicly funded programs provide services for free or at a reduced cost for any child who is eligible.

HOW DO YOU FIND OUT IF YOUR CHILD IS ELIGIBLE FOR EARLY INTERVENTION SERVICES?

Eligibility for early intervention services is oriented toward evaluating your child's skills and abilities.

If you, your child's doctor, or other care provider is concerned about your child's development, ask to be connected with your state or territory's early intervention program to find out if your child can get services to help. If your doctor cannot connect you, you can reach out yourself. A doctor's referral is not necessary.

If your child is under age three, call your state or territory's early intervention program and say you have concerns about your child's development and you would like to have your child evaluated to find out if she or he is eligible for early intervention services.

GOALS OF EARLY INTERVENTION
Early intervention programs help children gain the basic skills that they usually learn in the first two years of life, such as:
- Physical skills
- Thinking skills
- Communication skills
- Social skills
- Emotional skills

PREVENTION AND EARLY INTERVENTION
Considering the growing body of research, we now know that the better and more cost-effective place to stop the "cradle-to-prison pipeline" is as close to the beginning of that pipeline as possible. Early intervention prevents the onset of delinquent behavior and supports the development of a youth's assets and resilience. It also decreases rates of recidivism by a significant 16 percent when youth do go on to engage with the justice system. While many past approaches focus on remediating visible and/or long-standing disruptive behavior, research has shown that prevention and early intervention are more effective.

In addition to societal and personal benefits, research has demonstrated that delinquency prevention programs are a good financial investment. For example, a 2001 Washington State Institute for Public Policy (WSIPP) study found that the total benefits of effective prevention programs were greater than their costs. More recent research by WSIPP found that sound delinquency prevention programs can save taxpayers $7–10 for every dollar invested, primarily due to reductions in the amount spent on incarceration.

Intervening early "not only saves young lives from being wasted" but also prevents the onset of adult criminal careers and reduces the likelihood of youth perpetrating serious and violent offenses. This, in turn, reduces the burden of crime on society and saves taxpayers billions of dollars.

What Are Effective Programs?
Under this prevention and early intervention framework, an increasing body of research is being conducted to determine which

Early Intervention Strategies

existing programs are truly effective. Current literature indicates that effective programs are those that aim to act as early as possible and focus on known risk factors and the behavioral development of juveniles. In general, the Office of Juvenile Justice and Delinquency Prevention (OJJDP) recommends that the following types of school and community prevention programs be employed:
- Classroom and behavior management programs
- Multicomponent classroom-based programs
- Social competence promotion curriculums
- Conflict resolution and violence prevention curriculums
- Bullying prevention programs
- After-school recreation programs
- Mentoring programs
- School organization programs
- Comprehensive community interventions

Section 27.2 | Parent Notification and Consent in Early Intervention

This section includes text excerpted from "Parent Notification and Consent in Early Intervention," Center for Parent Information and Resources (CPIR), U.S. Department of Education (ED), July 1, 2021.

Parents are essential partners in early intervention. They have the right to be deeply involved at every step along the way, from the evaluation of their child to the writing of the Individualized Family Service Plan (IFSP) to help determine the early intervention services their child receives.

Not surprisingly, Part C of the Individuals with Disabilities Education Act (IDEA) includes specific provisions to support the informed involvement of parents in their child's early intervention program. Two notable requirements are as follows:
- Prior written notice, which the early intervention system must provide to parents at key points in time
- Parental consent, which must be obtained from parents, also at key points in time

The right to be informed and the right to give or refuse consent for pivotal activities are important procedural safeguards for parents and recognize their authority and responsibility in making decisions about their child's involvement in early intervention and that of the family.

PRIOR WRITTEN NOTICE: PARENTS' RIGHT TO BE FULLY INFORMED

Prior written notice refers to the notification that must be provided to parents a reasonable time before the lead agency or an early intervention service (EIS) provider proposes (or refuses) to "initiate or change the identification, evaluation, or placement of their infant or toddler, or the provision of early intervention services to the infant or toddler with a disability" and her or his family.

- **Purpose of prior written notice.** The purpose of prior written notice is always the same—to ensure that parents are fully informed regarding whatever action the lead agency or EIS provider is proposing to take (or not) with their infant or toddler or with the family. Parental consent is often needed before the lead agency or EIS provider may proceed and that consent must be informed. Even if parental consent is not required, parents still have the right to know when something about their child's (or family's) involvement in early intervention is being proposed, refused, about to start, or about to change.
- **Content of the notice.** The content of the notice must be in sufficient detail to inform parents about the following:
    - The action that is being proposed or refused
    - The reasons for taking (or refusing to take) the action
    - All procedural safeguards that are available to parents, should they disagree with the early intervention system (e.g., mediation, filing a state complaint or a due process complaint, relevant timelines)

Early Intervention Strategies

- **Examples for prior written notice**. Prior written notice to parents is required in the circumstances like the following:
  - The early intervention system wants to evaluate their infant or toddler and is seeking parental consent for the evaluation.
  - The early intervention system refuses to evaluate an infant or toddler when parents have requested an evaluation.
  - The early intervention system intends to change the child's identification as an eligible "infant or toddler with a disability."
  - The early intervention system wants to provide early intervention services to infants, toddlers, and families.
  - A service provider wants to change the services provided to an infant or toddler with a disability.
- **Native language**. To ensure that a parent can understand the notice, it must be written in a language understandable to the general public and provided in the parent's native language (or another mode of communication) unless it is not feasible to do so. If the parent's language is not a written one, the lead agency or EIS provider must ensure that:
  - The prior written notice is translated orally to the parent.
  - The parent understands the notice.
  - There is written evidence that these requirements have been met.

PARENTAL CONSENT

Consent within the IDEA has a very specific meaning that is closely tied to prior written notice. Consent, in IDEA, means informed written consent. The notice provided to parents informs them by completely describing a proposed or refused action and its reasons. This builds the foundation of understanding upon which informed consent may be given (or not).

The term consent is defined in the Part C regulations as follows:
- **§303.7 Consent.** Consent means that:
  - The parent has been fully informed of all information relevant to the activity for which consent is sought in the parent's native language as defined in §303.25.
  - The parent understands and agrees in writing to the carrying out of the activity for which the parent's consent is sought, and the consent form describes that activity and lists the early intervention records (if any) that will be released and to whom they will be released.
  - The parent understands that the granting of consent is voluntary on the part of the parent and may be revoked at any time. If a parent revokes consent, that revocation is not retroactive (i.e., it does not apply to an action that occurred before the consent was revoked).

The definitions make it clear that:
- The early intervention system must use the parents' native language (or another mode of communication) when seeking their consent for an activity.
- Parents must give consent in writing.
- There is a consent form describing the activity for which consent is sought.
- The consent form also lists the early intervention records that will be released (if any) and to whom.
- Giving consent is voluntary on the part of parents.
- Parents may revoke their consent at any time.

Process of Consent
- **Consent during the evaluation process.** It will be no surprise that prior written notice and parental consent are required repeatedly throughout the evaluation process. These times are:
  - Before administering screening procedures to see if an infant or toddler is suspected of having a disability

Early Intervention Strategies

- Before evaluating the infant or toddler to determine eligibility for Part C
- Before conducting all assessments of the infant or toddler
- **Consent before services are provided**. Parental consent is also required before the early intervention services listed in the child's IFSP may be provided. To ensure that parents understand what they are being asked to consent to, the Part C regulations require that the contents of the IFSP be fully explained to the parents. The Part C regulations also clarify that parents have the right to give or refuse consent for each service (one by one) and to revoke consent at any time for any service. Those regulations read:
  - The parents of an infant or toddler with a disability:
    - Determine whether they, their infant or toddler with a disability, or other family members will accept or decline any early intervention service under this part at any time by state law.
    - May decline service after first accepting it without jeopardizing other early intervention services under this part.

Each early intervention service must be provided as soon as possible after the parent provides consent for that service.
- **Other times when consent is required**. Other times, parental consent may be required, depending on state policy. Two are mentioned in §303.420(a) and stipulate that parental consent must be obtained before the lead agency:
  - May use the family's public benefits or insurance or private insurance if such consent is required under §303.520.
  - Discloses personally identifiable information.
- **May the lead agency challenge or try to override a parent's refusal to give consent?** No. The lead agency may not challenge a parent's refusal to consent, not even through the due process procedures that Parts C and B provide for resolving disputes.

Section 27.3 | Writing the Individualized Family Service Plan for Your Child

This section contains text excerpted from the following sources: Text beginning with the heading "What Is an Individualized Family Service Plan?" is excerpted from "Writing the IFSP for Your Child," Center for Parent Information and Resources (CPIR), U.S. Department of Education (ED), July 1, 2021; Text under the heading "Individualized Family Service Plans Tips" is excerpted from "Individualized Family Service Plans (IFSPs) Tips," Early Childhood Learning and Knowledge Center (ECLKC), June 7, 2022.

WHAT IS AN INDIVIDUALIZED FAMILY SERVICE PLAN?

The Individualized Family Service Plan (IFSP) is a written document that, among other things, outlines the early intervention services that your child and family will receive.

One guiding principle of the IFSP is that the family is a child's greatest resource and that a young child's needs are closely tied to the needs of her or his family. The best way to support children and meet their needs is to support and build upon the individual strengths of their family. So the IFSP is a whole family plan with the parents as major contributors to its development. The involvement of other team members will depend on what the child needs. These other team members could come from several agencies, including medical people, therapists, child development specialists, social workers, and so on. Each state has specific guidelines for the IFSP. Your service coordinator can explain what the IFSP guidelines are in your state.

WHAT IS INCLUDED IN THE INDIVIDUALIZED FAMILY SERVICE PLAN?

Your child's IFSP must include the following:
- Your child's present levels of functioning and need in the areas of her or his physical, cognitive, communication, social/emotional, and adaptive development
- Family information (with your agreement), including the resources, priorities, and your concerns, as parents, and other family members closely involved with the child

Early Intervention Strategies

- The major results or outcomes expected to be achieved for your child and family
- The specific early intervention services your child will be receiving
- Where in the natural environment (e.g., home, community) the services will be provided (if the services are not provided in the natural environment, the IFSP must include a statement justifying why not)
- When and where your son or daughter will receive services
- The number of days or sessions she or he will receive each service and how long each session will last
- Who will pay for the services?
- The name of the service coordinator overseeing the implementation of the IFSP
- The steps to be taken to support your child's transition out of early intervention and into another program when the time comes

The IFSP may also identify services in which your family may be interested, such as financial information or information about raising a child with a disability.

The IFSP must be fully explained to you, and the parents and your suggestions must be considered. You must give written consent before services can start. If you do not give your consent in writing, your child will not receive services.

WHO DEVELOPS THE INDIVIDUALIZED FAMILY SERVICE PLAN?

The meeting to develop the child's first IFSP (and each annual meeting thereafter to review the IFSP) must include the following participants:

- The parent or parents of the child
- Other family members, as requested by the parent, if feasible to do so
- An advocate or person outside of the family, if the parent requests the person to participate

- The service coordinator designated by the system to be responsible for implementing the IFSP
- A person or persons directly involved in conducting the evaluations and assessments of the child and family
- Persons who will provide early intervention services under this part to the child or family (as appropriate)

WHAT HAPPENS NEXT?

With your written consent, the IFSP is then implemented, meaning that the services described in the IFSP are provided to your child in the manner described in the IFSP. In other words, all that information you included in the IFSP now serves as a roadmap for the early intervention system as it provides services to your child and family.

About Parental Consent

You, as parents, have the right to decline any early intervention service without jeopardizing your child's eligibility for other early intervention services. Parents may also revoke their consent for one or more services at any time.

Review and Update of the Individualized Family Service Plan

The IFSP is reviewed every six months and is updated at least once a year. You, as parents, are also part of that review and revision process. Together, you and the team will look at your child's progress and decide how (or if) the IFSP needs to be changed to reflect your child's growth toward the goals you have set, the family's current situation, and so on.

INDIVIDUALIZED FAMILY SERVICE PLANS TIPS

Tips for Educators is a series of practical guides that education staff can use in early learning settings. Each guide is oriented on research evidence and professional knowledge.

Early Intervention Strategies

The IFSP is a written plan created to meet the individual needs, concerns, and priorities of individual children, from birth to age three, and their families. The plan states the family's desired outcomes for their child and themselves and lists the early intervention services and supports to help meet those outcomes. It also describes when, where, and how the services will be delivered.

A team of key members develops the IFSP. This team includes the family, educators and caregivers, the disability services coordinator, and any specialists who offer support and services identified in the plan. Working together, this team considers the child's strengths and needs, evaluation and assessment results, and the family's ideas, concerns, and priorities. All team members have access to the IFSP and use it to plan learning experiences and environments that support the child in achieving the identified outcomes.

Every state has its own system of early intervention services, and a few have expanded age limits for IFSP eligibility. It is important for all team members to become familiar with the specifics of the state agency.

Tips for Educators
- Get familiarized with your state's specific early intervention agency and services. The Infant and Toddler Coordinators Association state guide of the Individuals with Disabilities Education Act (IDEA) is a helpful starting point.
- Conduct development screenings to determine if a child has developmental concerns that require a complete evaluation.
- Include children with disabilities and other special needs in natural environments with their peers, where experiences and environments that promote children's learning are offered.
- Collect ongoing assessment information to individualize teaching and learning.
- Give children with disabilities or other special needs the comprehensive services (e.g., nutrition, dental) that all children and families receive.

- Work with other agencies' specialists to ensure the child and family receive the services and supports outlined in the IFSP.
- Share support strategies between educators and specialists on the IFSP team to promote continuity between settings and services.

Section 27.4 | Providing Early Intervention Services in Natural Environments

This section includes text excerpted from "Providing Early Intervention Services in Natural Environments," Center for Parent Information and Resources (CPIR), U.S. Department of Education (ED), July 1, 2021.

INDIVIDUALS WITH DISABILITIES EDUCATION ACT'S DEFINITION OF "NATURAL ENVIRONMENT"

Part C of the Individuals with Disabilities Education Act (IDEA) requires that eligible infants and toddlers with disabilities receive needed early intervention services in natural environments to the maximum extent appropriate. The 2011 regulations for Part C define the term as follows:

- **§303.26 Natural environments.** Natural environments mean natural or typical settings for a same-aged infant or toddler without a disability, may include the home or community settings, and must be consistent with the provisions of §303.126.

It is a straightforward, easily understood definition—except for how it ends ("must be consistent with the provisions of §303.126"). What might the provisions of §303.126 require?

Let us have a look. Here they are:

- **§303.126 Early intervention services in natural environments.** Each system must include policies and procedures to ensure, consistent with §303.13(a)(8) (early intervention services), §303.26 (natural environments), and §303.344(d)(1)(ii) (the content of

Early Intervention Strategies

an IFSP), that early intervention services for infants and toddlers with disabilities are provided:
- To the maximum extent appropriate in natural environments
- In settings other than the natural environment that are most appropriate, as determined by the parent and the Individualized Family Service Plan (IFSP) team, only when early intervention services cannot be achieved satisfactorily in a natural environment

Combining these two sets of provisions makes it clear that early intervention services:
- Must be provided in settings that are natural or typical for a same-aged infant or toddler without a disability to the maximum extent appropriate.
- May be provided in other settings only when the services cannot be achieved satisfactorily in a natural environment.

WHO DECIDES WHERE SERVICES WILL BE PROVIDED?

The Part C regulations also make it clear that the IFSP team determines the appropriate setting for providing early intervention services to a child or toddler. The IFSP team may determine that a service will not be provided in a natural environment only "when early intervention services cannot be achieved satisfactorily in a natural environment."

Note: The team refers broadly to the people who write the child's IFSP. More specifically, as described in the Part C regulations:
- The child's parents are members of the IFSP team. They may also invite other family members to participate in the team (if it is feasible). They may also request an advocate or person from outside the family to be part of the team.
- The IFSP team must include two or more individuals from separate disciplines or professions, one of which must be the family's service coordinator.

- The IFSP team must also include a person directly involved in conducting the evaluations and assessments of the child and family.
- As appropriate, people who will be providing early intervention services to the child may also serve on the IFSP team (§303.343).

This, then, is the group of well-informed individuals that makes the decision as to where early intervention services will be provided to the baby or toddler.

ON WHAT BASIS DOES THE TEAM DECIDE THE SETTING?
- **The short answer.** The IFSP team decides where each early intervention service (EIS) will be oriented on the measurable results or outcomes expected to be achieved by the child. Those results or outcomes have been identified by the IFSP team and listed in the IFSP.
- **The longer answer.** Again, the Part C regulations provide the necessary guidance. At §303.344(d)(1)(ii)(B), the regulations state that:
  - The determination of the appropriate setting for providing early intervention services to an infant or toddler with a disability, including any justification for not providing a particular early intervention service in the natural environment for that infant or toddler with a disability and service, must be:
    - Made by the IFSP team (which includes the parent and other team members)
    - Consistent with the provisions in §303.13(a)(8), §303.26, and §303.126
    - Based on the child's outcomes that the IFSP team identifies in paragraph (c) of this section
- **An example.** The Department of Education (ED) provides an example of how it may not always be practicable or appropriate for an infant or toddler with a disability to receive an early intervention service in the natural

environment oriented either on the nature of the service or the child's specific outcomes. The ED states that:
- For example, the IFSP team may determine that an eligible child needs to receive speech services in a clinical setting that serves only children with disabilities to meet a specific IFSP outcome. When the natural environment is not chosen concerning an early intervention service, the IFSP team must provide, in the IFSP, with an appropriate justification for that decision.

WHAT MUST BE INCLUDED ABOUT NATURAL ENVIRONMENTS IN THE CHILD'S INDIVIDUALIZED FAMILY SERVICE PLAN?

The Part C regulations indicate that the IFSP must include the following:
- A statement that each early intervention service is provided in the natural environment for that child or service to the maximum extent appropriate
- A justification for why an early intervention service will not be provided in the natural environment

If the IFSP team determines that an early intervention service will not be provided in the natural environment, it must document in the IFSP the justification for why not—in other words, why the alternative service setting is needed for the child to meet the developmental outcomes identified for the child in her or his IFSP.

TWO POINTS FROM THE U.S. DEPARTMENT OF EDUCATION

When the ED released the 2011 Part C implementing regulations, it included the often fascinating analysis of comments and changes. The ED's "natural environments" discussion includes two interesting and illuminating observations that ED shares with you:
- **Why not include a list of settings considered "natural environments" and those not considered "natural environments"?** The ED declined to add a fuller list of settings that may be considered (or would not be

considered) "natural environments." The current regulations only mention that natural environments "may include home and community settings." Why did the ED decline to include a fuller list? According to the ED:
- It would not be appropriate or practicable to include a list of every setting that may be the natural environment for a particular child or those settings that may not be natural in these regulations.
- In some circumstances, a setting that is natural for one eligible child oriented on that child's outcomes, family routines, or the nature of the service may not be natural for another child.
- The decision about whether an environment is a natural environment is an individualized decision made by an infant's or toddler's IFSP team, which includes the parent.

- **Are clinics, hospitals, or a service provider's office considered "natural environments"?** Some of the department's responses are as follows:
  - The ED appreciates the commenters' requests for clarification as to whether clinics, hospitals, or a service provider's office may be considered the natural environment in cases when specialized instrumentation or equipment that cannot be transported to the home is needed.
  - Natural environments mean settings that are natural or typical for an infant or toddler without a disability. The ED does not believe that a clinic, hospital, or service provider's office is a natural environment for an infant or toddler without a disability; therefore, such a setting would not be natural for an infant or toddler with a disability.
  - However, §303.344(d)(1) requires that the identification of the early intervention service needed, as well as the appropriate setting for providing each service to an infant or toddler with a disability, be individualized decisions

made by the IFSP team oriented on that child's unique needs, family routines, and developmental outcomes. Suppose a determination is made by the IFSP team that is oriented on a review of all relevant information regarding the unique needs of the child; the child cannot satisfactorily achieve the identified early intervention outcomes in natural environments. In that case, services could be provided in another environment (e.g., clinic, hospital, service provider's office). In such cases, a justification must be included in the IFSP.

Section 27.5 | Response to Intervention

This section includes text excerpted from "Essential Components of RTI—a Closer Look at Response to Intervention," U.S. Department of Education (ED), April 2010. Reviewed October 2022.

DEFINITION OF RESPONSE TO INTERVENTION

The National Center on Response to Intervention (NCRTI) offers a definition of response to intervention that reflects what is currently known from research and evidence-based practice. Response to intervention (RTI) integrates assessment and intervention within a multilevel prevention system to maximize student achievement and reduce behavioral problems. With RTI, schools use data to identify students at risk for poor learning outcomes, monitor student progress, provide evidence-based interventions and adjust the intensity and nature of those interventions depending on a student's responsiveness, and identify students with learning disabilities or other disabilities.

LEVELS, TIERS, AND INTERVENTION

The tertiary, secondary, and primary levels of prevention explain the progression of support across the multilevel prevention system. Although discussions in the field frequently refer to "tiers" to designate different interventions, NCRTI intentionally avoids using this term when describing the RTI framework and instead uses "levels" to refer to three prevention foci: primary, secondary, and tertiary levels. Within each of these levels of prevention, there can be more than one intervention. Regardless of the number of interventions a school or district implements, each should be classified under one of the three levels of prevention: primary, secondary, or tertiary. This will allow for a common understanding across schools, districts, and states.

For example, a school may have three interventions of approximately the same intensity at the secondary prevention level, while another may have one at that level. While there are differences in the number of interventions, these schools will have a common understanding of the nature and focus of the secondary prevention level.

THE CENTER'S DEFINITION OF RESPONSE TO INTERVENTION: THE "WHAT"

The RTI integrates student assessment and instructional intervention. RTI is a framework for providing comprehensive support to students and is not an instructional practice. RTI is a prevention-oriented approach to linking assessment and instruction that can inform educators' decisions about how best to teach their students. A goal of RTI is to minimize the risk of long-term negative learning outcomes by responding quickly and efficiently to documented learning or behavioral problems and ensuring the appropriate identification of students with disabilities.

Response to Intervention Employs a Multilevel Prevention System

A rigorous prevention system provides for the early identification of learning and behavioral challenges and timely intervention for students at risk for long-term learning problems. This system includes three levels of intensity or three levels of prevention, representing a continuum of supports. Many schools use more than one intervention within a given level of prevention.

- **Primary prevention**. High-quality core instruction that meets the needs of most students.

Early Intervention Strategies

- **Secondary prevention**. Evidence-based intervention(s) of moderate intensity that addresses the learning or behavioral challenges of most at-risk students.
- **Tertiary prevention**. Individualized intervention(s) of increased intensity for students who show minimal response to secondary prevention.

At all levels, attention is on the fidelity of implementation, considering cultural and linguistic responsiveness and recognizing student strengths.

The Response to Intervention Can Be Used to Both Maximize Student Achievement and Reduce Behavioral Problems

The RTI framework provides a system for delivering instructional interventions of increasing intensity. These interventions effectively integrate academic instruction with positive behavioral supports. The Center on Positive Behavioral Interventions and Supports (PBIS; www.pbis.org) provides a school-wide model similar to the framework described herein. The two can be combined to provide a school-wide academic and behavioral framework.

The Response to Intervention Can Be Used to Ensure the Appropriate Identification of Students with Disabilities

By encouraging practitioners to implement early intervention, RTI implementation should improve academic performance and behavior, simultaneously reducing the likelihood that students are wrongly identified as having a disability.

THE CENTER'S DEFINITION OF RESPONSE TO INTERVENTION: THE "HOW"
Identify Students at Risk for Poor Learning Outcomes or Challenging Behavior

Struggling students are identified by implementing a two-stage screening process. The first stage, universal screening, is a brief assessment for all students conducted at the beginning of the school year; however, some schools and districts use it twice. For students who score below the cut point on the universal screen, a second screening stage is conducted to more accurately predict which students are at risk for poor learning outcomes. This second stage involves additional, more in-depth testing or short-term progress monitoring to confirm a student's at-risk status. Screening tools must be reliable and valid, demonstrating diagnostic accuracy for predicting which students will develop learning or behavioral difficulties.

Provide Research-Based Curricula and Evidence-Based Interventions

Classroom instructors are encouraged to use research-based curricula in all subjects. Evidence-based interventions of moderate intensity are provided when a student is identified via screening as requiring additional intervention. These interventions, in addition to the core primary instruction, typically involve small group instruction to address specific identified problems. These evidenced-based interventions are well defined in terms of duration, frequency, and length of sessions, and the intervention is conducted as it was in the research studies. Students who respond adequately to secondary prevention return to primary prevention (the core curriculum) with ongoing progress monitoring. Students who show minimal response to secondary prevention move to tertiary prevention, where more intensive and individualized support is provided. All instructional and behavioral interventions should be selected with attention to their evidence of effectiveness and with sensitivity to culturally and linguistically diverse students.

Monitor Student Progress

Progress monitoring is used to assess students' performance over time, quantify student rates of improvement or responsiveness to instruction, evaluate instructional effectiveness, and formulate effective individualized programs for students who are least responsive to effective instruction. Progress monitoring tools must accurately represent students' academic development and must be useful for instructional planning and assessing student learning. In

Early Intervention Strategies

tertiary prevention, educators use progress monitoring to compare a student's expected and actual learning rates. If a student is not achieving the expected learning rate, the educator experiments with instructional components to improve the learning rate.

Adjust the Intensity and Nature of Interventions Depending on a Student's Responsiveness

Progress monitoring data determine when a student has or has not responded to instruction at any level of the prevention system. Increasing the intensity of an intervention can be accomplished in several ways, such as lengthening instructional time, increasing the frequency of instructional sessions, reducing the size of the instructional group, or adjusting the level of instruction. Also, intensity can be increased by providing intervention support from a teacher with more experience and skill in teaching students with learning or behavioral difficulties (e.g., a reading specialist or a special educator).

Identify Students with Learning Disabilities or Other Disabilities

If a student fails to respond to intervention, the student may have a learning disability or other disability that requires further evaluation. Progress monitoring and other data collected over the course of the provided intervention should be examined during the evaluation process, along with data from appropriately selected measures (e.g., tests of cognition, language, perception, and social skills).

In this way, effectively implemented RTI frameworks contribute to the process of disability identification by reducing inappropriate identification of students who might appear to have a disability because of inappropriate or insufficient instruction.

Use Data to Inform Decisions at the School, Grade, or Classroom Levels

Screening and progress monitoring data can be aggregated and used to compare and contrast the adequacy of the core curriculum and the effectiveness of different instructional and behavioral strategies for various groups of students within a school. For example, if 60 percent of the students in a particular grade score below the cut point on a screening test at the beginning of the year, school personnel might consider the appropriateness of the core curriculum or whether differentiated learning activities need to be added to better meet the needs of the students in that grade.

RESPONSE TO INTERVENTION 101: FREQUENTLY ASKED QUESTIONS

The NCRTI has received numerous questions about RTI from state and local educators, families, and other stakeholders across the country.

What Is at the Heart of Response to Intervention?

The purpose of RTI is to provide all students with the best opportunities to succeed in school, identify students with learning or behavioral problems, and ensure that they receive appropriate instruction and support. The goals of RTI are to:
- Integrate all the resources to minimize the risk of the long-term negative consequences associated with poor learning or behavioral outcomes.
- Strengthen the process of appropriate disability identification.

What Impact Does Response to Intervention Have on Students Who Are Not Struggling?

An important component of an effective RTI framework is the quality of the primary prevention level (i.e., the core curriculum), where all students receive high-quality instruction that is culturally and linguistically responsive and aligned to a state's achievement standards. This allows teachers and parents to be confident that a student's need for more intensive intervention or referral for special education evaluation is not due to ineffective classroom instruction. In a well-designed RTI system, primary prevention should be effective and sufficient for about 80 percent of the student population.

Early Intervention Strategies

What Is the Response to Intervention Prevention Framework?

The RTI has three levels of prevention: primary, secondary, and tertiary. Through this framework, student assessment and instruction are linked for data-based decision-making. If students move through the framework's specified levels of prevention, their instructional program becomes more intensive and individualized to target their specific areas of learning or behavioral need.

Why Is a Common Framework for Response to Intervention Helpful?

A common RTI framework may strengthen RTI implementation by helping schools understand how programming becomes increasingly intensive. This helps schools accurately classify practices as primary, secondary, or tertiary. These distinctions should assist building-level administrators and teachers in determining how to deploy staff sensibly and efficiently.

What Does Response to Intervention Do to Identify Students for Special Education?

The Individuals with Disabilities Education Act (IDEA) 2004 allows states to use a process oriented on a student's response to scientific, research-based interventions to determine if the child has a specific learning disability (SLD). In an RTI framework, a student's response to or success with instruction and interventions received across the levels of RTI would be considered part of the comprehensive evaluation for SLD eligibility.

Chapter 28 | The Special Education Process: An Overview

THE TEN BASICS OF THE SPECIAL EDUCATION PROCESS UNDER THE INDIVIDUALS WITH DISABILITIES EDUCATION ACT

When a child is having trouble in school, it is important to find out why. The child may have a disability. By law, schools must provide special help to eligible children with disabilities. This help is called "special education and related services."

There is much to know about how children are identified as having a disability and needing special education and related services. This chapter distilled the process into 10 basic steps. Once you have the big picture of the process, it is easier to understand the many details under each step.

Step 1: A Child Is Identified as Possibly Needing Special Education and Related Services

There are two primary ways in which children are identified as possibly needing special education and related services: the system known as "Child Find" (which operates in each state; sites.ed.gov/idea/regs/b/b/300.111), and by referral of a parent or school personnel.

This chapter contains text excerpted from the following sources: Text under the heading "The Ten Basics of the Special Education Process under the Individuals with Disabilities Education Act" is excerpted from "10 Basic Steps in Special Education," Center for Parent Information & Resources (CPIR), U.S. Department of Education (ED), April 2022; Text under the heading "Education Programs for People with Disabilities" is excerpted from "Jobs and Education for People with Disabilities," USA.gov, June 21, 2022.

- **Child Find**. The Individuals with Disabilities Education Act (IDEA) requires each state to identify, locate, and evaluate all children with disabilities in the state who need special education and related services. To do so, states conduct what are known as "Child Find activities." When Child Find identifies a child as possibly having a disability and as needing special education, parents may be asked for permission to evaluate their child. Parents can also call the Child Find office and ask that their child be evaluated.
- **Referral or request for evaluation**. A school professional may ask that a child be evaluated to see if she or he has a disability. Parents may also contact the child's teacher or another school professional to ask that their child be evaluated. This request may be verbal, but it is best to write it.

Parental consent is needed before a child may be evaluated. Under the federal IDEA regulations, the evaluation must be completed within 60 days after the parent gives consent. However, if a state's IDEA regulations give a different timeline for completing the evaluation, the state's timeline is applied.

Step 2: A Child Is Evaluated

Evaluation is an essential early step in the special education process for a child. It is intended to answer the following questions:
- Does the child have a disability that requires the provision of special education and related services?
- What are the child's specific educational needs?
- What special education services and related services, then, are appropriate for addressing those needs?

By law, the initial evaluation of the child must be full and individual—which is to say, focused on that child and that child alone. The evaluation must assess the child in all areas related to the suspected disability.

The Special Education Process: An Overview

The evaluation results will be used to decide the child's eligibility for special education and related services and make decisions about an appropriate educational program.

If the parents disagree with the evaluation, they have the right to take their child for an independent educational evaluation (IEE). They can ask that the school system pays for this IEE.

Step 3: Eligibility Is Decided

A group of qualified professionals and the parents look at the child's evaluation results. Together, they decide if the child is a "child with a disability," as defined by IDEA. If the parents do not agree with the eligibility decision, they may ask for a hearing to challenge the decision.

Step 4: A Child Is Found Eligible for Services

If the child is found to be a child with a disability, as defined by IDEA, she or he is eligible for special education and related services. Within 30 calendar days after a child is determined eligible, a team of school professionals and the parents must meet to write an individualized education program (IEP) for the child.

Step 5: Individualized Education Program Meeting Is Scheduled

The school system schedules and conducts the IEP meeting. School staff must:
- Contact the participants, including the parents.
- Notify parents early enough to make sure they have an opportunity to attend.
- Schedule the meeting at a time and place agreeable to parents and the school.
- Tell the parents the purpose, time, and location of the meeting.
- Tell the parents who will be attending.
- Tell the parents they may invite people to the meeting with specific knowledge or expertise about the child.

Step 6: Individualized Education Program Meeting Is Held, and the Individualized Education Program Is Written

The IEP team gathers to talk about the child's needs and write the student's IEP. Parents and the student (when appropriate) are full participating team members. If the child's placement (meaning where the child will receive her or his special education and related services) is decided by a different group, the parents must also be part of that group.

Before the school system may provide special education and related services to the child for the first time, the parents must consent. The child begins to receive services as soon as possible after the IEP is written and this consent is given.

If the parents do not agree with the IEP and placement, they may discuss their concerns with other IEP team members and try to work out an agreement. Parents can ask for mediation if they still disagree, or the school may offer mediation. Parents may file a state complaint with the state education agency or a due process complaint, which is the first step in requesting a due process hearing, at which time mediation must be available.

Step 7: After the Individualized Education Program Is Written, Services Are Provided

The school ensures that the child's IEP is carried out as it was written. Parents are given a copy of the IEP. Each child's teacher and service provider has access to the IEP and knows her or his specific responsibilities for carrying out the IEP. This includes the accommodations, modifications, and supports that must be provided to the child, keeping with the IEP.

Step 8: Progress Is Measured and Reported to Parents

The child's progress toward the annual goals is measured, as stated in the IEP. Parents are regularly informed of their child's progress and whether that progress is enough for the child to achieve the goals by the end of the year. These progress reports must be given to parents at least as often as parents are informed of their nondisabled children's progress.

Step 9: Individualized Education Program Is Reviewed

The child's IEP is reviewed by the IEP team at least once a year or more often if the parents or school ask for a review. If necessary, the IEP is revised. Parents, as team members, must be invited to participate in these meetings. Parents can make suggestions for changes and agree or disagree with the IEP and the placement.

If parents do not agree with the IEP and placement, they may discuss their concerns with other IEP team members and try to work out an agreement. Several options include additional testing, an independent evaluation, asking for mediation, or a due process hearing. They may also file a complaint with the state education agency.

Step 10: A Child Is Re-evaluated

At least every three years, the child must be re-evaluated. This evaluation is sometimes called a "triennial." Its purpose is to determine if the child continues to be a child with a disability, as defined by IDEA, and what the child's educational needs are. However, the child must be re-evaluated more often if conditions warrant it or the child's parent or teacher asks for a new evaluation.

EDUCATION PROGRAMS FOR PEOPLE WITH DISABILITIES

Learn how to find government education programs and financial aid for people with disabilities.

- Your state department of education or your local school board can tell you about the following:
  - Nearby programs
  - The state's education rights for people with disabilities
- An IEP is a plan developed by teachers and parents to meet that child's needs. It is essential to the IDEA. The IDEA guarantees a free, appropriate public education to eligible children with disabilities.
- College-bound students with intellectual disabilities may be eligible for financial aid programs. The office for Federal Student Aid (FSA) has information on loans, grants, and scholarships.
- Contact the school you want to attend for more information on what help they offer.

Chapter 29 | Understanding Your Child's Right to Special Education Services

Chapter Contents
Section 29.1—Section 504 299
Section 29.2—The Individuals with Disabilities
    Education Act 303
Section 29.3—Every Student Succeeds Act 307

Section 29.1 | **Section 504**

This section contains text excerpted from the following sources: Text beginning with the heading "Discrimination on the Basis of Disability" is excerpted from "Discrimination on the Basis of Disability," U.S. Department of Health and Human Services (HHS), June 8, 2020; Text under the heading "What Is Section 504, and How Does It Relate to Section 508?" is excerpted from "What Is Section 504 and How Does It Relate to Section 508?" U.S. Department of Health and Human Services (HHS), August 19, 2015. Reviewed November 2022.

DISCRIMINATION ON THE BASIS OF DISABILITY

This is a list and an explanation of the laws and regulations the Office for Civil Rights (OCR) enforces related to discrimination on disability. The target audience is individuals and advocates. As they apply to entities under the jurisdiction of the OCR enforces:

- Section 504 of the Rehabilitation Act of 1973 includes programs and activities that are conducted by the U.S. Department of Health and Human Services (HHS) or receiving federal financial assistance from the HHS.
- Section 508 of the Rehabilitation Act of 1973 covers access to electronic and information technology provided by the HHS.
- Title II of the Americans with Disabilities Act (ADA) of 1990 covers all health-care and social services programs and activities of public entities.
- Section 1557 of the Patient Protection and Affordable Care Act (ACA) ensures that an individual is not excluded from participating in, denied benefits because of, or subjected to discrimination as prohibited under Section 504 of the Rehabilitation Act of 1973 (disability), under any health program or activity, any part of which is receiving federal financial assistance, or any program or activity that an executive agency administers or any entity established under Title I of the ACA or its amendments.

RIGHTS AND RESPONSIBILITIES UNDER SECTION 504 AND THE AMERICANS WITH DISABILITIES ACT

Section 504 and the ADA protect qualified individuals with disabilities from discrimination based on disability in providing benefits and services. Covered entities must not, based on disability:

- Exclude a person with a disability from a program or activity.
- Deny a person with a disability the benefits of a program or activity.
- Afford a person with a disability an opportunity to participate in or benefit from a benefit or service that is not equal to what is afforded to others.
- Provide a benefit or service to a person with a disability that is not as effective as what is provided to others.
- Provide different or separate benefits or services to a person with a disability unless necessary to provide benefits or services that are as effective as what is provided to others.
- Apply eligibility criteria that tend to screen out persons with disabilities unless necessary for the provision of the service, program, or activity.

Covered entities must:

- Provide services and programs in the most integrated setting appropriate to the needs of the qualified individual with a disability.
- Ensure that programs, services, activities, and facilities are accessible.
- Make reasonable modifications in their policies, practices, and procedures to avoid discrimination based on disability unless it would result in a fundamental alteration of the program.
- Provide auxiliary aids to persons with disabilities, at no additional cost, where necessary to afford an equal opportunity to participate in or benefit from a program or activity.
- Designate a responsible employee to coordinate their efforts to comply with Section 504 and the ADA.

- Adopt grievance procedures to handle complaints of disability discrimination in their programs and activities.
- Provide notice that indicates:
  - That the covered entity does not discriminate based on disability
  - How to contact the employee who coordinates the covered entity's efforts to comply with the law
  - Information about the grievance procedures

SECTION 508 OF THE REHABILITATION ACT

Section 508 requires that any electronic and information technology used, maintained, developed, or procured by the federal government allow persons with disabilities comparable access to information and technology. This applies to persons with disabilities who use assistive technology to read and navigate electronic materials.

WHAT IS SECTION 504, AND HOW DOES IT RELATE TO SECTION 508?

Responsibilities under Sections 504 and 508 can overlap. Both statutes impose different but somewhat related obligations on the HHS's operating divisions (OPDIVs) and staff divisions (STAFFDIVs) that are intended to protect individuals with disabilities from discrimination based on their disabilities. Agencies must comply with both provisions when they distribute information.

Section 508 requires federal agencies to ensure that persons with disabilities (employees and public members) have comparable access to and use electronic information technology. Any electronic and information technology used, maintained, developed, or procured by the HHS must be accessible to persons with disabilities.

Section 504 requires agencies to provide individuals with disabilities an equal opportunity to participate in their programs and benefit from their services, including providing information to employees and public members. Agencies must provide appropriate auxiliary aids where necessary to ensure equal opportunity. Types of auxiliary aids may include Braille or large print versions of materials, electronic diskettes, audiotapes, qualified interpreters or readers, telecommunications devices for deaf persons (TDDs), captioning of video, and other methods of making information available and accessible to persons with disabilities. In considering what type of auxiliary aid to provide, agencies must give primary consideration to the request of the individual with a disability and shall honor that request unless it can demonstrate that another effective means of communication exists.

What Does This Mean for Managing Websites?

Agencies must ensure that all published electronic information is compatible with assistive technology devices commonly used by people with disabilities for information and communication. This applies to persons with disabilities who use assistive technology to read and navigate electronic materials. If an electronic publication cannot be compliant, then OPDIVs/STAFFDIVs must provide a reasonable alternative to the document.

An agency may, in some instances, be able to meet its Section 504 obligation to provide equal opportunity to persons with disabilities and ensure effective communication by making information available in a Section-508-compliant form on its external-facing website or intranet(s). However, in other cases, to meet its Section 504 obligation, an agency may need to provide appropriate auxiliary aid to an individual with a disability, regardless of whether the information on its website meets accessibility requirements under Section 508.

The following are examples of situations where an agency would be required to provide information to a person with disabilities in an alternate format:

- A person who is blind requests an audio or Braille version of a publicly available report posted on an agency's Section-508-compliant website. If necessary, to provide the person equal access to the information, the agency must provide the report in an alternate format, such as an audio file or Braille.
- A person with a manual impairment that limits her or his ability to effectively use a computer requests

an agency to provide web-based information about seasonal influenza in print. If a printed version of the information is necessary for the person to have equal access to the information, the agency must provide the information in print.

Section 29.2 | The Individuals with Disabilities Education Act

This section contains text excerpted from the following sources: Text beginning with the heading "What Is the Individuals with Disabilities Education Act?" is excerpted from "About—IDEA," U.S. Department of Education (ED), December 15, 2015. Reviewed November 2022; Text beginning with the heading "Individuals with Disabilities Education Act (IDEA) Services" is excerpted from "Individuals with Disabilities Education Act (IDEA) Services," Centers for Disease Control and Prevention (CDC), May 2, 2022.

WHAT IS THE INDIVIDUALS WITH DISABILITIES EDUCATION ACT?

The Individuals with Disabilities Education Act (IDEA) is a law that makes available free appropriate public education to eligible children with disabilities throughout the nation and ensures special education and related services to those children.

The IDEA governs how states and public agencies provide early intervention, special education, and related services to more than 7.5 million (as of the school year 2018–2019) eligible infants, toddlers, children, and youth with disabilities.

Infants and toddlers, from birth through age two, with disabilities and their families receive early intervention services under IDEA Part C. Children and youth aged 3–21 receive special education and related services under IDEA Part B.

Additionally, the IDEA authorizes:
- **Formula grants** to states to support special education and related services and early intervention services
- **Discretionary grants** to state educational agencies, institutions of higher education, and other nonprofit organizations to support research, demonstrations, technical assistance and dissemination, technology development, personnel preparation and development, and parent training and information centers

Congress reauthorized the IDEA in 2004 and most recently amended the IDEA through Public Law 114–95, the Every Student Succeeds Act (ESSA), in December 2015.

In the law, Congress states:
- Disability is a natural part of the human experience and in no way diminishes the right of individuals to participate in or contribute to society. Improving educational results for children with disabilities is an essential element of our national policy of ensuring equality of opportunity, full participation, independent living, and economic self-sufficiency for individuals with disabilities.

WHAT IS THE PURPOSE OF THE INDIVIDUALS WITH DISABILITIES EDUCATION ACT?

The stated purpose of the IDEA is:
- To ensure that all children with disabilities have available to them a free appropriate public education that emphasizes special education and related services designed to meet their unique needs and prepare them for further education, employment, and independent living.
- To ensure that the rights of children with disabilities and parents of such children are protected.
- To assist states, localities, educational service agencies, and federal agencies in providing for the education of all children with disabilities.
- To assist states in the implementation of a statewide, comprehensive, coordinated, multidisciplinary, interagency system of early intervention services for infants and toddlers with disabilities and their families.
- To ensure that educators and parents have the necessary tools to improve educational results for children with disabilities by supporting system improvement activities; coordinated research and personnel preparation; coordinated technical

assistance, dissemination, and support; and technology development and media services.
- To assess and ensure the effectiveness of efforts to educate children with disabilities.

HISTORY OF THE INDIVIDUALS WITH DISABILITIES EDUCATION ACT

On November 29, 1975, President Gerald Ford signed into law the Education for All Handicapped Children Act (EHA; Public Law 94-142), now known as the IDEA. In adopting this landmark civil rights measure, Congress opened public school doors for millions of children with disabilities and laid the foundation of the country's commitment to ensuring that children with disabilities have opportunities to develop their talents, share their gifts, and contribute to their communities.

The law guaranteed access to a free appropriate public education (FAPE) in the least restrictive environment (LRE) to every child with a disability. Subsequent amendments, as reflected in the IDEA, have led to an increased emphasis on access to the general education curriculum, the provision of services for young children from birth through five, transition planning, and accountability for the achievement of students with disabilities. The IDEA upholds and protects the rights of infants, toddlers, children, and youth with disabilities and their families.

In the past 40+ years, IDEA has advanced our expectations for all children, including children with disabilities. Classrooms have become more inclusive, and the future of children with disabilities is brighter. Significant progress has been made toward protecting the rights of, meeting the individual needs of, and improving educational results and outcomes for infants, toddlers, children, and youths with disabilities.

Since 1975, IDEA has progressed from excluding nearly 1.8 million children with disabilities from public schools to providing special education and related services designed to meet their individual needs to more than 7.5 million children with disabilities in 2018–2019.

In 2018–2019, more than 64 percent of children with disabilities were in general education classrooms 80 percent or more of their school day (IDEA Part B Child Count and Educational Environments Collection), and early intervention services were being provided to more than 400,000 infants and toddlers with disabilities and their families (IDEA Part C Child Count and Settings).

INDIVIDUALS WITH DISABILITIES EDUCATION ACT SERVICES

Both early intervention and school-aged services are available through our nation's special education law—the IDEA. Part C of IDEA deals with early intervention services (birth through 36 months of age), while Part B applies to services for school-aged children (3–21 years of age). Even if your child has not been diagnosed with cerebral palsy (CP), she or he may be eligible for IDEA services.

PART C OF THE INDIVIDUALS WITH DISABILITIES EDUCATION ACT: EARLY INTERVENTION FOR BABIES AND TODDLERS

Early intervention services can help children from birth through 36 months of age learn new skills, whether they have been identified with motor and movement delays or already have a CP diagnosis. Early intervention services can start even before a CP diagnosis is made.

Depending on the child's needs, early intervention services might include family training, counseling, and home visits; occupational, physical, or speech therapy; hearing loss services; health, nutrition, social work, and assistance with service coordination; assistive technology devices and services; and transportation.

Before Part C services start, an Individual Family Service Plan (IFSP) is developed by a team, which includes the parents and all providers who work with the child and the family. The IFSP describes the child's present level of development, the family's strengths and needs, the specific services to be provided to the child and the family, and a plan to transition to public school.

PART B OF THE INDIVIDUALS WITH DISABILITIES EDUCATION ACT: SERVICES FOR SCHOOL-AGED CHILDREN

Services for school-aged children with developmental disabilities (3–21 years of age) are provided free of charge through the public school system. Among the services covered under IDEA are special education; related services such as physical, occupational, and speech therapy; and supplementary aids and services, such as adaptive equipment or special communication systems.

Before Part B services start, an Individualized Education Plan (IEP) is developed for children 3–21 years of age who qualify for special education services from school districts. An IEP is similar to an IFSP but more focused on the child's goals rather than on the family's goals.

Section 29.3 | Every Student Succeeds Act

This section contains text excerpted from the following sources: Text under the heading "What Is the Every Student Succeeds Act?" is excerpted from "What Is the Every Student Succeeds Act?" U.S. Department of Education (ED), October 28, 2020; Text beginning with the heading "A New Education Law" is excerpted from "Every Student Succeeds Act (ESSA)," U.S. Department of Education (ED), June 23, 2022.

WHAT IS THE EVERY STUDENT SUCCEEDS ACT?

The Every Student Succeeds Act (ESSA) is the federal K-12 education law of the United States. ESSA was signed into law in 2015 and replaced the previous education law called "No Child Left Behind" (NCLB). The ESSA extended more flexibility to states in education and laid out expectations of transparency for parents and for communities.

The ESSA requires every state to measure performance in reading, math, and science. Each state determines the way students are assessed. Every school in each state must inform parents about their standards and their results. It requires every state to develop a concise and easily understandable "state report card" that is accessible online and provides parents with important information on test performance in reading, math, and science. The report cards must also provide data on graduation rates, suspensions, absenteeism, teacher qualifications, and many other areas. It increases transparency to empower parents with information to help them make the best choices for their children. For the first time ever, states are required to report how much money, on average, they spend per student. This is called "per pupil expenditures." The ESSA also requires states to list their lowest-performing five percent of schools. These schools require "comprehensive support and improvement."

The ESSA extends flexibility for funds to be invested in career and technical education and even toward transportation for students to attend higher-performing schools.

A NEW EDUCATION LAW

Then the ESSA was signed by President Obama on December 10, 2015, and represents good news for our nation's schools. This bipartisan measure reauthorizes the 50-year-old Elementary and Secondary Education Act (ESEA), the nation's national education law and long-standing commitment to equal opportunity for all students.

The new law builds on key areas of progress in recent years, made possible by the efforts of educators, communities, parents, and students across the country.

For example, nowadays, high school graduation rates are at all-time highs. Dropout rates are at historic lows. And more students are going to college than ever before. These achievements provide a firm foundation for further work to expand educational opportunities and improve student outcomes under the ESSA.

The previous version of the law, the NCLB Act, was enacted in 2002. The NCLB represented a significant step forward for our nation's children in many respects, particularly as it shined a light on where students were making progress and where they needed additional support, regardless of race, income, zip code, disability, home language, or background. The law was scheduled for revision in 2007, and over time, the NCLB's prescriptive requirements became increasingly unworkable for schools and educators. Recognizing this fact, in 2010, the Obama administration joined a call from educators and families to create a better law that focused on the clear goal of fully preparing all students for success in college and careers. Congress has now responded to that call. The ESSA reflects many of the priorities of this administration.

HIGHLIGHTS OF THE EVERY STUDENT SUCCEEDS ACT
President Obama signed the ESSA into law on December 10, 2015.
  The ESSA includes provisions that will help ensure success for students and schools. Below are just a few. The law:
- Advances equity by upholding critical protections for America's disadvantaged and high-need students.
- Requires—for the first time—that all students in America be taught to high academic standards that will prepare them to succeed in college and careers.
- Ensures that vital information is provided to educators, families, students, and communities through annual statewide assessments that measure students' progress toward those high standards.
- Helps support and grow local innovations—including evidence- and place-based interventions developed by local leaders and educators—consistent with our investment in innovation and promised neighborhoods.
- Sustains and expands this administration's historic investments in increasing access to high-quality preschool.
- Maintains an expectation that there will be accountability and action to effect positive change in our lowest-performing schools, where groups of students are not making progress and where graduation rates are low over extended periods of time.

HISTORY OF THE ELEMENTARY AND SECONDARY EDUCATION ACT
The ESEA was signed into law in 1965 by President Lyndon Baines Johnson, who believed that "full educational opportunity" should be "our first national goal." From its inception, the ESEA was a civil rights law.

The ESEA offered new grants to districts serving low-income students, federal grants for textbooks and library books, funding for special education centers, and scholarships for low-income college students. Additionally, the law provided federal grants to state educational agencies to improve the quality of elementary and secondary education.

NO CHILD LEFT BEHIND ACT AND ACCOUNTABILITY

The NCLB put in place measures that exposed achievement gaps among traditionally underserved students and their peers and spurred an important national dialogue on education improvement. This focus on accountability has been critical in ensuring a quality education for all children, yet it also revealed challenges in the effective implementation of this goal.

Parents, educators, and elected officials across the country recognized that a strong, updated law was necessary to expand opportunity to all students; support schools, teachers, and principals; and strengthen our education system and economy.

In 2012, the Obama administration began granting flexibility to states regarding specific requirements of the NCLB in exchange for rigorous and comprehensive state-developed plans designed to close achievement gaps, increase equity, improve the quality of instruction, and increase outcomes for all students.

Chapter 30 | Individualized Education Programs

WHAT IS AN INDIVIDUALIZED EDUCATION PROGRAM?
An individualized education program (IEP) is a written statement of the educational program designed to meet a child's individual needs. Every child who receives special education services must have an IEP. That is why the process of developing this vital document is of great interest and importance to educators, administrators, and families alike.

WHAT IS THE INDIVIDUALIZED EDUCATION PROGRAM'S PURPOSE?
The IEP has two general purposes:
- To set reasonable learning goals for a child.
- To state the services that the school district will provide for the child.

WHO DEVELOPS THE INDIVIDUALIZED EDUCATION PROGRAM?
The IEP is developed by a team of individuals that includes key school staff and the child's parents. The team meets, reviews the assessment information available about the child, and designs an educational program to address the child's educational needs that result from her or his disability.

This chapter includes text excerpted from "The Short-and-Sweet IEP Overview," Center for Parent Information & Resources (CPIR), U.S. Department of Education (ED), April 2022.

WHEN WAS THE INDIVIDUALIZED EDUCATION PROGRAM DEVELOPED?

An IEP meeting must be held within 30 calendar days after it is determined, through a full and individual evaluation, that a child has one of the disabilities listed in the Individuals with Disabilities Education Act (IDEA) and needs special education and related services. A child's IEP must also be reviewed annually to determine whether the annual goals are being achieved and must be revised as appropriate.

WHAT IS IN AN INDIVIDUALIZED EDUCATION PROGRAM?

Each child's IEP must contain specific information, as listed within the IDEA, our nation's special education law. This includes (but is not limited to):

- The child's present levels of academic achievement and functional performance, describing how the child is currently doing in school and how the child's disability affects her or his involvement and progress in the general curriculum
- Annual goals for the child, meaning what parents and the school team think she or he can reasonably accomplish in a year
- The special education and related services to be provided to the child, including supplementary aids and services (such as a communication device) and changes to the program or support for school personnel
- How much of the school day the child will be educated separately from nondisabled children or not participate in extracurricular or other nonacademic activities such as lunch or clubs
- How (and if) the child is to participate in state- and district-wide assessments, including what modifications to tests the child needs
- When services and modifications will begin, how often they will be provided, where they will be provided, and how long they will last
- How school personnel will measure the child's progress toward the annual goals

Individualized Education Programs

CAN STUDENTS BE INVOLVED IN DEVELOPING THEIR OWN INDIVIDUALIZED EDUCATION PROGRAMS?

Yes, they certainly can be! IDEA requires that the student be invited to any IEP meeting where transition services will be discussed. These are services designed to help the student plan for her or his transition to adulthood and life after high school.

Chapter 31 | Supports, Modifications, and Accommodations for Students with Disabilities

For many students with disabilities—and many without—the key to success in the classroom lies in having appropriate adaptations, accommodations, and modifications made to the instruction and other classroom activities.

Some adaptations are as simple as moving a distractible student to the front of the class or away from the pencil sharpener or the window. Other modifications may involve changing how the material is presented or how students respond to show their learning.

Adaptations, accommodations, and modifications need to be individualized for students oriented on their needs and personal learning styles and interests. It is not always obvious what adaptations, accommodations, or modifications would benefit a particular student or how changes to the curriculum, its presentation, the classroom setting, or student evaluation might be made. This chapter is intended to help teachers and others find information that can guide them in making appropriate changes in the classroom oriented on what their students need.

This chapter includes text excerpted from "Supports, Modifications, and Accommodations for Students," Center for Parent Information & Resources (CPIR), U.S. Department of Education (ED), March 1, 2020.

A QUICK LOOK AT TERMINOLOGY
You might wonder if the terms support, modifications, and adaptations all mean the same thing. The simple answer is: no, not completely, but yes for the most part. To be sure, people tend to use the terms interchangeably, and it will be done here, for ease of reading, but distinctions can be made between the terms.

Sometimes, people get confused about what it means to have a modification and what it means to have an accommodation. Usually, a modification means a change in what is being taught or expected from the student. Making an assignment easier, so the student is not doing the same work as other students, is an example of a modification.

An accommodation is a change that helps a student overcome or work around the disability. Allowing a student who has trouble writing to give her or his answers orally is an example of an accommodation. This student is still expected to know the same material and answer the same questions as fully as the other students, but she or he does not have to write her or his answers to show that she or he knows the information.

What is most important to know about modifications and accommodations is that both are meant to help a child learn.

DIFFERENT TYPES OF SUPPORTS
Special Education
Special education is "specially designed instruction." And the Individuals with Disabilities Education Act (IDEA) defines it as follows:
- Specially designed instruction means adapting, as appropriate to the needs of an eligible child under this part, the content, methodology, or delivery of instruction:
  - To address the unique needs of the child that result from the child's disability.
  - To ensure access of the child to the general curriculum so that the child can meet the educational standards within the jurisdiction of the public agency that apply to all children.

Supports, Modifications, and Accommodations for Students with Disabilities

Thus, special education involves adapting the "content, methodology, or delivery of instruction." The special education field can take pride in the knowledge base and expertise it is developed in the past 30+ years of individualizing instruction to meet the needs of students with disabilities. It is a pleasure to share some of that knowledge with you now.

Adapting Instruction

Sometimes, a student may need to change class work or routines because of her or his disability. Modifications can be made to:
- What a child is taught
- How a child works at school

Modifications or accommodations are most often made in the following areas:
- **Scheduling**. For example:
  - Giving the student extra time to complete assignments or tests.
  - Breaking up testing over several days.
- **Setting**. For example:
  - Working in a small group.
  - Working one-on-one with the teacher.
- **Materials**. For example:
  - Providing audiotaped lectures or books.
  - Giving copies of the teacher's lecture notes.
  - Using large print books, Braille, or books on compact disc (CD—digital text).
- **Instruction**. For example:
  - Reducing the difficulty of assignments.
  - Reducing the reading level.
  - Using a student/peer tutor.
- **Student response**. For example:
  - Allowing answers to be given orally or dictated.
  - Using a word processor for written work.
  - Using sign language, a communication device, Braille, or a native language if it is not English.

Because adapting the content, methodology, and/or delivery of instruction is an essential element in special education and extremely valuable support for students, it is equally essential to know as much as possible about how instruction can be adapted to address the needs of an individual student with a disability. The special education teacher who serves on the individualized education program (IEP) team can contribute her or his expertise in this area, which is the essence of special education.

Related Services

A look at the IDEA's definition of related services at §300.34 makes it clear that these services are supportive in nature although not in the same way that adapting the curriculum is. Related services support children's special education and are provided when necessary to help students benefit from special education. Thus, related services must be included in the treasure chest of accommodations and support exploring. The definition begins:

- **General**. Related services mean transportation and such developmental, corrective, and other supportive services as are required to assist a child with a disability to benefit from special education.

Here is the list of related services in the law:
- Speech-language pathology and audiology services
- Interpreting services
- Psychological services
- Physical and occupational therapy
- Recreation, including therapeutic recreation
- Early identification and assessment of disabilities in children
- Counseling services, including rehabilitation counseling
- Orientation and mobility services
- Medical services for diagnostic or evaluation purposes
- School health services and school nurse services
- Social work services in schools

Supports, Modifications, and Accommodations for Students with Disabilities

This is not an exhaustive list of possible related services. There are others (not named here or in the law) that states and schools routinely make available under the umbrella of related services. The IEP team decides which related services a child needs and the specificities of the child's IEP.

Supplementary Aids and Services
One of the most powerful types of support available to children with disabilities is the other kinds of support or services (other than special education and related services) that a child needs to be educated with nondisabled children to the maximum extent appropriate. Some examples of these additional services and supports, called "supplementary aids and services" in the IDEA, are as follows:
- Adapted equipment, such as a special seat or a cutout cup for drinking
- Assistive technology, such as a word processor, special software, or a communication system
- Training for staff, students, and/or parents
- Peer tutors
- A one-on-one aide
- Adapted materials, such as books on tape, large print, or highlighted notes
- Collaboration/consultation among staff, parents, and/or other professionals

The IEP team, which includes the parents, is the group that decides which supplementary aids and services a child needs to support her or his access to and participation in the school environment. The IEP team must work together to ensure that a child gets the supplementary aids and services that she or he needs to succeed. Team members talk about the child's needs, the curriculum, and school routine and openly explore all options to ensure the right supports for the specific child are included.

Program Modifications and Supports for School Staff
If the IEP team decides that a child needs a particular modification or accommodation, this information must be included in the IEP.

Supports are also available for those who work with the child to help them help that child be successful. Support for school staff must also be written into the IEP. Some of these supports might include:
- Attending a conference or training related to the child's needs.
- Getting help from another staff member or administrative person.
- Having an aide in the classroom.
- Getting special equipment or teaching materials.

Accommodations in Large Assessments
The IDEA requires that students with disabilities take part in state- or district-wide assessments. These are tests that are periodically given to all students to measure achievement. It is one way that schools determine how well and how much students learn. The IDEA now states that students with disabilities should have as much involvement in the general curriculum as possible. This means that if a child receives instruction in the general curriculum, she or he could take the same standardized test that the school district or state gives to nondisabled children. Accordingly, a child's IEP must include all modifications or accommodations that the child needs to participate in state- or district-wide assessments.

The IEP team can decide that a particular test is inappropriate for a child. In this case, the IEP must include the following:
- An explanation of why that test is not suitable for the child
- How the child will be assessed instead (often called "alternate assessment")

Ask your state and/or local school district for a copy of their guidelines on the types of accommodations, modifications, and alternate assessments available to students.

This concludes that even a child with many needs must be involved with nondisabled peers to the maximum extent appropriate. Just because a child has severe disabilities or needs modifications to the general curriculum does not mean that she or he may

Supports, Modifications, and Accommodations for Students with Disabilities

be removed from the general education class. If a child is removed from the general education class for any part of the school day, the IEP team must include in the IEP an explanation for the child's nonparticipation.

Because accommodations can be so vital to helping children with disabilities access the general curriculum, participate in school (including extracurricular and nonacademic activities), and be educated alongside their peers without disabilities, IDEA reinforces their use again and again, in its requirements, definitions, and principles.

Chapter 32 | Specialized Teaching Techniques

Chapter Contents
Section 32.1—Differentiated Instruction 325
Section 32.2—Speech-Language Therapy 329

Section 32.1 | Differentiated Instruction

This section includes text excerpted from "Teal Center Fact Sheet No. 5: Differentiated Instruction," Literacy Information and Communication System (LINCS), October 14, 2015. Reviewed November 2022.

Differentiated instruction is an approach that enables instructors to plan strategically to meet the needs of every learner. It is rooted in the belief that there is variability among any group of learners and that instructors should adjust instruction accordingly. The approach encompasses the planning and delivery of instruction, classroom management techniques, and expectations of learners' performance that consider the diversity and varying levels of readiness, interests, and learning profiles of the learners.

Differentiated instruction can be looked at as an instructor's response to learner differences by adapting curriculum and instruction on six dimensions, including:
- How the instructor approaches:
  - Content (the what of the lesson)
  - Process (the how of the lesson)
  - Expected product (the learner-produced result)
- How the instructor takes into consideration the learner's:
  - Interest
  - Profile (learning strengths, weaknesses, and gaps)
  - Readiness

These adaptations can be planned to happen simultaneously, in sequence, or as needed depending on the circumstance and goals of instruction. Teaching small groups of learners, groups oriented on instructional approach and learner profile, is a cornerstone of differentiated instruction.

HOW DOES IT WORK IN ADULT EDUCATION?

Here is an example. An instructor who is teaching writing (the content) in an adult basic education (ABE) class needs to understand the various learners' readiness to write independently or collaboratively, the supports they might need to engage in the process oriented on their learning profiles, the quality and quantity of the learner product to be expected, and the learners' interests. This understanding will come from professional observation of the learners over time; some will come from informal assessments gathered from previous writing assignments.

Planning is critical. For instance, knowing that some learners need templates, prompts, or advance organizers to prepare them to write or software to assist them with spelling means that the necessary supports, such as the use of the computer lab with concept-mapping software and word processors, need to be planned for in advance. Perhaps a colleague with more experience with a particular level or type of learner can collaborate, or the team teaches a small group to better meet their needs. Perhaps a more advanced peer learner can run a small group or provide technical assistance.

An instructor teaching persuasive essays (the content) may begin with a study of various models, such as op-ed pieces from the local newspaper, to identify the elements of such an essay. The class may spend time brainstorming to elicit learners' interests in various "hot topics" of the day while creating lists of vocabulary to support composition. Deciding on a couple of key topics, learners may be grouped to continue to generate possible argument points. A scribe in the group can generate a web or advance organizer that captures the discussion. Learners can then be regrouped according to the level of support they need (their profile and readiness) for composition (the process).

Those who can compose on their own can work independently or in dyads to conduct further research on the Internet to provide evidence for their argument; those who need technical support can work in the computer lab with the instructor and an advanced peer, possibly with a precreated outline or template; and those who cannot compose on their own can work in a smaller group with a tutor or the instructor to generate a group essay that learners can each then work on for editing and revising. Conferencing with each learner can be another opportunity to accommodate learners' readiness by focusing only on the mechanics, grammar,

Specialized Teaching Techniques

or organizational elements the writer can master. Final products can be shared in various ways: published by the learners on a blog or submitted to a newspaper, posted in the classroom, read to the class, and so on. The essays, and the products, which result from the group, will vary in complexity and sophistication. Yet all learners will have engaged in a persuasive essay's process and basic key elements (brainstorming, planning, outlining, composing, editing, revising, and sharing).

HOW CAN TECHNOLOGY HELP?

Technology tools can help make this coordination more efficient by providing productivity support for instructors, providing support for learners at varying readiness levels, and offering learners options for demonstrating their understanding and mastery of the material.

Managing Differentiated Instruction

Classroom management to coordinate flexible groupings and projects is a key component of differentiated instruction. Here are some ideas for creating and coordinating groups in a multilevel, differentiated class:
- Set up stations in the classroom where different learning groups can work simultaneously. Such stations naturally invite flexible grouping.
  - Encourage peer-to-peer learning and mentoring and help learners learn to be tutors.
  - Ask volunteers to lead small-group instruction stations.
- Structure problem-based learning (PBL) to have learners actively solve problems, either individually or in small groups.
  - Use WebQuests (webquest.org/index.php) as PBL for teams of learners; these inquiry-based projects are prearranged, and many have teaching supports (lesson plans, tips, handouts, and additional materials) linked to them.

- Share reflections with other instructors leading problem-based learning at www.Edutopia.org.
- Assign tiered activities to allow learners to work on the same concepts but with varying complexity.
  - Find texts on a single, encompassing topic (i.e., climate change) in various levels of complexity and readability.
  - Encourage learners to find audiobooks and digital text at their interest level rather than their independent reading level.
- Employ compacting to assess learners' knowledge and skills before beginning a unit of study and allow learners to move to advanced work oriented on their preassessment.
  - Find ways to give credit for independent study and advancement if a learner is particularly motivated or interested in a topic.
  - Help learners supplement class instruction with online classes or learning opportunities such as webinars, online chats, blogs, social networks, or daily content blasts.
- Chunk or break assignments and activities into smaller, more manageable parts and provide more structured directions for each part.
  - Have learners make personalized lists of tasks to complete the chunks in a specified but flexible time frame.
  - Encourage self-study, especially when learners must "stop out" of regular attendance.
- Model differentiation by keeping grades and scores in a variety of ways.
  - Use portfolios to reflect on learner growth over time and encourage learners to critique their growth.
  - Keep scores and observations in a spreadsheet that can be sorted flexibly to reveal natural groups.

Specialized Teaching Techniques

Section 32.2 | Speech-Language Therapy

This section contains text excerpted from the following sources: Text begins with excerpts from "Speech-Language Therapy for Autism," Eunice Kennedy Shriver National Institute of Child Health and Human Development (NICHD), April 20, 2021; Text under the heading "What Speech-Language Pathologists Do" is excerpted from "Speech-Language Pathologists," U.S. Bureau of Labor Statistics (BLS), U.S. Department of Labor (DOL), September 28, 2022.

Speech-language therapy can help people with autism spectrum disorder (ASD) improve their abilities to communicate and interact with others.

VERBAL SKILLS

This type of therapy can help some people improve their spoken or verbal skills, such as:
- Correctly naming people and things.
- Better explaining feelings and emotions.
- Using words and sentences better.
- Improving the rate and rhythm of speech.

NONVERBAL COMMUNICATION

Speech-language therapy can also teach nonverbal communication skills, such as:
- Using hand signals or sign language.
- Using picture symbols to communicate (Picture Exchange Communication System® (PECS®)).

Speech-language therapy activities can also include ways to improve social skills and social behaviors. For example, a child might learn how to make eye contact or stand at a comfortable distance from another person. These skills make it a little easier to interact with others.

WHAT SPEECH-LANGUAGE PATHOLOGISTS DO

Speech-language pathologists (called "speech therapists") assess, diagnose, treat, and help prevent communication and swallowing disorders in children and adults. Speech, language, and swallowing disorders result from various causes, such as a stroke, brain injury, hearing loss, developmental delay, Parkinson disease (PD), a cleft palate, or autism.

Duties
Speech-language pathologists typically do the following:
- Evaluate levels of speech, language, or swallowing difficulty.
- Identify treatment options.
- Create and carry out an individualized treatment plan that addresses specific functional needs.
- Teach children and adults how to make sounds and improve their voices and maintain fluency.
- Help individuals improve vocabulary and sentence structure used in oral and written language.
- Work with children and adults to develop and strengthen the muscles used to swallow.
- Counsel individuals and families on how to cope with communication and swallowing disorders.

Speech-language pathologists work with children and adults with speech and language problems, including related cognitive or social communication problems. They may be unable to speak at all, speak with difficulty, or have rhythm and fluency problems, such as stuttering. Speech-language pathologists may work with people who are unable to understand language or with those who have voice disorders, such as inappropriate pitch or a harsh voice.

Speech-language pathologists must also complete administrative tasks, including keeping accurate records and documenting billing information. They record their initial evaluations and diagnoses, track treatment progress, and note changes in an individual's condition or treatment plan.

Some speech-language pathologists work with specific age groups, such as children or the elderly. Others focus on treatment programs for specific communication or swallowing problems, such as strokes, trauma, or a cleft palate.

Specialized Teaching Techniques

In medical facilities, speech-language pathologists work with physicians, surgeons, social workers, psychologists, occupational therapists, physical therapists, and other health-care workers. Schools evaluate students for speech and language disorders and work with teachers, other school personnel, and parents to develop and carry out individual or group programs, provide counseling, and support classroom activities.

Chapter 33 | Coping with School-Related Challenges

Chapter Contents
Section 33.1—Building a Good Relationship with
  Your Child's Teacher 335
Section 33.2—Parental Involvement in Child's Success
  in School and Life 339

Section 33.1 | Building a Good Relationship with Your Child's Teacher

This section includes text excerpted from "Working with Teachers and Schools—Helping Your Child Succeed in School," U.S. Department of Education (ED), September 1, 2003. Reviewed November 2022.

Many teachers say they do not often receive information from parents about problems at home. Many parents say they do not know what the school expects from their children. Sharing information is essential, and teachers and parents are responsible for making it happen.

TALKING TO YOUR CHILD'S TEACHER

The following questions and answers can help you get the most out of talking to your child's teacher or other school staff members.

What Do You Do First?

Learn everything that you can about your child's school. The more you know, the easier your job as a parent will be. Ask for a school handbook. This will answer many questions that will arise over the year. If your school does not have a handbook, ask questions. Ask the principal and teachers: What classes does the school offer? Which classes are required? What are your expectations for your child? How does the school measure student progress? Does it meet state standards? What are the school's rules and regulations?

Ask about specific teaching methods and materials—are the methods oriented on evidence about what works best in teaching reading or math? Are the science and history textbooks up to date?

Ask if the school has a website and, if so, get the address. School websites can provide you with reading access to all kinds of information—schedules of events, names of people to contact, rules and regulations, and so forth.

Keep informed throughout the school year. If your schedule permits, attend parent–teacher association (PTA) or parent–teacher organization (PTO) meetings. If you cannot attend, ask that the minutes of the meetings be sent to you. Or find out if the school makes these minutes available on its website.

When Should You Talk with Your Child's Teacher?

Early and often. Contact your child's teacher or teachers at the beginning of the year or as soon as possible. Get acquainted and show your interest.

Tell teachers what they need to know about your child. If she or he has special needs, make these known from the beginning.

Contact the teacher immediately if you notice a big change in your child's behavior, school performance, or attitude during the school year.

Report cards indicate how well your child is doing in school. But you also need to know how things are going between report cards. For example, if your child is having trouble in math, contact the teacher to find out when he has his next math test and when it will be returned to him. This allows you to address a problem before it mushrooms into something bigger. Call the teacher if your child does not understand an assignment or if she or he needs extra help to complete an assignment. You may also want to know if your child's teachers use e-mail to communicate with parents. Using e-mail will allow you to send and receive messages at times that are most convenient for you.

What If Your Child Has a Problem with Homework or Does Not Understand What Is Happening in Class?

Contact the teacher as soon as you suspect your child has trouble with her or his schoolwork. Schools are responsible for keeping you informed about your child's performance and behavior, and you have a right to be upset if you do not find out until report card time that your child is having difficulties. On the other hand, you may figure out that a problem exists before the teacher does. By alerting the teacher, you can work together to solve a problem in its early stages.

Request a meeting with the teacher to discuss problems. Tell her or him briefly why you want to meet. If English is your second

Coping with School-Related Challenges

language, you may need to make special arrangements, such as including in the meeting someone bilingual.

Approach the teacher with a cooperative spirit. Believe that the teacher wants to help you and your child, even if you disagree about something. Do not go to the principal without first giving the teacher a chance to work out the problem with you and your child.

How Do You Get the Most out of Parent–Teacher Conferences?

Be prepared to listen as well as to talk. It helps if you write down questions before you leave home. Also, jot down what you want to tell the teacher. Be prepared to take notes during the conference and ask for an explanation if you do not understand something.

The teacher should offer specific details about your child's work and progress in conferences. If your child has already received some grades, ask how your child is being evaluated.

Talk about your child's talents, skills, hobbies, study habits, and any special sensitivities, such as concern about weight or speech difficulties.

Tell the teacher if you think your child needs special help and about any special family situation or event that might affect your child's ability to learn. Mention a new baby, an illness, or a recent or upcoming move. Ask about specific ways to help your child at home. Try to have an open mind.

At home, think about what the teacher said and follow up. If the teacher has told you that your child needs to improve in certain areas, check back in a few weeks to see how things are going.

What If You Do Not Agree with a School Rule or Teacher's Assignments?

First, do not argue with the teacher in front of your child. Set up a meeting to talk about the issue. Before the meeting, plan what you will say—why you think a rule is unfair or what you do not like about an assignment. Get your facts straight and do not rely on anger to win your argument. Try to be positive and remain calm. Listen carefully.

If the teacher's explanation does not satisfy you, arrange to talk with the principal or the school superintendent. Do not feel intimidated by titles or personalities. An educator's primary responsibility is to ensure the success of each and every student in her or his classroom, school, or district.

What Is the Best Way for You to Stay Involved in Your Child's School Activities?

Attend school events. Go to sports events, concerts, back-to-school nights, parent–teacher meetings, and awards events, such as a "perfect attendance" breakfast.

Volunteer at your child's school. If your schedule permits, look for ways to help out at your child's school. Schools often send home lists of ways in which parents can get involved. Chaperones are needed for school trips or dances (and if your child thinks it is embarrassing to have you on the dance floor, sell soft drinks down the hall from the dance). School committees need members, and the school newsletter may need an editor. The school may have councils or advisory committees that need parent representatives. If work or other commitments make it impossible for you to volunteer in the school, look for ways to help at home. For example, you can call other parents to tell them about school-related activities or maybe help translate a school newsletter from English into another language.

What If You Do Not Have Time to Volunteer as Much as You Would Like?

Even if you cannot volunteer to do work at the school building, you can help your child learn when you are at home. The key question is, "What can you do at home, easily and in a few minutes a day, to reinforce and extend what the school is doing?" This is the involvement that every family can and must provide. The schools also need to take steps, so parents feel good about what they are doing at home and know they are helping.

Coping with School-Related Challenges

Section 33.2 | Parental Involvement in Child's Success in School and Life

This section includes text excerpted from "Intellectual Disability," Center for Parent Information & Resources (CPIR), U.S. Department of Education (ED), June 1, 2017. Reviewed November 2022.

A child with an intellectual disability can do well in school but will likely need the individualized help available as special education and related services. The level of help and support that is needed will depend upon the degree of intellectual disability involved.

- **General education.** It is important that students with intellectual disabilities be involved in, and make progress in, the general education curriculum. It is the same curriculum learned by those without disabilities. Be aware that the Individuals with Disabilities Education Act (IDEA) does not permit a student to be removed from education in age-appropriate general education classrooms solely because she or he needs modifications to be made in the general education curriculum.
- **Supplementary aids and services.** Given that intellectual disabilities affect learning, supporting students with an identity document (ID) in the classroom is often crucial. This includes making accommodations appropriate to the needs of the student. It also includes providing what the IDEA calls "supplementary aids and services." Supplementary aids and services are supports that may include instruction, personnel, equipment, or other accommodations that enable children with disabilities to be educated with nondisabled children to the maximum extent appropriate.

Thus, for families and teachers alike, it is important to know what changes and accommodations are helpful to students with intellectual disabilities. If appropriate, these need to be discussed

by the individual education program plan (IEP) team and included in the IEP.
- **Adaptive skills**. Many children with intellectual disabilities need help with adaptive skills, which are skills needed to live, work, and play in the community. Teachers and parents can help a child work on these skills at school and home. Some of these skills include:
  - Communicating with others
  - Taking care of personal needs (dressing, bathing, going to the bathroom)
  - Health and safety
  - Home living (helping to set the table, cleaning the house, or cooking dinner)
  - Social skills (manners, knowing the rules of conversation, getting along in a group, playing a game)
  - Reading, writing, and basic math
  - As they get older, skills that will help them in the workplace
- **Transition planning**. It is extremely important for families and schools to begin planning early for the student's transition into the world of adulthood. Because intellectual disability affects how quickly and well an individual learns new information and skills, the sooner transition planning begins, the more the student can do before leaving high school.

The IDEA requires that at the latest, transition planning for students with disabilities begin no later than the first IEP to be in effect when they turn 16. The IEP teams of many students with intellectual disabilities feel that it is important for these students to begin earlier than that. And they do.

TIP FOR TEACHERS
- **Recognize that you can make an enormous difference in this student's life!** Find out the student's strengths and

Coping with School-Related Challenges

interests and emphasize them. Create opportunities for success.
- **If you are not part of the student's IEP team, ask for a copy of her or his IEP**. The student's educational goals will be listed there, as well as the services and classroom accommodations she or he is to receive. As necessary, talk to others in your school (e.g., special educators). They can help you identify effective methods of teaching this student, ways to adapt the curriculum, and how to address the student's IEP goals in your classroom.
- **Be as concrete as possible**. Demonstrate what you mean rather than giving verbal directions. Rather than just relating new information verbally, show a picture. And, rather than just showing a picture, provide the student with hands-on materials and experiences and the opportunity to try things out.
- **Break longer, new tasks into small steps**. Demonstrate the steps. Have the student do the steps, one at a time. Assist, as necessary. Give the student immediate feedback.
- Teach the student life skills such as daily living, social skills, and occupational awareness and exploration, as appropriate. Involve the student in group activities or clubs.
- **Work together with the student's parents and other school personnel to create and implement an IEP tailored to meet the student's needs**. Regularly share information about how the student is doing at school and home.

TIPS FOR PARENTS
- **Learn about intellectual disability**. The more you know, the more you can help yourself and your child.
- **Be patient, be hopeful**. Your child, like every child, has a whole lifetime to learn and grow.
- **Encourage independence in your child**. For example, help your child learn daily care skills, such as dressing, feeding herself or himself, using the bathroom, and grooming.

- **Give your child chores**. Keep her or his age, attention span, and abilities in mind. Break down jobs into smaller steps. For example, if your child's job is to set the table, first ask her or him to get the right number of napkins. Then have her or him put one at each family member's place at the table. Do the same with the utensils, going one at a time. Tell her or him what to do, step by step, until the job is done. Demonstrate how to do the job. Help her or him when she or he needs assistance.
- **Give your child frequent feedback**. Praise your child when she or he does well. Build your child's abilities.

Chapter 34 | Alternative Educational Options

Chapter Contents
Section 34.1—Homeschooling 345
Section 34.2—Choosing a Tutor 353

Section 34.1 | Homeschooling

This section includes text excerpted from "Home Schooling in the United States: Trends and Characteristics," United States Census Bureau, April 16, 2022.

THE IMPACT OF HOMESCHOOLING

According to widely repeated estimates, as many as two million American children are schooled at home, growing at 15–20 percent per year. Compared with other recent changes in the educational system, such as the growth of charter schools, homeschooling has received relatively little attention. It could be argued, however, that homeschooling may have a much larger impact on the educational system in the short and long run. This is because homeschooling seems to be taking place on a larger scale than other educational innovations.

After all, homeschooling may have a greater immediate impact on educational practices in existing schools because homeschooling has brought new institutional forms that have the potential to grow over the longer term.

DATA ON HOMESCHOOLING

The National Household Education Surveys Program (NHES) are nationally representative telephone survey administered by the National Center for Education Statistics (NCES). The two surveys included homeschooling questions in 1996 and 1999. The number of children 6–17 was 16,257 in 1996 and 10,718 in 1999. In both years, the same question was asked of all children: "Some parents decide to educate their children at home rather than sending them to school. Is ... being schooled at home?"

The data sets also provide several types of information on the characteristics of homeschoolers and their families. All provide race, Hispanic ethnicity, age, and sex of children. They also provide information on the household: number of adults in the household, their education, labor force participation, and household income. In both the current population survey (CPS) and national health service (NHS), income was given in ranges. For regression analyses, these were recoded to the midpoints and differenced from the mean. The CPS provided state of residence, metropolitan status, and urban/rural location. Although it is traditional to use census-defined regions for analyses, it was felt that homeschooling might not follow traditional patterns. Dr. William H. Frey, Ph.D., population studies professor at the University of Michigan, developed a regional taxonomy that reflects the major migration patterns of recent years, and these are probably more closely related to the types of social trends that would affect homeschooling decisions. The states were recoded to regions following this migration taxonomy. An urban–rural division was developed from metropolitan and urban/rural variables in CPS. In both 1996 and 1999, the NHES asked parents of homeschoolers about their motivations for teaching their children at home. Respondents were asked to select reasons from a list of 16.

All analyses in this paper use weighted data, adjusted to reflect an assumed design effect of 2.0, except that the standard errors associated with the total number of homeschoolers were estimated using the Taylor-series linearization method available in the safety assurance system (SAS) statistical package. Specific types of analysis are described as they appear in the paper.

EXTENT AND GROWTH OF HOMESCHOOLING

Table 34.1 lists the projected number of children aged 6–17 who are homeschooled according to these data sources. Taken at face value, they show growth at face value from 360,000 in 1994 to 790,000 in 1999. Unfortunately, the point estimates from these data cannot be used directly to make such inferences. The 1994 CPS estimate of 360,000 is not much more than half the size of the 1996 NHES estimate of 640,000. This difference is statistically significant but is too large to be explained by growth in the homeschool population. Hemke et al. noted that the gap is implausibly large but could not pinpoint an explanation. A likely reason for the discrepancy is the difference in question wording between CPS and NHES.

In the CPS, the form of the homeschooling question depended on the previous answer to the question on school enrollment. If a household reported children were attending school, they were not asked directly about homeschooling but had to choose it from a

Alternative Educational Options

Table 34.1. Estimates of the Number of U.S. Children Schooled at Home: Current Population Survey and National Household Education Surveys

	Estimate	Standard Err
CPS 1994	356,000	40,000
NHES 1996	636,000	54,000
NHES 1999	791,000	62,000

list. This lower response is evident from the extremely low rate of homeschooling observed in the subset of CPS respondents who responded affirmatively to the enrollment question. In the CPS, only 190,000 children were reported in school and homeschooled. In the 1996 NHES, 450,000 children were reported this way. By contrast, people who initially indicated nonenrollment faced similar yes/no questions on homeschooling in both surveys. They were much closer in number—170,000 homeschoolers in CPS and 190,000 in the 1996 NHES.

The 1999 NHES data also seem to show growth in homeschooling. However, the growth is not quite statistically significant from 1996, given the sample size (the p value is between 0.05 and 0.10). Since the two NHES surveys are nearly identical in content and methodology, the trend oriented on these two data points provides the best estimate of growth, but the range is wide. A 95 percent confidence interval ranges from a three percent annual decline to a 15 percent annual growth.

Therefore, NHES cannot say much about the growth of the homeschooling population at the first level of analysis. However, NHES can refute some of the grander claims advocates have made. The number of homeschooled children was well under one million in 1999, and the growth rate from 1996 to 1999 was unlikely to have exceeded 15 percent per year.

CHARACTERISTICS OF HOMESCHOOLED CHILDREN

To better understand trends in homeschooling, it is helpful to know what similarities and differences exist between homeschooled children and those in regular school. If homeschoolers are currently limited to a portion of the population with distinct characteristics, it is possible that the phenomenon will be self-contained. On the other hand, if those characteristics are becoming more prevalent in the population, then homeschooling might grow along with the group in which it is found.

Homeschoolers are like their peers in many respects. Homeschoolers are not especially likely to be young or old. They are about as likely to be of one sex or the other, with perhaps a slightly greater percentage female. In some ways, however, homeschoolers do stand out. Homeschooled children are more likely to be non-Hispanic White; they are likely to live in households headed by a married couple with moderate-to-high levels of education and income. They are likely to live in a household with an adult, not in the labor force.

Data show these relationships in a multiple regression framework. This regression cannot be interpreted as causal, as they include several factors probably endogenous to the homeschooling decision (e.g., parental work status and household income). However, the relative magnitude of different influences can be seen when taken together. Automatic model selection routines were used to develop a pared-down regression equation because some coefficients were sensitive to the inclusion or exclusion of other variables in the model. The initial set of variables included all those, along with interactions of all variables with the survey year. Two of the effects (the main effect of being Black and the effect of a father's education) were retained even though they did not meet the cutoff criterion in the selection routine because of their possible substantive importance.

Most of the same variables that showed differences across homeschool status in cross-tabulations were also significant in the regression analysis. Sex was retained as marginally significant, but age was not. Girls seem slightly more likely to be homeschooled than boys. Household variables had stronger effects—family structure, mother's education, father's education, and region of residence. The main effect of income was not significant. However, the square of income had a relatively strong effect. This indicates that the

Alternative Educational Options

families most likely to homeschool their children are of middle income—neither rich nor poor. Race and ethnicity had strong effects. Hispanics were less likely to be homeschooled, and Blacks were much less likely to be homeschooled—especially in the two earlier years under study, 1994 and 1996. Convergence between Blacks and Whites occurred from 1994 to 1999, but the effect is marginally significant. The U.S. Census Bureau will have to await new rounds of surveys to see if this is a sustained trend.

One of the strongest influences on homeschooling is having a nonworking adult in the household. The coefficient of there being a nonworking adult is large and highly significant. The cross-tabular results hinted that this relationship was diminishing across years, but the interaction with years was insignificant in the multiple regression framework. However, the main effect of nonworking remains. Sixty percent of homeschooled children have a nonworking adult in the home, compared with 30 percent of other children. If homeschooling is limited to a particular subgroup, it is probably this.

A major issue arising from the association of homeschooling with the presence of a nonworking adult is the possible limitations this presents to future growth. Although 40 percent of homeschoolers lived with working adults, at least one adult was in the labor force only part-time in most cases. Fewer than 10 percent lived with two full-time working adults. If two-parent families with a nonworking parent primarily undertake homeschooling, it could be a self-limiting phenomenon. However, even if homeschooling does remain mainly within this group, it has not come close to exhausting its constituency. Seven and one-half million two-adult households have a nonworking adult at home, and the number has remained stable in recent years despite declines in previous decades. More broadly, of 36 million women with children under 18, 10 million do not work, and another 6.5 million work part-time. Homeschooled children could grow from 790,000 to over 30 million without exhausting this core constituency.

Is it possible that homeschooling may spread beyond this core group of two-parent families with a parent at home? Must it also be limited to households where parents have moderate-to-high education? While it would seem that having a (well-educated) parent at home would be a prerequisite for engaging in homeschooling, this is not an absolute requirement. Many homeschool households have working adults and adults with low education. In all three surveys, a small number of homeschooled children lived full-time with a single parent or two adults in the labor force. In addition, a small number had no adult in the home with a high school diploma. A follow-up question in the 1999 NHES on participation in regular school by homeschoolers showed that many homeschooled children who lived with working adults also attended school at least part of the time. Still, a portion of parents remained who seemed to be defying logic by schooling their children at home without being home themselves.

Further exploration of these cases might turn up special circumstances (home businesses, odd working hours, cooperative instructional arrangements) that could explain. Alternatively, these families could use Internet courseware or other technologies to avoid the need for direct instruction. Many advice books and curricula promise home education can be successful even when parents have little time or training for the job.

DISCUSSION AND CONCLUSION

Although the evidence on characteristics of homeschoolers is still incomplete, it is important that you take account of these characteristics now rather than waiting for further data collection to provide additional detail. Homeschooling, despite being smaller and slower-growing than claimed by advocates, is still an important emerging phenomenon. What it portends for the current system of schools is still unknown.

Homeschooling has emerged with, and indeed is linked to, other emerging educational trends—online education and other systems that allow families and individuals to choose their own educational paths (school vouchers, charter schools). At the same time, it flies in the face of trends toward educational standardization, such as national curricula and systems of assessment. Another type of standardization results from establishing increasingly detailed occupational credentialing and licensure systems. These trends might

Alternative Educational Options

not be easily reconciled. High-stakes testing, especially, has come under strong attack from homeschooling groups.

The period of institutional flux now reigning in education may be derived from a breakdown in the traditional education model designed with the regimentation of instruction for students entering an industrializing world. Schools seem to have lost some legitimacy as they have lost a clear functional role in preparing youth for their role in the larger economic system. Rather than representing a definite trend toward "individualizing" instruction, however, homeschooling may represent an attempt by parents to reclaim a schooling process—to make schooling valuable in ways that are understandable to them through the cultural means at their disposal. This is not incompatible with Apple's description of homeschooling as part of "conservative modernization." Yet homeschooling may not be linked to a unified conservative agenda in quite the way he describes. There is a true tension between home educators and the school standards movement, just as there is between homeschooling and the increasing demand by employers for occupationally specific training and credentials. These movements do not have a conservative agenda in common but an attempt by each sector with interest in schooling to gain greater control over the system.

It may be that homeschoolers come to create their own new schools, as predicted by Hill. It may be that homeschoolers remain independent. In either case, however, as homeschooling grows, calls will continue for existing public schools to provide services that homeschool families cannot provide easily, such as advanced courses and extracurricular activities. A class of families will be allowed to pick and choose among school offerings. The pressures on schools that might result in an environment with increasing competition from other instructional providers are easily envisioned.

The alternative to accommodating homeschoolers would involve political difficulties. First, homeschoolers making no use of regular school facilities could not be counted on to provide political support for school funding. Second, the schools would lose an ally in fighting battles against standardization, test requirements, and credentialing, making it increasingly difficult to provide a broad, general education to children. Dealing with homeschoolers will require a difficult balance of competing claims. The success of traditional schools in dealing with the homeschool phenomenon will depend on school leadership.

Although some stronger claims about the extent of homeschooling are probably overstated, the data examined in this section show that it has established itself as an alternative to regular school for a small set of families and is poised to continue its growth. In 1999, around 790,000 children between the ages of six and 17 were being schooled at home, and in the late 1990s, the number was growing.

Homeschoolers and their families differed from regular school attendees, but the differences were not large. Some of the distinctive characteristics of homeschoolers seemed to be decreasing. Homeschoolers were likely to be non-Hispanic White, but there was some evidence of fading racial differences over time. Some distinctive characteristics of homeschoolers seemed not to be changing very rapidly, but the characteristics need not be thought of as limitations to future growth. Households with homeschooled children had moderate-to-high education and income and were located in the rural or suburban West. Homeschoolers were likely to live with two adults, with one not in the labor force or working part-time.

We have just begun to see the emergence of homeschooling as an important national phenomenon. Unless the needs of parents are met in different ways, homeschooling will likely have a large impact on the school as an institution in the coming decades.

Alternative Educational Options

Section 34.2 | Choosing a Tutor

This section includes text excerpted from "The Perceived Success of Tutoring Students with Learning Disabilities: Relations to Tutee and Tutoring Variables," U.S. Department of Education (ED), 2016. Reviewed November 2022.

Students with learning disabilities face difficulties on university and college campuses. The difficulties encountered include:
- Deficits in study skills, such as test preparation, note-taking, listening comprehension
- Problems with organizational skills
- Difficulties with social interaction
- Deficits in specific academic areas, with reading and written composition being the most frequent
- Low self-esteem
- Higher dropout rates

The growth in the number of college students with learning disabilities and the recognition that these students experience various difficulties have led to an increase in the support services offered in institutions of higher learning. In addition to providing legally required accommodations, an increasing number of colleges now offer a variety of optional support programs for students with disabilities. These programs provide services such as specialized academic advising, personal counseling, time management and study skills training, and individualized academic programs. One service commonly provided in support centers is peer assistance in the form of tutoring.

This section will present results from a survey that evaluated the PERACH (a national program for social impact) peer tutoring project for students with learning disabilities at 29 universities, regional colleges, and teacher training colleges in Israel. The survey aimed to identify variables that may influence the perceived success of the tutoring project for college students with learning disabilities.

PEER TUTORING STUDENTS WITH LEARNING DISABILITIES

Peer tutoring is a class of practices and strategies that employ peers as one-on-one teachers to provide individualized instruction, practice, repetition, and clarification of concepts. This type of support exists in many settings, such as classrooms and the home, and includes cross-age individual tutoring, small group, and class-wide configurations. Studies have shown that moderate-to-large academic benefits can be attributed to peer tutoring in general and to students with learning disabilities.

Despite its prevalence, the effectiveness of peer tutoring in general and tutoring college students with learning disabilities, in particular, has not been thoroughly examined. Past research has suggested that since typically there are fewer differences in age and status, more mutuality of interaction, and relationships of a longer duration, peer relationships may serve in a supportive capacity related to career advancement and psychosocial functioning. As for tutoring college students with learning disabilities, some of the authors found that participation in a peer tutoring program contributed to a general feeling of efficacy and greater use of learning strategies and skills. Barbara Kirshenblatt-Gimblett, M.A., is professor Emerita of performance studies at New York University, reported improving self-image and a smooth transition to college life among the tutees. Gila Vogel, lecturer in the Department of Special Education at Beit Berl College in Israel; Barbara Fresko, associate professor of education, Beit Berl College, Israel; and Cheruta Wertheim, researcher at Beit Berl College in Israel, found that both tutees and tutors perceived tutoring as very beneficial to the tutees, and the level of satisfaction with the tutoring program for both groups was high. However, little is known regarding the variables contributing to the success of the tutoring process. This is aimed at identifying variables that may influence the perceived success of the tutoring project for college students with learning disabilities. Specifically, two variables were examined: tutoring-related (the degree of engagement in different tutoring activities and difficulties encountered during tutoring) and tutee-related (learning difficulties and academic self-efficacy).

ANTECEDENTS OF TUTORING SUCCESS FOR STUDENTS WITH LEARNING DISABILITIES

According to Dr. Colette Daiute, is professor in the Ph.D. programs in psychology and and M.A. in childhood and youth Studies, and

Alternative Educational Options

Dr. Bridget Dalton, B.A, M.A., associate professor of literacy studies at the University of Colorado, Boulder, having a companion with whom to talk and exchange points of view permits development in peer tutoring settings. This claim is per that propounded by Dr. Jean E. Rhodes Ph.D., American psychologist, author, and director of The Center for Evidence-Based Mentoring at the University of Massachusetts, Boston, and Dr. David L. DuBois, Ph.D., professor of Community Health Sciences in the School of Public Health, University of Illinois, Chicago, who suggested a model connecting various characteristics of the mentor–mentee relationship to mentoring success. Since mentoring is similar to tutoring (both can involve students from colleges and universities helping other students on a sustained and systematic basis under direction and supervision), it is plausible that Rhodes and DuBois' model is also relevant to the tutoring process. Specifically, the model mentioned attributes such as companionship, genuine caring and support, and the provision of enrichment activities. Nonetheless, it should be noted that whereas mentoring tends to focus on life skills and often is held outside the academic setting, tutoring generally focuses on academic learning and is usually held in the educational institution. Consequently, the contribution of tutoring-related variables to the success of the tutoring process needs further examination.

Daiute, Dalton, Rhodes, and DuBois emphasized only one aspect of the mentoring/tutoring process, the aspect of relationships. They did not consider other possible influences, such as the tutee's characteristics. This may be especially important when the tutees are students with disabilities. When considering students with learning disabilities, one should remember that these students continuously confront academic challenges. Many have significant deficiencies in reading, writing, and/or mathematics, as well as in memory, time management, and organization. In the academic realm, where students are expected to learn largely via lecture format and to read a great amount of literature, these demands are magnified for students with learning disabilities. Furthermore, some students with learning disabilities face greater difficulties than their nondisabled counterparts in concentrating on the task at hand, determining the salience of information presented in class, and applying test strategies, all potentially contributing to higher levels of anxiety and lower grade point average (GPA) scores.

The various challenges students encounter with learning disabilities may impact their self-efficacy, especially in the academic domain. As suggested by Bandura, efficacy expectations are hypothesized to be acquired and modified via four types of sources of information: past performance accomplishment, exposure to and identification with efficacious role models (vicarious learning), access to verbal persuasion and support from others, and experience of emotional or physiological arousal in the context of task performance. Students with learning disabilities may be expected, as a group, to have lower self-efficacy than students without disabilities, partially because of less access to sources of efficacy information. When repeated failure becomes internalized, beliefs about one's ability to achieve in the academic domain are likely to suffer. This weakened sense of efficacy may limit the level of future performance these students are willing to try to achieve and their persistence under stressful conditions. Low perceptions of ability, thereby, become reinforced by experience.

Self-efficacy studies indicate that compared to peers without learning disabilities, students with learning disabilities have lower academic self-efficacy and decreased academic competence. In addition, surveys examining the self-efficacy beliefs of students with learning disabilities have revealed that self-efficacy plays a primary role in predicting academic achievement. However, several studies found that students with learning disabilities tend to overestimate their efficacy. Furthermore, individuals with strong efficacy beliefs are more likely to exert effort in the face of difficulty and persist in working on tasks when they believe they have the requisite skills. Students feel differently about themselves and cope differently with challenges depending on what they believe they are capable of and what they hope they will be able to achieve. It should be noted that most studies on students with learning disabilities focused on younger students rather than on college students. Nonetheless, in light of the findings, the research assumption in the present study was that similar results will also be found in this

group. Specifically, the hypotheses were those college students' difficulties will be related to their academic self-efficacy and this sense of efficacy will predict the degree to which they perceive tutoring to be beneficial to them, alongside other variables related to the tutoring process such as tutoring activities and difficulties encountered during tutoring sessions. In sum, this study addressed three research questions:
- What are the characteristics of tutoring college students with learning disabilities in terms of tutees' difficulties, tutoring activities, difficulties encountered during tutoring, and the perceived success of the tutoring process?
- Are tutees' difficulties related to their academic self-efficacy?
- Do tutees' self-efficacy, engagement in different tutoring activities, and difficulties encountered during tutoring sessions contribute to their perceptions regarding the success of the tutoring process?

INSTRUMENTS
Tutees' Difficulties

A measure was used that was developed by Vogel. Participants are asked to rate how they cope with difficulties in 12 different domains. These domains are divided into three subgroups as follows:
- **General study skills** (attention and concentration, studying for exams, use of time, memory, and mathematics)
- **Language-related skills** (reading materials in English, writing papers, summarizing articles, finding information, and reading materials in Hebrew)
- **Nonacademic skills** (emotional areas and social areas)

Possible answers range from one ("very difficult") to five ("no problem"). Vogel and colleagues did not report Cronbach's alphas; however, in the study, they were 0.73 for the general study skills and 0.82 for the language-related skills. A significant positive correlation was found between the two items that comprised the nonacademic skills domain (r = 0.73, p < 0.001).

Academic Self-Efficacy

A five-item measure based on the subject-level academic self-efficacy scale of Mimi Bong, professor of Educational Psychology, Korea University, was administered. Instead of mentioning a particular subject area (such as mathematics), as in the original questionnaire, general statements were used. For example, the item "I can master even the hardest material in [a specific subject] if I try" was rephrased as "I can master even the hardest material in my studies if I try." Participants are asked to rate each item on a response scale ranging from one ("not at all true") to five ("very true"). Cronbach's alphas ranged between 0.86 and 0.91 in the original study (depending on the subject matter) and in the current study $\alpha = 0.86$.

Engagement in Tutoring Activities

A list of eight different tasks was developed by Vogel and colleagues. Participants are asked to rate how each task was dealt with during the tutoring sessions. Possible answers range from one ("not at all") to five ("very much"). Varimax factor analysis of the data in the current study revealed three distinct factors: general academic activities (four items, e.g., "reading articles"), review of material (two items, e.g., "studying for exams"), and nonacademic activities (two items, e.g., "discussion of personal matters"). Cronbach's alphas were 0.73 for the general academic activities and 0.80 for the whole list. Significant positive correlations emerged between the two reviews of material activities items (r = 0.62, p < 0.001) and the two nonacademic activities items (r = 0.77, p < 0.001).

Difficulties Encountered during Tutoring

This measure was also developed by Vogel and colleagues. Participants are asked to rate the extent to which seven different situations occurred during the tutoring period that hindered tutoring (e.g., "sessions were ineffective"). Possible answers range from one ("not at all") to five ("very much"). Varimax factor analysis of the data in the current study revealed only one factor with an internal consistency of 0.84.

Perceived Success of Tutoring

A scale was developed specifically for the present study based on a literature review, prior research questionnaires used in the evaluation of the PERACH program, in-depth knowledge of tutoring in the context of PERACH, and several consultations with colleagues in the field of tutoring. The scale includes six items measuring tutees' perceptions regarding the contribution of the tutoring process to their academic functioning, including improvement in grades, preparation, and organization before lectures; participation during lectures; in writing papers and doing exercises; in studying for exams; and in learning habits (e.g., "the tutoring program helped me improve my grades"). Participants are asked to rate the extent to which each statement is true for them on a scale ranging from one ("not at all") to five ("very much"). Varimax factor analysis of the data revealed only one factor. Cronbach's alpha was 0.88.

Chapter 35 | Transition to High School

Chapter Contents
Section 35.1—Transition to High School: An Overview 363
Section 35.2—Frequently Asked Questions about
　　　　　　Transition to High School 369

Section 35.1 | Transition to High School: An Overview

This section contains text excerpted from the following sources: Text begins with excerpts from "Transition of Students with Disabilities to Postsecondary Education: A Guide for High School Educators," U.S. Department of Education (ED), January 10, 2020; Text under the heading "Transition Planning Process Develops over Time" is excerpted from "Transition Planning for Students with Disabilities," U.S. Department of Education (ED), November 2004. Reviewed November 2022.

For students with disabilities, accurate knowledge about their civil rights is a big factor in their successful transition from high school to postsecondary education. This aims to provide high school educators with answers to questions students with disabilities may have as they prepare to move to the postsecondary education environment.

The Office for Civil Rights (OCR) of the U.S. Department of Education (ED) has enforcement responsibilities under Section 504 of the Rehabilitation Act of 1973 (Section 504), as amended, and Title II of the Americans with Disabilities Act (ADA) of 1990, as amended (Title II), which prohibit discrimination oriented on disability. Every school district and college and university in the United States is subject to one or both of these laws, which have similar requirements. Private postsecondary institutions that do not receive federal financial assistance are not subject to Section 504 or Title II. They are, however, subject to Title III of the ADA, which is enforced by the U.S. Department of Justice (DOJ) and prohibits discrimination oriented on disability by private entities that are not private clubs or religious entities.

This also refers to Part B of the Individuals with Disabilities Education Act (IDEA), which provides funds to states to assist in making free appropriate public education (FAPE) available to eligible children with disabilities. The IDEA requirements apply to state education agencies, school districts, and other public agencies that serve IDEA-eligible children. Institutions of postsecondary education have no legal obligations under the IDEA.

Similarly, this guide references the state vocational rehabilitation (VR) services program, authorized by the Rehabilitation Act, which provides funds to state VR agencies to assist eligible individuals with disabilities in obtaining employment. State VR agencies provide a wide range of employment-related services, including services designed to facilitate the transition of eligible students with disabilities from school to postschool activities.

This section highlights the significant differences between the rights and responsibilities of students with disabilities in the high school setting and the rights and responsibilities these students will have once they are in the postsecondary education setting. The following set of frequently asked questions provides practical suggestions that high school educators can share with students to facilitate their successful transition to postsecondary education.

THE TRANSITION PLANNING PROCESS DEVELOPS OVER TIME

Transition planning is not a uniform experience for students as they age; indeed, several aspects of the process are different for older students. Some of the differences, such as the role youth take in the process, may occur because of the increased maturity that comes with age. Other differences may reflect an increasing sense of urgency on everyone's part as high school exit approaches.

Initial Transition Planning

The mean age for the initiation of transition planning is 14.4 years. Three-fourths of 14-year-olds have started transition planning, and the process is increasingly likely for older students. By the time students are 17 or 18 years old, 96 percent have had transition planning, reflecting a 20-percentage-point increase over 14-year-olds.

Participants in Transition Planning

Older students appear to exhibit greater responsibility for postschool goals than younger students, which may partly explain their greater likelihood of participating actively in transition planning. School staff reported on the participants participating in the transition planning process.

- One-third of 14-year-old students with disabilities are present for transition planning but do not participate—a passive role taken by only one-fifth of 17- and 18-year-olds.

Transition to High School

- Providing active input into planning increases for older students, with more than 60 percent of 17- and 18-year-olds providing input, compared with 45 percent of younger students.
- The transition planning process's student leadership is also more likely among older students; more than 15 percent of 17- and 18-year-olds take this role.

Although the participation of parents (85%), special education teachers (97%), and general education teachers (59%) vary little for students across the age range, the participation of general education vocational teachers in transition planning is greater for older students; this difference reflects the increased likelihood of older students' taking vocational education courses and the approach of students' transition to postsecondary vocational training and employment. About 40 percent of 17- and 18-year-old students have a general education vocational teacher involved in their transition planning, twice as many as 14-year-olds.

Consistent with the increasing emphasis on vocational goals and services for older students, the participation of a state vocational rehabilitation counselor is more common for these students. One in four 17- and 18-year-old students have such an individual involved in their transition planning, compared with one in ten 14-year-olds. Similarly, the active participation of representatives from various other outside organizations increases as early adulthood approaches from one in ten 15-year-olds to one in five 17- and 18-year-old students.

Supports for Transition

Instruction focused specifically on transition planning (e.g., a specialized curriculum designed to help students assess options and develop strategies for leaving secondary school and transitioning to adult life) is one way to help students reach their goals. According to school staff, 64 percent of students have received such instruction, and older students (76% for 17- and 18-year-olds) are more likely than younger students (48% for 14-year-olds) to have had it.

Generally, according to the school staff reports, more post-high-school service needs are identified as part of transition planning as students approach the transition to adult service systems. Most notably, vocational training and employment service needs are more commonly identified for older and younger students. Parents of older students are more likely to receive information from the schools about adult services, and school contacts with many outside organizations on behalf of students with disabilities intensify as school exit nears.

TRANSITION PLANNING REFLECTS A DIVERSITY OF NEEDS AND ABILITIES

The goals and needs specified in students' transition plans, the participants in the planning process, and many transition-related activities differ markedly across the disability categories. School staff provided information on the following aspects of students' transition plans.

- **Students' goals**. Students with disabilities have multiple goals that reflect their future plans. The various transition goals shared by some students in all disability categories mask a large range across categories in the percentages of students who have each goal. For example:
  - Although about half of students with disabilities plan to go to college, that plan varies from 10 percent of students with mental retardation to more than 70 percent with visual impairments.
  - Postsecondary vocational training is planned for about 40 percent of students with disabilities overall; however, almost 60 percent of students with other health impairments have this goal, compared with about 20 percent of students with visual impairments.
  - Supported employment is the transition goal for fewer than 10 percent of students with disabilities overall, but it is the goal of almost 40 percent of students with autism.

Supports for Transition

The percentages of students for whom a variety of supports are in place (i.e., a course of study students should pursue to meet their transition goals, instruction focused on transition planning skills, and a list of postschool service needs consistent with students' goals) vary with students' disability category.

- Specification of the student's course of study in the individualized education program (IEP) relative to transition goals varies from 65 percent of students with hearing impairments to 75 percent of students with learning disabilities.
- Instruction for transition planning is designed to assist students in assessing their options, and developing strategies for transition is received by 55–70 percent of students across categories. Students with autism or multiple disabilities are the most likely to receive this type of instruction; students with other health impairments are the least likely to do so.

Students' transition plans also identify a wide range of service and program needs for the post-high-school period.

- The transition plans for students with learning disabilities or hearing, orthopedic, or other health impairments are the most likely to specify postsecondary education accommodations.
- The plans for students with autism, multiple disabilities, or deaf-blindness typically specify a constellation of postschool services, including vocational training, support living arrangements, and behavioral interventions, as well as transportation, social work, mental health, and communication services.
- The plans for students with emotional disturbances are very likely to specify behavioral interventions and mental health services.
- For students with specific sensory or physical disabilities, the plans typically suggest corresponding services such as audiology, vision and mobility services, and occupational or physical therapy.

The types of organizations that schools contact regarding programs or employment for students when they leave high school reflect the students' postschool goals and identified needs. Schools typically make more contacts for students in the disability categories that have more identified needs. Schools are also more likely to provide parents of students in the disability categories with multiple identified service needs with information about appropriate services than parents in disability categories with fewer identified needs.

Perceptions of the Processes

Parents and school staff of students in each disability category hold various views regarding transition planning and the school programs designed to meet students' transition goals. For example:
- School staff report that more than half of students with visual impairments have programs that are very well suited to help them achieve their transition goals, whereas only one-third of students with emotional disturbances have such highly rated school programs.
- More than four in 10 students with mental retardation or visual impairments have parents who report that the transition planning process is very useful. However, less than three in 10 students with autism have parents who feel this way.
- Parents report that one in four students with emotional disturbances or other health impairments has transition plans that are not very or not at all useful for their children, compared to one in 12 students with mental retardation whose parents report limited usefulness of transition planning.

Transition to High School

Section 35.2 | Frequently Asked Questions about Transition to High School

This section includes text excerpted from "Transition of Students with Disabilities to Postsecondary Education: A Guide for High School Educators," U.S. Department of Education (ED), January 10, 2020.

THE ADMISSIONS PROCESS
Are Students with Disabilities Entitled to Changes in Standardized Testing Conditions on Entrance Exams for Institutions of Postsecondary Education?

It depends. In general, tests may not be selected or administered in a way that tests the disability rather than the achievement or aptitude of the individual. In addition, federal law requires changes to the testing conditions necessary to allow a student with a disability to participate as long as the changes do not fundamentally alter the examination or create undue financial or administrative burdens. Although some postsecondary education institutions may have their own entrance exams, many use a student's score on commercially available tests.

In general, to request one or more changes in standardized testing conditions, which test administrators may also refer to as "testing accommodations," the student will need to contact the institution of postsecondary education or the entity that administers the exam and provide documentation of a disability and the need for a change in testing conditions. The issue of documentation is discussed below. Examples of changes in testing conditions that may be available include but are not limited to:
- Braille
- Large print
- Fewer items on each page
- Tape-recorded responses
- Responses on the test booklet
- Frequent breaks
- Extended testing time
- Testing over several sessions
- Small group setting
- Private room

- Preferential seating
- The use of a sign language interpreter for spoken directions

Are Institutions of Postsecondary Education Permitted to Ask an Applicant If She or He Has a Disability before an Admission Decision Is Made?

Generally, postsecondary education institutions are not permitted to make what is known as a "preadmission inquiry" about an applicant's disability status. Preadmission inquiries are permitted only if the institution of postsecondary education is taking remedial action to correct the effects of past discrimination or taking voluntary action to overcome the effects of conditions that limit the participation of individuals with disabilities.

Examples of impermissible preadmission inquiries include: "Are you in good health?" "Have you been hospitalized for a medical condition in the past five years?" Postsecondary education institutions may inquire about an applicant's ability to meet essential program requirements, provided such inquiries are not designed to reveal disability status. For example, if physical lifting is an essential requirement for a degree program in physical therapy, an acceptable question that could be asked is, "with or without reasonable accommodation, can you lift 25 pounds?" After admission, in response to a student's request for "academic adjustments," reasonable modifications, or auxiliary aids and services, postsecondary education institutions may ask for documentation regarding disability status.

May Postsecondary Education Institutions Deny an Applicant Admission Because She or He Has a Disability?

No. If an applicant meets the essential requirements for admission, an institution may not deny that applicant admission simply because she or he has a disability, nor may an institution categorically exclude an applicant with a particular disability as not being qualified for its program. For instance, an institution may not automatically assume that all applicants with hearing or visual impairments would be unable to meet the essential eligibility requirements of its music program. An institution may require an applicant to meet any essential technical or academic standards for admission to, or participation in, the institution and its program. An institution may deny admission to any student, disabled or not, who does not meet essential requirements for admission or participation.

Are Institutions Obligated to Identify Students with Disabilities?

No. Institutions do not have a duty to identify students with disabilities. Students in postsecondary education institutions are responsible for notifying institution staff of their disability should they need academic adjustments. High schools, in contrast, are obligated to identify students within their jurisdiction who have a disability and may be entitled to services.

Are Students Obligated to Inform Institutions That They Have a Disability?

No. A student has no obligation to inform an institution of postsecondary education that she or he has a disability; however, if the student wants an institution to provide an academic adjustment or assign the student to accessible housing or other facilities or if a student wants other disability-related services, the student must identify herself or himself as having a disability. The disclosure of a disability is always voluntary. For example, a student who has a disability that does not require services may choose not to disclose her or his disability.

POSTADMISSION: DOCUMENTATION OF A DISABILITY
What Are Academic Adjustments and Auxiliary Aids and Services?

Academic adjustments are defined in the Section 504 regulations at 34 CFR §104.44(a) as follows:
- Such modifications to the academic requirements are necessary to ensure that such requirements do not discriminate or have the effect of discriminating, oriented on (disability) against a qualified applicant or student (with a disability). Academic requirements

that the recipient can demonstrate are essential to the instruction being pursued by such student or to any directly related licensing requirement and will not be regarded as discriminatory within the meaning of this section. Modifications may include changes in the length of time permitted to complete degree requirements, the substitution of specific courses required to complete degree requirements, and adaptation of how specific courses are conducted.

Academic adjustments may also include a reduced course load, extended time on tests, and the provision of auxiliary aids and services. Auxiliary aids and services are defined in the Section 504 regulations at 34 CFR §104.44(d) and the Title II regulations at 28 CFR §35.104. They include notetakers, readers, recording devices, sign language interpreters, screen-readers, voice recognition and other adaptive software or hardware for computers, and other devices designed to ensure the participation of students with impaired sensory, manual, or speaking skills in an institution's programs and activities.

Institutions are not required to provide personal devices and services such as attendants; individually prescribed devices, such as eyeglasses; readers for personal use or study; or other services of a personal nature, such as tutoring. If institutions offer to tutor the general student population, however, they must ensure that tutoring services are also available to students with disabilities. In some instances, a state vocational rehabilitation (VR) agency may provide auxiliary aids and services to support an individual's postsecondary education and training once that individual has been determined eligible to receive services under the VR program.

What Documentation Is Necessary for Students with Disabilities to Receive Academic Adjustments from Postsecondary Education Institutions?

Institutions may set their own requirements for documentation so long as they are reasonable and comply with Section 504 and Title

Transition to High School

II. It is not uncommon for documentation standards to vary from institution to institution; thus, students with disabilities should research documentation standards at those institutions that interest them.

Upon request, a student must provide documentation that she or he has a disability, an impairment that substantially limits a major life activity and supports the need for an academic adjustment. The documentation should identify how a student's ability to function is limited as a result of her or his disability. The primary purpose of the documentation is to establish a disability to help the institution work interactively with the student to identify appropriate services. The focus should be on whether the information adequately documents the existence of a current disability and the need for an academic adjustment.

Who Is Responsible for Obtaining the Necessary Testing to Document the Existence of a Disability?

The student is responsible. Postsecondary education institutions are not required to conduct or pay for an evaluation to document a student's disability and need for an academic adjustment although some institutions do. If a student with a disability is eligible for services through the state VR services program, she or he may qualify for an evaluation at no cost. High school educators can assist students with disabilities in locating their state VR agency (rsa.ed.gov). If students with disabilities cannot find other funding sources to pay for necessary evaluation or testing for postsecondary education, they are responsible for paying for it themselves.

At the elementary and secondary school levels, a school district's duty to provide a free appropriate public education (FAPE) encompasses the responsibility to provide, at no cost to the parents, an evaluation of suspected areas of disability for any of the district's students who are believed to need special education or related aids and services. Under Section 504 or Title II, school districts are not required to conduct evaluations to obtain academic adjustments once a student graduates and goes on to postsecondary education.

Is a Student's Most Recent Individualized Education Program or Section 504 Plan Sufficient Documentation to Support the Existence of a Disability and the Need for an Academic Adjustment in a Postsecondary Setting?

Generally, no. Although an individualized education program (IEP) or Section 504 plan may help identify services that the student in the past has used, they generally are not sufficient documentation to support the existence of a current disability and need for an academic adjustment from an institution of postsecondary education. Assessment information and other material used to develop an IEP or Section 504 plan may be helpful to document a current disability or the need for an academic adjustment or auxiliary aids and services.

In addition, a student receiving services under Part B of the individuals with disabilities education act (IDEA) must be provided with a summary of her or his academic achievements and functional performance that includes recommendations on how to assist in meeting the student's postsecondary goals. This information may provide helpful information about disability and the need for academic adjustment.

What Can High School Personnel, Such as School Psychologists and Counselors, Transition Specialists, Special Education Staff, and Others, Do to Assist Students with Disabilities with Documentation Requirements?

By the time most students with disabilities are accepted into a postsecondary institution, they will likely have a transition plan and/or be receiving transition services, which may include evaluations and services provided by the state VR agency. High school personnel can help a student with disabilities identify and address the specific documentation requirements of the postsecondary institution that the student will be attending. This may include assisting the student in identifying existing documentation in her or his education records that would satisfy the institution's criteria, such as evaluation reports and a summary of the student's academic achievement and functional performance.

Transition to High School

School personnel should be aware that postsecondary education institutions typically do not accept brief conclusory statements for which no supporting evidence is offered as sufficient documentation of a disability and the need for an academic adjustment. School personnel should also be aware that some colleges may delay or deny services if the diagnosis or the documentation is unclear.

Will a Medical Diagnosis from a Treating Physician Help Document Disability?

An impairment diagnosis alone does not establish an individual's disability within Section 504 or Title II. Rather, the impairment must substantially limit a major life activity, or the individual must have a record of such an impairment or be regarded as having such an impairment. A diagnosis from a treating physician and information about how the disability affects the student may suffice. As noted above, postsecondary education institutions may set their own requirements for documentation so long as they are reasonable and comply with Section 504 and Title II.

If It Is Clear That a Student Has a Disability, Why Does an Institution Need Documentation?

Students with the same disability may not necessarily require the same academic adjustment. Section 504 and Title II require that postsecondary education institutions make individualized determinations regarding appropriate academic adjustments for each student. If the student's disability and need for an academic adjustment are obvious, less documentation may be necessary.

How Will the Student Know If an Institution Thinks the Documentation Is Insufficient?

If the documentation a student submitted for the institution's consideration does not meet the institution's requirements, an official should notify the student promptly of what additional documentation the student needs to provide. As noted above, a student may need a new evaluation to provide documentation of a current disability.

POSTADMISSION: OBTAINING SERVICES
Must Institutions Provide Every Academic Adjustment a Student with a Disability Wants?

It depends. Institutions are not required to provide an academic adjustment that would alter or waive essential academic requirements. They also do not have to provide an academic adjustment that would fundamentally alter the nature of a service, program, or activity or result in undue financial or administrative burdens considering the institution's resources. For example, an appropriate academic adjustment may be to extend the time a student with a disability is allotted to take tests.

Still, an institution is not required to change the substantive content of the tests. In addition, an institution is not required to make modifications that would result in undue financial or administrative burdens. Public institutions are required to give primary consideration to the auxiliary aid or service that the student requests but can opt to provide alternative aids or services if they are effective. They can also opt to provide an effective alternative if the requested auxiliary aid or service would fundamentally alter the nature of a service, program, or activity or result in undue financial or administrative burdens.

For example, if it would be a fundamental alteration or undue burden to provide a disability with a notetaker for oral classroom presentations and discussions and a tape recorder would be an effective alternative, a postsecondary institution may provide the student with a tape recorder instead of a notetaker.

If Students Want to Request Academic Adjustments, What Must They Do?

Institutions may establish reasonable procedures for requesting academic adjustments; students are responsible for knowing these procedures and following them. Institutions usually include information on the procedures and contacts requesting an academic adjustment in their general information publications and websites. If students cannot locate the procedures, they should contact an institution official, such as an admissions officer or counselor.

What Should Students Expect in Working with a Disability Coordinator at an Institution of Postsecondary Education?

A high school counselor, a special education teacher, or a VR counselor may meet with high school students with disabilities to provide services or monitor their progress under their education plans periodically. The role of the disability coordinator at an institution of postsecondary education is very different.

At many institutions, there may be only one or two staff members to address the needs of all students with disabilities attending the institution. The disability coordinator evaluates documentation, works with students to determine appropriate services, assists students in arranging services or testing modifications, and deals with problems as they arise. A disability coordinator may have contact with a student with a disability only two or three times a semester.

Disability coordinators usually will not directly provide educational services, tutoring, or counseling or help students plan or manage their time or schedules. Students with disabilities are generally expected to be responsible for their own academic programs and progress as nondisabled students.

When Should Students Notify the Institution of Their Intention to Request an Academic Adjustment?

It should be done as soon as possible. Although students may request academic adjustments at any time, students needing services should be advised to notify the institution as early as possible to ensure that the institution has enough time to review their request and provide an appropriate academic adjustment. Some academic adjustments, such as interpreters, may take time to arrange. In addition, students should not wait until after completing a course or activity or receiving a poor grade to request services and then expect the grade to be changed or to be able to retake the course.

How Do Institutions Determine What Academic Adjustments Are Appropriate?

Once a student has identified herself or himself as an individual with a disability, requested an academic adjustment, and provided appropriate documentation upon request, institution staff should discuss with the student what academic adjustments are appropriate in light of the student's individual needs and the nature of the institution's program.

Students with disabilities possess unique knowledge of their individual disabilities and should be prepared to discuss the functional challenges they face and, if applicable, what has or has not worked for them in the past. Institution staff should be prepared to describe the barriers students may face in individual classes that may affect their full participation and discuss academic adjustments that might enable students to overcome those barriers.

Who Pays for Auxiliary Aids and Services?

Once the needed auxiliary aids and services have been identified, institutions may not require students with disabilities to pay part or all of the costs of such aids and services, nor may institutions charge students with disabilities more for participating in programs or activities than they charge students who do not have disabilities.

Institutions generally may not condition their provision of academic adjustments on the availability of funds, refuse to spend more than a certain amount to provide academic adjustments, or refuse to provide academic adjustments because they believe other providers of such services exist. In many cases, institutions may meet their obligation to provide auxiliary aids and services by assisting students in obtaining them or obtaining reimbursement for their costs from an outside agency or organization, such as a state VR agency. Such assistance notwithstanding, institutions retain ultimate responsibility for providing necessary auxiliary aids and services and for any costs associated with providing such aids and services or utilizing outside sources.

However, as noted above, if the institution can demonstrate that providing a specific auxiliary aid or service would result in undue

Transition to High School

financial or administrative burdens, considering the institution's resources as a whole, it can opt to provide another effective one.

What If the Academic Adjustments the Institution Provides Are Not Working?

If the academic adjustments are not meeting the student's needs, it is the student's responsibility to notify the institution as soon as possible. It may be too late to correct the problem if the student waits until the course or activity is completed. The student and the institution should work together to resolve the problem.

Chapter 36 | Transition to College and Vocational Programs

As a student approaches the time to leave high school, it is important that preparations for adult life are well underway. For early transition planning and active participation in decision-making for students with disabilities, members of the planning team need to be well-informed about the student's abilities, needs, and available services. This chapter highlights educational opportunities, credentials, and employment strategies designed to assist students with disabilities while in school to prepare for meaningful postsecondary education and/or thriving careers.

TRANSITION PLANNING

A successful transition process results from comprehensive team planning driven by youth's dreams, desires, and abilities. A transition plan provides the basic structure for preparing an individual to live, work, and play in the community as fully and independently as possible.

Local educational agencies (LEAs) and state vocational rehabilitation (VR) agencies participate in planning meetings to assist students and family members make critical decisions about this stage of the student's life and future postschool goals. During the planning process, schools and VR agencies work together to identify

This chapter includes text excerpted from "A Transition Guide to Postsecondary Education and Employment for Students and Youth with Disabilities," U.S. Department of Education (ED), August 24, 2020.

the transition needs of students with disabilities, such as the need for assistive or rehabilitation technology, orientation and mobility services or travel training, and career exploration through vocational assessments or work experience opportunities.

The individualized education program (IEP), developed under the Individuals with Disabilities Education Act (IDEA), for each student with a disability, must address transition services requirements beginning not later than the first IEP to be in effect when the child turns 16, or younger if determined appropriate by the IEP Team, and must be updated annually thereafter. The IEP must include the following:

- Appropriate measurable postsecondary goals oriented upon age-appropriate transition assessments related to training, education, employment, and, where appropriate, independent living skills
- The transition services (including courses of study) that are needed to assist the student with a disability in reaching those goals

While the IDEA statute and regulations refer to courses of study, they are but one example of appropriate transition services. Examples of independent living skills to consider when developing postsecondary goals include self-advocacy, management of the home and personal finances, and the use of public information.

EDUCATION AND TRAINING OPPORTUNITIES

Several opportunities and programs are available for students preparing to exit secondary school. Many of these education and training opportunities involve formal or informal connections between educational, VR, employment, training, social services, and health services agencies. Specifically, high schools, career centers, community colleges, four-year colleges, universities, and state technical colleges are key partners. These partners offer federal, state, and local funds to assist a student in preparing for postsecondary education.

Furthermore, research suggests that enrollment in more rigorous, academically intense programs (e.g., advanced placement

(AP), international baccalaureate (IB), or dual enrollment) in high school prepares students, including those with low achievement levels, to enroll and persist in postsecondary education at higher rates than similar students who pursue less challenging courses of study.

The following are examples of exciting options, programs, and activities that may be available as IEP teams develop IEPs to prepare the student for the transition to adult life.

Regular High School Diploma

The term "regular high school diploma" means the standard high school diploma awarded to the preponderance of students in the state that is fully aligned with state standards, or a higher diploma, except that a regular high school diploma shall not be aligned to the alternate academic achievement standards, and does not include a recognized diploma equivalent, such as a general equivalency diploma, certificate of completion, certificate of attendance, or similar lesser credentials.

The vast majority of students with disabilities should have access to the same high-quality academic coursework as all other students in the state that reflects grade-level content for the grade in which the student is enrolled, enabling them to participate in assessments aligned with grade-level achievement standards.

Alternate High School Diploma

Some students with the most significant cognitive disabilities may receive a state-defined high school diploma oriented on alternate academic achievement standards, but that diploma must be standards-based.

Working toward an alternate diploma sometimes causes delays or keeps the student from completing the requirements for a regular high school diploma. However, students with the most significant cognitive disabilities working toward an alternate diploma must receive instruction aligned with the state's challenging academic content standards, promoting their involvement and progress in the general education curriculum, consistent with the IDEA.

Furthermore, states must continue to make free appropriate public education (FAPE) available to any student with a disability who graduates from high school with a credential other than a regular high school diploma, such as an alternate diploma, General Educational Development (GED), or certificate of completion. While FAPE under the IDEA does not include education beyond grade 12, states and school districts are required to continue to offer to develop and implement an IEP for an eligible student with a disability who graduates from high school with a credential other than a regular high school diploma until the student has exceeded the age of eligibility for FAPE under state law.

Depending on a state law that sets the state's upper age limit for FAPE, the entitlement to FAPE under IDEA of a student with a disability who has not graduated high school with a regular high school diploma could last until the student's 22nd birthday. However, some state laws may address providing educational services to individuals with disabilities beyond their 22nd birthday.

The IEPs for students with disabilities could include transition services in the form of coursework at a community college or other postsecondary institution, provided that the state recognizes the coursework as secondary school education under state law. Secondary school education does not include beyond grade 12 and must meet state education standards.

DUAL OR CONCURRENT ENROLLMENT PROGRAM

Increasingly, states and school districts permit students to participate in dual or concurrent enrollment programs while still in high school. The term "dual or concurrent enrollment program" refers to a partnership between a postsecondary education institution and a local school district in which the student who has not yet graduated from high school with a regular high school diploma can enroll in one or more postsecondary courses and earn postsecondary credit. The credit(s) can be transferred to the college or university in the partnership and applied toward completing a degree or recognized educational credential, which the student would earn after leaving high school.

Transition to College and Vocational Programs

Programs are offered both on campuses of colleges or universities or in high school classrooms. As with all students taking classes at postsecondary institutions, students with disabilities who have IEPs must meet the postsecondary institution's criteria to take the class.

Comprehensive transition programs (CTPs) are a type of postsecondary education. CTPs offered at institutions of higher education institutions (IHEs) provide inclusive, academic, social, and career and technical education programs for individuals with intellectual disabilities seeking a postsecondary or college experience and career path. Participation in a CTP may generate academic credit leading to a postsecondary credential or degree. These programs embrace high expectations and provide valuable opportunities for individuals with intellectual disabilities to gain skills that will maximize their opportunities for achieving employment, including competitive integrated employment. After exiting high school, students can enroll in CTPs full-time.

Additionally, since CTPs are a type of postsecondary education program, students may be able to dually enroll in CTPs while still attending secondary school if the IHE enrolls high school students to take CTP classes. If under state law, attending classes at a postsecondary institution, whether auditing or for credit, is considered secondary school education for students in grade 12 or below and the education provided meets applicable state standards, those services can be designated as transition services on a student's IEP and paid for with IDEA Part B funds consistent with the student's entitlement to FAPE. Dual enrollment can be a helpful option for students in facilitating their transition from secondary school to postsecondary education and the workforce.

EARLY COLLEGE HIGH SCHOOL

The term "early college high school" refers to a partnership between at least one school district and at least one college or university that allows a student to simultaneously complete requirements toward earning a regular high school diploma and earn not less than 12 credits that are transferable to the college or university within the partnership as part of her or his course of study toward a postsecondary degree or credential at no cost to the student or student's family.

Summary of Performance

A summary of performance (SOP) is required for each student with an IEP whose eligibility for services under IDEA terminates due to graduation from secondary school with a regular high school diploma or exceeding the age of eligibility for FAPE under state law. The school district must provide the student with a summary of the student's academic achievement and functional performance that includes recommendations on how to assist the student in meeting the student's postsecondary goals. This summary of the student's achievement and performance can be used to assist the student in accessing postsecondary education and/or employment services.

Chapter 37 | Employment and Postsecondary Education

TRANSITIONING FROM SCHOOL TO EMPLOYMENT
As a student approaches the time to leave high school, it is important that preparations for adult life are well underway. For youth with disabilities, as with all youth, the transition from school to adulthood is an important time to prepare for future employment and being able to support oneself. Supports may be needed in education, vocational training, income support, health insurance coverage, health care, transportation, life skills, housing, and so on.

Moving from adolescence to adulthood is a critical time period for all youth. Those with disabilities will benefit most when continuity of services can be provided for them during this transition. The federal partners in transition (youth.gov/feature-article/federal-partners-transition) workgroup on youth transition services for students and youth with disabilities provides a more in-depth discussion on providing continuity of services for this population. The federal partners in transition workgroup, which includes representatives from several federal agencies, was formed to support all youth, including youth with disabilities, in successfully transitioning from school to adulthood. Another helpful resource is a transition guide to postsecondary education and employment for

---

This chapter contains text excerpted from the following sources: Text beginning with the heading "Transitioning from School to Employment" is excerpted from "Employment and Postsecondary Education," Youth.gov, March 17, 2018. Reviewed November 2022; Text beginning with the heading "Employment Considerations for Youth with Disabilities" is excerpted from "Employment Considerations for Youth with Disabilities," Youth.gov, June 15, 2022.

students and youth with disabilities, with information for students, youth, and families.

The Individuals with Disabilities Education Act (IDEA) and its implementing regulations address secondary transition services for students with disabilities. Secondary transition services help students with a disability successfully prepare for life after high school. Transition services may be special education provided as specially designed instruction or a related service if required to assist a child with a disability to benefit from special education. Beginning no later than the first individualized education programs (IEPs) to be in effect when the child turns 16 and younger if determined appropriate by the IEP team, and updated annually thereafter, the IEP must include postsecondary goals and the transition services needed to assist the student in reaching those goals.

Individualized learning plans (ILPs) are another helpful tool often used to aid the transition from school to employment for all youth, including those with a disability. ILPs are state-based transition planning tools currently used in 38 states. Working with their counselors and other supportive adults, students can develop ILPs to walk through the process of developing self-knowledge, relating that knowledge to career options, and laying out goals and skill-building activities to help achieve these goals.

This transition can be difficult for all youth, especially those with disabilities. Recent research has found that in comparison with their peers who did not have a disability, transitioning youth with disabilities were found:

- To be less likely to have enrolled in postsecondary programs.
- To be less likely to have attended a four-year university.
- To have lower completion rates of postsecondary education.

Additionally, findings from the National Longitudinal Transition Study (NLTS) 2012 have found that in comparison to youth who do not have an IEP, youth with an IEP are:

- More likely to be socioeconomically disadvantaged and face problems with health, communication, and completing typical tasks independently

Employment and Postsecondary Education

- More likely to struggle academically and yet are less likely to receive some form of school-based support
- Lagging behind their peers when planning and taking steps to obtain postsecondary education and jobs

However, it was also found that almost all of these young adults with disabilities, up to eight years after high school, were employed, and more than half were living independently. This study also found that the most common post-high-school goals for this population included:
- Secure independent living
- Attending a two- or four-year college
- Attending a postsecondary vocational training program
- Enhancing social and interpersonal relationships
- Obtaining more functional independence

Two factors are crucial for youth with disabilities to transition successfully into employment:
- Employment training and work experiences while in high school
- High parental expectations

Students with paid work experience during high school are likely to develop workplace socialization skills. Career awareness training and attendance at a vocational school are also associated with a greater likelihood of post-high-school employment. Parents' high expectations are connected to high school academic achievement, goal persistence in college, and employment outcomes.

In the hiring process, the main factors that drive employers' decisions to hire a youth with a disability focus on their perception of the youth, including the applicant's soft skills, such as:
- Preparedness for the interview
- Professionalism
- Ability to perform on the job (i.e., prior paid work experience)

Additionally, through a survey completed by employers in the United States, it was found that the assistance of a job developer in making the job match is more likely to be highly valued by small and medium-sized employers compared to larger companies. A job developer is a human resources professional who can help find job opportunities, perform outreach with potential places of employment, and provide training in soft skills. A job developer can also help demonstrate the unique contributions the youth can offer the employer. This is useful information to consider when working with youth preparing for employment after high school and finding the right fit for the youth and the employer.

A WORKFORCE DEVELOPMENT SYSTEM

The Workforce Innovation and Opportunity Act (WIOA) was designed to strengthen and improve the nation's public workforce development system by helping people who have traditionally faced barriers to employment overcome those hurdles, including individuals with disabilities, out-of-school and at-risk youth, and others. The WIOA is also intended to help employers hire and retain skilled workers. By providing a one-stop service delivery system, known as the "American Job Centers," it is hoped that job seekers will have seamless access to a system of high-quality career services, education, and job-based training in areas employers are seeking to hire. The U.S. Department of Labor (DOL), the U.S. Department of Education (ED), and the U.S. Department of Health and Human Services (HHS) are working together to support WIOA.

EMPLOYMENT CONSIDERATIONS FOR YOUTH WITH DISABILITIES

Although efforts have been taken to help improve employment opportunities for people with disabilities, research continues to suggest that youth with disabilities are less likely than their nondisabled peers to graduate from high school, attend and complete four-year colleges and universities, and be employed.

Guideposts for Transitions

Through an extensive literature search, the National Collaborative on Workforce and Disability for Youth (NCWD/Youth) identified guideposts for the successful transition to adulthood that are

important for all youth, particularly those with disabilities. The guideposts are oriented on the following assumptions:
- Access to high-quality, standards-based education, regardless of the setting
- Information about career options and exposure to the world of work, including structured internships
- Opportunities to develop social, civic, and leadership skills
- Strong connections to caring adults
- Access to safe places to interact with their peers
- Support services and specific accommodations to allow them to become independent adults

The guideposts focus on school-based experiences, career preparation, and work-based learning experiences, connecting activities, youth development and leadership, and family involvement and support.

EDUCATION

For youth with disabilities, access to high-quality education with the necessary support and high expectations helps ensure that they are prepared for postsecondary and career opportunities. The College and Career Readiness and Success Center (CCRS) of the ED developed an issue brief that discusses issues and strategies related to preparation and readiness for postsecondary education and careers. The brief includes examples of current programs and policies that help students with disabilities successfully transition to college and careers.

DISCLOSING DISABILITIES

As youth with disabilities transition from K–12 education, they must recognize that they are no longer entitled to the support that they had received during school. Instead, they must make their needs known in order to receive accommodations that are covered by the law. Youth with disabilities must determine whether or not to disclose their disability within employment or postsecondary education experiences. It may be necessary to support youth as they determine whether it will be beneficial to disclose their disability, when they should disclose it, and what information they need to disclose.

ACCOMMODATIONS ON THE JOB

The Americans with Disabilities Act (ADA) defines an accommodation as "any modification or adjustment to a job or the work environment that will enable a qualified applicant or employee with a disability to participate in the application process or to perform essential job functions. Reasonable accommodation also includes adjustments to assure that a qualified individual with a disability has rights and privileges in employment equal to those of employees without disabilities."

Providing reasonable accommodations when individuals with disabilities disclose their disability and their needed accommodations is a key nondiscrimination requirement in the ADA's employment provisions. It is important for youth and employers to recognize that the accommodations that youth with disabilities need often are not costly for employers. A survey conducted in the fall of 2005 found that the median cost for accommodations was just $600, with about 72 percent of individuals reporting that necessary accommodations were free.

Part 5 | Living with Learning Disabilities

Chapter 38 | Coping with a Learning Disability

Learning disabilities have no cure, but early intervention can lessen their effects. People with learning disabilities can develop ways to cope with their disabilities. Getting help earlier increases the chance of success in school and later in life. If learning disabilities remain untreated, a child may feel frustrated, leading to low self-esteem and other problems.

Experts can help a child learn skills by building on the child's strengths and finding ways to compensate for the child's weaknesses. Interventions vary depending on the nature and extent of the disability.

TIPS FOR MANAGING A LEARNING DISABILITY IN ADULTHOOD

Support from schools can improve elementary and secondary students' math, reading, and other language skills. But how can people with learning disabilities prepare for the demands of university or working life?

Dr. Brett Miller, M.D., directs the reading, writing, and related learning disabilities program within the Child Development and Behavior Branch (CDBB) of the National Institute of Child Health and Human Development (NICHD).

This chapter includes text excerpted from "What Are the Treatments for Learning Disabilities?" *Eunice Kennedy Shriver* National Institute of Child Health and Human Development (NICHD), September 11, 2018. Reviewed November 2022.

Be Your Own Advocate
It is important to know and speak up for what you need. Understand your learning challenges, identify possible solutions, and ask for the resources that will allow you to reach your goals.

Ensure That Your Surroundings Facilitate Success
Work with your school or employer to create a supportive learning environment, such as access to software that will help you succeed now and in the future.

Take Advantage of Assistive Technology
Use computer tools customized to your own pace and needs that can read text aloud, help you articulate your thoughts, and provide structure to your writing.

WAYS TO COPE WITH LEARNING DISABILITIES
Special Education Services
Children diagnosed with learning disabilities can receive special education services. The Individuals with Disabilities Education Act (IDEA) requires that public schools provide free special education supports to children with disabilities.

In most states, each child is entitled to these services beginning at age three and extending through high school or until age 21, whichever comes first. The IDEA rules for each state are available from the Early Childhood Technical Assistance Center (ECTA).

The IDEA requires that children be taught in the least restrictive environment. This means the teaching environment should meet a child's needs and skills while minimizing restrictions to typical learning experiences.

Individualized Education Programs
Children who qualify for special education services will receive an individualized education program (IEP). This personalized and written education plan:
- Lists goals for the child.

Coping with a Learning Disability

- Specifies the services the child will receive.
- Lists the specialists who will work with the child.

Qualifying for Special Education

To qualify for special education services, a child must be evaluated by the school system and meet federal and state guidelines. Parents and caregivers can contact their school principal or special education coordinator to find out how to have their child evaluated.

Interventions for Specific Learning Disabilities

Below are a few ways in which schools help children with specific learning disabilities.

Dyslexia

- **Intensive teaching techniques**. These can include specific, step-by-step, and very methodical approaches to teaching reading to improve spoken and written language skills. These techniques are generally more intensive regarding how often they occur and how long they last and involve small group or one-on-one instruction.
- **Classroom modifications**. Teachers can give students with dyslexia extra time to finish tasks and provide taped tests that allow the child to hear the questions instead of reading them.
- **Use of technology**. Children with dyslexia may benefit from listening to audiobooks or using word-processing programs.

Dysgraphia

- **Special tools**. Teachers can offer oral exams, provide a notetaker, or allow the child to videotape reports instead of writing them. Computer software can facilitate children being able to produce written text.
- **Use of technology**. A child with dysgraphia can be taught to use word processing programs, including

speech-to-text translation, or an audio recorder instead of writing by hand.
- **Reducing the need for writing.** Teachers can provide notes, outlines, and preprinted study sheets.

Dyscalculia
- **Visual techniques.** Teachers can draw pictures of word problems and show the student how to use colored pencils to differentiate parts of problems.
- **Memory aids.** Rhymes and music can help a child remember math concepts.
- **Computers.** A child with dyscalculia can use a computer for drills and practice.

Chapter 39 | Self-Esteem and Children with Learning Disabilities

WHAT IS SELF-ESTEEM?
Self-esteem has to do with the value and respect you have for yourself. Simply put, it is your opinion of yourself.

If you have healthy self-esteem, you feel good about yourself and are proud of what you can do. Having healthy self-esteem can help you feel positive overall. And it can make you brave enough to tackle serious challenges, such as trying out for a school play or standing up to a bully.

If you have low self-esteem, you may not think very highly of yourself. Of course, it is normal to feel down about yourself sometimes. But you may have low self-esteem if you feel bad about yourself more often than good. You can read about rating your self-esteem.

How can low self-esteem hurt? Low self-esteem may stop you from doing things you want to do or from speaking up for yourself. Low self-esteem may even lead you to try to feel better in unhealthy ways, such as using drugs or alcohol. Also, some people may feel so sad or hopeless about themselves that they develop mental health problems such as depression and eating disorders.

This chapter contains text excerpted from the following sources: Text beginning with the heading "What Is Self-Esteem?" is excerpted from "Self-Esteem and Self-Confidence," girlshealth.gov, Office on Women's Health (OWH), February 11, 2015. Reviewed November 2022; Text beginning with the heading "Relationship between Social Support and Self-Esteem" is excerpted from "Perceived Social Support and Self-Esteem in Adolescents with Learning Disabilities at a Private School," U.S. Department of Education (ED), 2008. Reviewed November 2022.

A lot of things can affect self-esteem. These include how others treat you, your background and culture, and your experiences at school. For example, being put down by your boyfriend, classmates, or family or being bullied can affect how you see yourself. But one of the biggest influences on your self-esteem is you!

RELATIONSHIP BETWEEN SOCIAL SUPPORT AND SELF-ESTEEM

The role of perceived social support in developing adolescent self-esteem has become an increasingly important line of research. Researchers believe that social support, or the behaviors and general support from others, can enhance self-esteem and is a critical source of self-worth for developing adolescents. Social support has also been shown to positively affect the adaptations of adolescents at risk of school failure. Research has confirmed the positive relationship between support from friends and family and self-esteem.

Conversely, there is strong evidence that a lack of adequate social support has detrimental effects on self-esteem. Perceptions of familial support may be the most powerful predictor of adolescent self-esteem and remain "the best indicator of emotional problems during adolescence." According to Forman, "The child who … experiences a lack of social support from significant others is likely to demonstrate a considerable degree of emotional distress."

Although the relationship between self-esteem and social support has been validated in numerous investigations involving students with and without learning disabilities, most literature concerning these variables has focused solely on adolescents in public schools. The lack of empirical investigations on adolescent self-esteem and perceived social support among individuals with learning disabilities who attend private schools is unfortunate, considering the potential benefits to the self-esteem of settings where individualized instruction and positive feedback are present.

LEARNING DISABILITIES AND SELF-ESTEEM

While there is wide documentation that compared to their non-learning disabilities peers, students with learning disabilities report a lower self-concept and self-efficacy, especially in the intellectual/

academic domain, and often report lower self-concepts in the social domain, an interesting theme has emerged from the literature. Although students with learning disabilities report a lower self-concept in the academic domain, they are often able to maintain a global self-perception relatively equivalent to that of their nonlearning disabilities peers. One might also expect that for an individual with a learning disability with a negative self-concept related to school achievement, a lower general self-perception would be generalized. However, the literature establishes that individuals with learning disabilities are able to maintain a positive sense of global self-worth despite lower perceptions in the academic domain.

Various explanations have been offered for the tendency of adolescents with learning disabilities to report a low self-concept in the academic domain yet maintain a global self-concept relatively equal to that of nonlearning disabilities students. Some researchers have attributed a positive global self-concept in students with learning disabilities to perceived personal competence in other domains, while others believe that the favorable learning environment created by encouraging feedback from and interaction with teachers or other supporters helps maintain self-esteem. Finally, a small number of investigations have associated attendance at specialized schools for learning disabilities with variances in self-esteem.

THE VALUE OF SPECIAL SCHOOLS FOR STUDENTS WITH LEARNING DISABILITIES

Three particularly relevant inquiries about the self-esteem of children with learning disabilities assert that there are positive benefits to self-esteem for students who attend private schools for learning disabilities. Specifically, Dr. Ruth Butler, Ph.D., senior lecturer at the School of Education, Hebrew University of Jerusalem, and Deganit Marinov Glassman, M.A., psychologist in Jerusalem Municipality, conducted research with students who attended a special school where all students shared a learning disability diagnosis to discover whether isolation from nondisabled peers ultimately undermines or enhances their self-esteem. These researchers supported their belief that students placed in self-contained classrooms, "where their salient reference group consists of other students with disabilities feel more positively about themselves than students who attend regular classes." The authors concluded that children with learning disabilities in special schools in Israel perceived themselves more favorably than students who attended classes in public schools.

Dr. Joep T.A. Bakker, Ph.D., and Dr. Anna M.T. Bosman, Ph.D., assistant professors at Radboud University Nijmegen, explored the well-being of children who attended schools for special education in the Netherlands, arguing against the potentially negative consequences of inclusive education in public schools. Finding that "the self-esteem of children with learning disabilities does not benefit from regular education attendance," the authors firmly concluded that the higher self-image of students in special education schools "warrants heightened attention."

Finally, through qualitative research, Narcie Kelly, a research fellow at the University of Exeter Medical School (UEMS), and Dr. Norwich, Ph.D., professor at the University of Exeter, also found that children with moderate learning disabilities in special schools reported more positive self-perceptions of their educational abilities. Overall, these three distinctive investigations agree and support the notion that students with learning disabilities in special schools exhibit positive outcomes in self-concept.

One theory about why students in an isolated or private school might exhibit high self-esteem is related to the potential support offered by teachers. That is, in classrooms specifically structured to meet the needs of students in small settings, positive support and feedback may foster positive self-perceptions. Given that children's self-perceptions are often affected by their academic achievement, it may be important to consider that in classrooms taught by teachers trained to address the unique academic and social needs of students with learning disabilities and where students of similar abilities attend, self-esteem would be enhanced. "Students may fare better in some classrooms than in others, partly due to different patterns of instructional interactions, and teacher beliefs and attitudes toward students with learning difficulties." Dr. Jordan and Dr. Stanovich from Department of Curriculum, Teaching and Learning, Ontario Institute for Studies in Education, University of Toronto, found that students who had teachers who saw themselves as responsible for their student's achievement reported significantly higher self-esteem scores than did students of teachers who do not maintain such a philosophy. The classroom environment, therefore, is particularly important for students with learning disabilities.

Another relevant investigation explored the importance of social support for self-concept in a private school. This study sought to determine whether supportive teachers exerted more influence on scholastic self-concept than classmates or friends or whether peers played an important role in determining nonacademic self-concepts. In this study, students who attended a private school for learning disabilities reported levels of general self-esteem no different from those who attended a university clinic. It is worthwhile to acknowledge that Forman used a very small sample of students in the private school, causing the researchers to express the possibility that "the small number of subjects in both resource and regular classroom placements made it difficult to achieve statistically significant differences." In the same research, Forman also compared students in a private school to students diagnosed in a university clinic and attending various placements. The finding that "school placement did not seem to affect self-concept in this sample of subjects" seems unclear, given there was no comparison between private and public per se. The limitations noted in Forman's investigation related to the small sample size and differing definitions of school placement warrant consideration when interpreting those findings and applying them to the current study.

In 2007, the learning disabilities resources listed over 260 independent kindergartens through grade 12 schools with learning disabilities support programs in the United States, not including learning centers, reading clinics, or tutors. However, to date, a limited number of investigators have chosen to focus on this population. The current investigation was an attempt to extend the findings of prior research on adolescents who attend private schools for students with learning disabilities outside of the United States by investigating a sample of students in the United States. If students with learning disabilities at a private school display greater levels of self-esteem than their peers with or without learning disabilities in public school, efforts should be undertaken to identify the students who would most benefit from a private setting.

The results of the investigation potentially impact the decision-making process for parents, practitioners, administrators, and researchers. Understanding that social support and school placement can influence self-esteem can help parents and practitioners provide the most supportive environment for their children at home and school and enable them to choose the most appropriate school environment for their children with learning disabilities. Furthermore, given the potentially damaging effects of low self-esteem, determining the most beneficial school environment offers a promising model for administrators who seek to foster favorable self-esteem in their students.

Chapter 40 | Parenting a Child with a Learning Disability

You all want to keep your children safe and secure and help them be happy and healthy. Preventing injuries and harm is not very different for children with disabilities compared to children without disabilities. However, finding the right information and learning about the kinds of risks children might face at different ages is often not easy for parents of children with disabilities. Each child is different—and the general recommendations available to keep children safe should be tailored to fit your child's skills and abilities. There are steps that parents and caregivers can take to keep children with disabilities safe.

To keep all children safe, parents and caregivers need to:
- Know and learn about what health concerns or special conditions are unique for their child.
- Plan ways to protect their child and share the plan with others.
- Remember that their child's needs for protection will change over time.

This chapter contains text excerpted from the following sources: Text begins with excerpts from "Keeping Children with Disabilities Safe," Centers for Disease Control and Prevention (CDC), September 17, 2019; Text under the heading "Suggestions and Considerations for Parents" is excerpted from "Learning Disabilities (LD)," Center for Parent Information & Resources (CPIR), U.S. Department of Education (ED), July 2015. Reviewed November 2022.

WHAT CAN PARENTS AND CAREGIVERS DO?

Parents or caregivers can talk to their child's doctor or health-care professional about keeping them safe. Your child's teacher or child-care provider might also have some good ideas. Once you have ideas about keeping your child safe, make a safety plan, explain it to your child, and share it with other adults who might be able to help if needed.

Following are some things to consider when making a safety plan for your child.

Moving Around and Handling Things

Does your child have challenges with moving around and handling things around them? Sometimes, children are faced with unsafe situations, especially in new places. Children with limited ability to move, see, hear, or make decisions and children who do not feel or understand pain might not realize that something is unsafe or have trouble getting away.

Take a look around the place where your child will be to make sure every area your child can reach is safe for your child. Check your child's clothing and toys—are they suitable for her or his abilities, not just age and size? For example, clothing and toys meant for older children might have strings that are not safe for a child who cannot easily untangle themselves, or toys might have small parts that are not safe for children who are still mouthing toys.

Safety Equipment

Do you have the right kind of safety equipment? Safety equipment is often developed for age and size and less for ability.

For example, a major cause of child death is motor vehicle crashes. Keeping your child safe in the car is important. When choosing the right car seat, you might need to consider whether your child has difficulties sitting up or sitting still in the seat, in addition to your child's age, height, and weight. If you have a child with disabilities, talk to your health-care professional about the best type of car seat or booster seat and the proper seat position for your child. You can also ask a certified child passenger safety technician trained in special needs.

Parenting a Child with a Learning Disability

Other examples of special safety equipment are as follows:
- Life jackets may need to be specially fitted for your child.
- Smoke alarms that signal with a light and vibration may be better in a home where there is a child who cannot hear.
- Handrails and safety bars can be put into homes to help a child who has difficulty moving around or is at a greater risk of falling.

Speak to your health-care professional about the right equipment for your child and have this equipment ready and available before you may need it.

Talking and Understanding

Does your child have problems with talking or understanding? Children who have problems communicating might have a limited ability to learn about safety and danger.

For example, children who cannot hear might miss spoken instructions. Children who have trouble understanding or remembering might not learn about safety as easily as other children. Children who have difficulty communicating might not be able to ask questions about safety. Adults might think children with disabilities are aware of dangers when they are not.

Parents and caregivers may need to find different ways to teach their children about safety, such as:
- Showing them what to do.
- Using pretend play to rehearse.
- Practicing regularly.

Parents and caregivers may need to find ways to let their children communicate that they are in danger. For example, you might teach your child to use a whistle, bell, or alarm that can alert others to danger. Tell adults who take care of your child about the ways to communicate with your child if there is any danger.

It is also useful to contact your local fire department and explain any special circumstances you have so that they do not have to rely on the child or others to explain their special needs in an emergency.

Making Decisions

Does your child have problems with making decisions? Children might have limited ability to make decisions either because of developmental delays or limits in their thinking skills or in their ability to stop themselves from doing things they want but should not do.

For example, children with attention deficit hyperactivity disorder (ADHD) or fetal alcohol spectrum disorders (FASDs) might be very impulsive and fail to think about the results of their actions. People often put more dangerous things higher up so that little child cannot reach them. Your older child might be able to reach something that she or he is not ready to handle safely. Check your child's environment, particularly new places.

Some children might also have problems distinguishing when situations and people are safe or dangerous. They might not know what to do. Parents and caregivers can give children specific instructions on how to behave in certain situations that might become dangerous.

Moving and Exploring

Does your child have enough chances to move and explore? Children with disabilities often need some extra protection. But, just like all children, they also need to move and explore to develop healthy bodies and minds.

Some parents of children with special needs worry about their children needing extra protection. It is not possible to protect children from every bump and bruise. Exploring can help children learn what is safe and what might be difficult or dangerous. Being fit and healthy can help children stay safe, and an active lifestyle is important for long-term health.

Children with disabilities might find it hard to take part in sports and active play—for example, equipment may need to be adjusted; coaches may need extra information and support to help a child with a disability; or a communication problem may make it more difficult for some children to play as part of a team.

Talk to your child's teachers, potential coaches, care providers, or health professionals about ways to find the right balance between being safe and being active.

Parenting a Child with a Learning Disability

OTHER CONCERNS

Do you have other concerns? Every child is different. This is not a complete list of questions and concerns; these are just examples. Your questions and concerns may be different. Speak with your health-care provider, teacher, or childcare provider to learn more about keeping your child safe.

SUGGESTIONS AND CONSIDERATIONS FOR PARENTS

A child with learning disabilities may need help at home and school. Here are several suggestions and considerations for parents:

- **Learn about learning disabilities**. The more you know, the more you can help yourself and your child. Take advantage of the excellent resources for parents.
- **Praise your child when she or he does well**. Children with learning disabilities are often very good at various things. Find out what your child enjoys doing, such as dancing, playing soccer, or working with computers. Give your child plenty of opportunities to pursue her or his strengths and talents.
- **Find out the ways your child learns best**. Does she or he learn by hands-on practice, looking, or listening? Help your child learn through her or his areas of strength.
- **Let your daughter or son help with household chores**. These can build self-confidence and concrete skills. Keep instructions simple, break down tasks into smaller steps, and reward your child's efforts with praise.
- **Make homework a priority**. Read more about how to help your child be a success at homework.
- **Pay attention to your child's mental health (and your own!)**. Be open to counseling, which can help your child deal with frustration, feel better about herself or himself, and learn more about social skills.
- **Talk to other parents whose children have learning disabilities**. Parents can share practical advice and

emotional support. You can identify parent groups in your area.
- **Meet with school personnel and help develop an individualized education plan (IEP) team to address your child's needs.** Plan what accommodations your child needs and do not forget to discuss accessible instructional materials (AIM) or assistive technology!
- **Establish a positive working relationship with your child's teacher.** Through regular communication, exchange information about your child's progress at home and school.

Chapter 41 | Bullying and Learning Disabilities: What Parents Need to Know

Bullying does not just happen to the smallest kid in the class. Children who bully others target those who seem to be less powerful or not as strong. Children who bully others also often target children who seem different. Children with disabilities or chronic diseases are sometimes more likely to be bullied than children without disabilities.

Bullying, teasing, and harassment should not be considered normal rites of passage or kids just being kids. The effects of bullying can be serious, including depression, low self-esteem, health problems, and even suicide. Adults can help prevent bullying by teaching children about bullying, giving them tools for what to do if they are being bullied, and taking steps to protect children's legal right not to be bullied.

WHAT IS BULLYING?

Bullying is unwanted, aggressive behavior involving a real or perceived power imbalance. The aggressive behavior is repeated, or has the potential to be repeated, over time.

This chapter contains text excerpted from the following sources: Text begins with excerpts from "People with Disabilities and Chronic Diseases: Information about Bullying," Centers for Disease Control and Prevention (CDC), June 25, 2020; Text under the heading "Parents' Responsibility in Preventing Bullying" is excerpted from "What You Can Do," StopBullying.gov, U.S. Department of Health and Human Services (HHS), November 10, 2021.

Types of Bullying
The following are three types of bullying:
- **Physical**. Physical bullying involves hurting a person's body or possessions. Physical bullying includes hitting/kicking/pinching, spitting, tripping/pushing, taking or breaking someone's things, and making mean or rude hand gestures.
- **Verbal**. Verbal bullying is saying or writing mean things. Verbal bullying includes teasing, name-calling, inappropriate sexual comments, taunting, and threatening to cause harm.
- **Social**. Social bullying, sometimes referred to as relational bullying, involves hurting someone's reputation or relationships. Social bullying includes leaving someone out on purpose, telling other children not to be friends with someone, spreading rumors about someone, or embarrassing someone in public.

Verbal and social bullying can also come in the form of electronic aggression (e.g., cyberbullying using the Internet or cell phones). It can include threatening, embarrassing, or insulting emails and texts.

THE EFFECTS OF BULLYING
Children and youth who are bullied are more likely than other children to:
- Be depressed, lonely, and anxious.
- Have low self-esteem.
- Experience headaches, stomachaches, tiredness, and poor eating.
- Be absent from school, dislike school, and have poorer school performance.
- Think about suicide or plan for suicide.

Some children with disabilities have low self-esteem or feel depressed, lonely, or anxious because of their disability, and bullying may worsen this. Bullying can cause serious, lasting problems

Bullying and Learning Disabilities: What Parents Need to Know

not only for children who are bullied but also for children who bully and those who witness bullying.

WAYS TO PREVENT BULLYING

Parents, school staff, and other caring adults can help prevent bullying. They can do the following:
- **Explain bullying**. Children do not always know when they are bullied. They might feel bad but do not know how to talk about it. Children with disabilities that affect how they think, learn, or interact with others might need a very detailed explanation about how to recognize bullying when it happens to themselves or others.
- **Teach children what to do**. Children need assistance learning what to do to protect themselves from bullying and help others who are being bullied. They might need the following:
  - Very specific instructions are tailored to them, particularly if they have disabilities that affect how they think, learn, or interact with others.
  - To be encouraged to always reach out to a trusted adult.
  - To learn to recognize and avoid situations where bullying occurs.

Here are ways to teach children how to respond to bullying:
- Talk with them often about what they have experienced and think about different ways to respond.
- Practice with them how to act and respond to bullying by using role plays.
- Suggest ways to respond to children who bully others, including telling them to stop, use humor, walk away, and get help.

Children might not always know when they are bullying another child. Children whose disabilities impact their thinking, learning, or social skills might need extra help learning how to express themselves concerning others.

- **Protect your child's legal rights.** Your child has the right not to be harassed by peers, school personnel, or other adults. Disability harassment is discrimination that violates Section 504 of the Individuals with Disabilities Education Act (IDEA) and its regulations. Titles II and III of the Americans with Disabilities Act (ADA) also address harassment.

PARENTS' RESPONSIBILITY IN PREVENTING BULLYING

Parents play a key role in preventing and responding to bullying. If you know or suspect that your child is involved in bullying, there are several resources that may help.

- **Recognize the warning signs that your child is involved in bullying.** They could be being bullied, bullying others, or witnessing bullying. Although these signs could signal other issues, you should talk to your child if they display any sort of behavioral or emotional changes. Many times kids will not ask for help, so it is important to know what to look for. If your child is at immediate risk of harming herself or himself or others, get help right away.
- **Learn what bullying is and what it is not.** Understanding what bullying is the first step in forming a plan to prevent or respond to bullying with your child. Many behaviors that look like bullying may be just as serious but may require different response strategies. You can also learn about the following:
  - The frequency of bullying
  - Who is at risk of being bullied and bullying others
  - The effects of bullying
- **Cyberbullying often requires different strategies than in-person bullying.** Learn how to work with your kids to prevent cyberbullying and how to respond when it occurs.
- **Utilize tips and tools to talk to your child about bullying.** Opening lines of communication before your child is involved in bullying makes it easier for them to

Bullying and Learning Disabilities: What Parents Need to Know

tell you when something happens. It is also important to work with a school to help prevent bullying before it starts.
- **If you know or suspect bullying has occurred, learn how to find out what has happened to your child.** Understanding what has happened can also help in communicating with school or community officials about the situation.
- **If you have determined bullying has occurred, learn how you and school or community officials can work together to support your child, whether they were bullied, bullied others, or witnessed bullying.** Learn also about considerations for specific groups.
- **If bullying is occurring at school, learn about what your state requires schools to do in your state's anti-bullying law.** Learn also about federal laws that require schools to address harassment based on race, color, national origin, sex, and disabilities and ways to report situations that have not been adequately addressed to the U.S. Departments of Education (ED) and the U.S. Departments of Justice (DOJ).
- **If you have worked with your child and your school and need additional assistance, find resources to help address the situation.**

Chapter 42 | Preparing for Adulthood: Tips for Adolescents with Learning Disabilities

Life is full of transitions; one of the more remarkable ones occurs when you get ready to leave high school and go out in the world as a young adult. When the student has a disability, planning ahead for that transition is especially helpful. In fact, the Individuals with Disabilities Education Act (IDEA) requires it.

QUICK SUMMARY OF THE TRANSITION
Transition services are intended to prepare students to move from the world of school to the world of adulthood. Transition planning begins during high school at the latest. The IDEA requires that transition planning starts when the student reaches the age of 16. Transition planning may start earlier (when the student is younger than 16) if the individualized education program (IEP) team decides it would be appropriate. Transition planning is part of developing the student's IEP. The IEP team (which includes the student and the parents) develops the transition plan.

The student must be invited to any IEP meeting where postsecondary goals and transition services needed to reach those goals

---

This chapter includes text excerpted from "Transition to Adulthood," Center for Parent Information & Resources (CPIR), U.S. Department of Education (ED), February 2018. Reviewed November 2022.

will be considered. The IEP team considers areas such as postsecondary education or vocational training, employment, independent living, and community participation in transition planning. Transition services must be a coordinated set of activities oriented toward producing results. Transition services are oriented on the student's needs and must take into account her or his preferences and interests.

INDIVIDUALS WITH DISABILITIES EDUCATION ACT'S DEFINITION OF TRANSITION SERVICES

Any discussion of transition services must begin with its definition in law. The IDEA's definition of transition services appears at §300.43. It is rather long, but let us see it in its entirety first and then discuss it in parts.

§300.43 Transition services:
- The term "transition services" mean a coordinated set of activities for a child with a disability that:
  - Is designed to be within a results-oriented process that is focused on improving the academic and functional achievement of the child with a disability to facilitate the child's movement from school to postschool activities, including postsecondary education, vocational education, integrated employment (including supported employment), continuing and adult education, adult services, independent living, or community participation.
  - Is oriented on the individual child's needs, taking into account the child's strengths, preferences, and interests. Includes instruction, related services, community experiences, the development of employment and other postschool adult living objectives, and, if appropriate, acquisition of daily living skills and provision of a functional vocational evaluation.
- Transition services for children with disabilities may be special education provided as specially designed instruction or a related service if required to assist a child with a disability to benefit from special education.

Preparing for Adulthood: Tips for Adolescents with Learning Disabilities

CONSIDERING THE DEFINITION
Several keywords in the definition above capture important concepts about transition services:
- Activities need to be coordinated with each other.
- The process focuses on results.
- Activities must address the child's academic and functional achievement.
- Activities are intended to smooth the young person's movement into the postschool world.

You can also see that the definition mentions independent and adult living domains: the community, employment, adult services, daily living skills, vocational, and postsecondary education. This acknowledges that adulthood involves a wide range of skill areas and activities. It also clarifies that preparing a child with a disability to perform functionally across this spectrum of areas and activities may involve considerable planning, attention, and focused coordinated services.

Note that word—coordinated. Transition activities should not be haphazard or scattershot. Services are to be planned in sync to drive toward a result.

What result might that be? From a federal perspective, the result sought can be found in the first finding of Congress in the IDEA, which refers to "our national policy of ensuring equality of opportunity, full participation, independent living, and economic self-sufficiency for individuals with disabilities" (20 U.S.C. 1400(c)(1)). Preparing children with disabilities to "lead productive and independent adult lives, to the maximum extent possible," is one of IDEA's stated objectives (20 U.S.C. 1400(c)(5)(A)(ii)).

STUDENTS AT THE HEART OF PLANNING THEIR TRANSITION
For the students themselves, transition activities are personally defined. This means that the postsecondary goals developed for a student must consider her or his interests, preferences, needs, and strengths. To make sure of this, the school:
- Must invite the youth with a disability to attend the IEP team meeting "if the purpose of the meeting will be the

consideration of the postsecondary goals for the child and the transition services needed to assist the child in reaching those goals under §300.320(b)."
- "Must take other steps to ensure that the child's preferences and interests are considered" if the child cannot attend.

Keep the importance of student involvement in mind because many excellent materials and guides are available to help students become involved in their own transition planning, and there are many good reasons to do so.

WHEN MUST TRANSITION SERVICES BE INCLUDED IN THE INDIVIDUALIZED EDUCATION PROGRAM?

What is not apparent in IDEA's definition of transition services but nonetheless critical to mention is the timing of transition-related planning and services: When must transition planning begin? The answer lies in a different provision related to the content of the IEP. From §300.320(b):

- **Transition services**. Beginning not later than the first IEP to be in effect when the child turns 16, or younger if determined appropriate by the IEP Team, and updated annually, thereafter, the IEP must include:
  - Appropriate measurable postsecondary goals oriented upon age-appropriate transition assessments related to training, education, employment, and, where appropriate, independent living skills
  - Transition services (including courses of study) needed to assist the child in reaching those goals

So the IEP must include transition goals by the time the student is 16. That age frame, though, is not cast in concrete. Note that in keeping with the individualized nature of the IEP, the IEP team has the authority to begin transition-related considerations earlier in a student's life if team members (which include the parent and the student with a disability) think it is appropriate, given the student's needs and preferences.

Preparing for Adulthood: Tips for Adolescents with Learning Disabilities

A CLOSER LOOK AT WHAT TO INCLUDE IN THE INDIVIDUALIZED EDUCATION PROGRAM

Breaking the provisions at §300.320(b) into their component parts is a useful way to see what needs to be included in the student's IEP. This is also where the rubber meets the road, so to speak because what is included in the IEP must:

- State the student's postsecondary goals (what she or he hopes to achieve after leaving high school).
- Be broken down into IEP goals that represent the steps along the way that the student needs to take while still in high school to get ready for achieving the postsecondary goals after high school.
- Detail the transition services that the student will receive to support her or his achieving the IEP goals.

Writing goal statements can be challenging because it is not always obvious what needs to be included in a goal statement. Goal writing is a topic worthy of an entire discussion on its own. This chapter is to shed light on how to write transition-related goals statements—both postsecondary goals and the corresponding IEP goals.

THE DOMAINS OF ADULTHOOD TO CONSIDER

The definition of transition services mentions specific domains of adulthood to be addressed during transition planning. To recap, these are:

- Postsecondary education
- Vocational education
- Integrated employment (including supported employment)
- Continuing and adult education
- Adult services
- Independent living
- Community participation

These are the areas to be explored by the IEP team to determine what types of transition-related support and services a student with a disability needs. It is easy to see how planning ahead in each of these areas, and developing goal statements and corresponding services for the student, can greatly assist that student in preparing for life after high school.

TYPES OF ACTIVITIES TO CONSIDER

Remember that the Individuals with Disabilities Education Act (IDEA) definition of transition services states that these are a "coordinated set of activities" designed within a results-oriented process. Specific activities are also mentioned, which gives the IEP team insight into the range of activities to be considered in each of the domains above:

- Instruction
- Related services
- Community experiences
- The development of employment and other postschool adult living objectives
- If appropriate, the acquisition of daily living skills and provision of a functional vocational evaluation

Confused by all these lists? Unnecessary and unclear. The IEP team must discuss and decide whether the student needs transition services and activities (e.g., instruction, related services, community experiences, etc.) to prepare for the different domains of adulthood (postsecondary education, vocational education, employment, adult services, independent living, etc.). That is a lot of ground to cover!

But it is essential if the student's transition to the adult world is to be facilitated. A spectrum of adult activities is evident here, from community to employment, from being able to take care of oneself (e.g., daily living skills) to considering other adult objectives and undertakings.

Chapter 43 | Overview of Independent Living

Independent living is about life, and it is about choice, seeing to your own affairs, and pursuing your talents, interests, passions, and selfhood as independently as possible. You all must see young people grow to adulthood and find their place in the world, doing for themselves to the best of their ability.

Disability can complicate independence, to be sure, which is why independent living can be an important part of helping a young person with a disability get ready for life after high school. The more involved the disability, the more likely it is that independent living will be a subject of serious discussion—and preparation.

This chapter is designed to help you and yours take apart the concept of independent living, examine its many elements, and put the concept back together with concrete plans and insight into what it takes to turn it into reality.

PHILOSOPHICAL UNDERPINNINGS

One search of the web using the term "independent living" clearly shows that a great deal of passion and commitment exists in the independent living movement and community. It is rather breathtaking. You will see phrases such as all people achieving their maximum potential, barrier-free society, self-determination, self-respect, dignity, equal opportunities, consumer-driven, and empowerment. At its heart, the passion in the independent

This chapter includes text excerpted from "Independent Living Connections," Center for Parent Information & Resources (CPIR), U.S. Department of Education (ED), March 2019.

living community is fueled by individuals with disabilities. And it is worldwide, this passion for selfhood.

Independent living does not mean that you want to do everything by yourself and do not need anybody or that you want to live in isolation. Independent living means that you demand the same choices and control in your everyday lives that your nondisabled brothers and sisters, neighbors, and friends take for granted. You want to grow up in your family, go to the neighborhood school, use the same bus as your neighbors, work jobs that align with your education and interests, and start families of your own. You are profoundly ordinary people sharing the same need to feel included, recognized, and loved.

You will find this sentiment, this fierce independence, echoed in a thousand websites, brochures, training materials, and resource guides because selfhood matters.

DEFINING INDEPENDENT LIVING

The Center on Transition Innovations (centerontransition.org) posts the following definition of independent living.

Independent living is "those skills or tasks that contribute to the successful independent functioning of an individual in adulthood." You often categorize these skills into the major areas related to your daily lives, such as housing, personal care, transportation, and social and recreational opportunities.

Each of these areas related to your daily life has its own aspects and concerns that the individual education program (IEP) team will want to consider and plan ahead for, as appropriate for the student's needs and plans.

DOES THE STUDENT NEED TRANSITION PLANNING AND SERVICES IN THE DOMAIN OF INDEPENDENT LIVING?

It is important to understand that not all students with disabilities will need an in-depth investigation of, and preparation for, independent living after high school. As the U.S. Department of Education (ED) stated in its analysis of comments and changes:
- The only area in which postsecondary goals are not required in the IEP is in the area of independent

Overview of Independent Living

living skills. Goals in the area of independent living are required only if appropriate. It is up to the child's IEP team to determine whether IEP goals related to developing independent living skills are appropriate and necessary for the child to receive free and appropriate public education (FAPE).

Whether or not will very much depend on the nature and severity of the student's disability. As the department notes, it is up to each student's IEP team to decide if planning for independent living is needed. If the team feels that the student can benefit from transition planning and services in this domain, then independent living will be an area of discussion during IEP meetings where the transition is discussed. If the student with whom you are involved will need transition planning and services in the domain of independent living, then keep reading.

WHAT IS INVOLVED IN INDEPENDENT LIVING?

Independent living clearly involves many activities, skills, and learning needs. Consider just the three mentioned in the definition posted at the National Secondary Transition Technical Assistance Center (NSTTAC):

- Leisure/recreation
- Home maintenance and personal care
- Community participation

Each of these can be broken down in its own turn to include more skills, activities, and learning needs. Just think about what is involved in "home maintenance and personal care" alone: everything from brushing teeth, to shopping for food, to cooking it, to cleaning up afterward, getting ready for bed, locking the front door, and setting the alarm clock for the next day. It is enough to boggle the mind, all the little facets and skills of taking care of ourselves as best you can, with support or solo.

So how is an IEP team take on the task of planning for a student's independent living in the future? Much will depend on the nature and severity of the student's disability. Some students will not need transition planning or services to prepare for independent living. Others will need a limited amount targeted at specific areas of need or interest. And still others, especially those with significant support needs, will need to give independent living their focused attention.

Fortunately, a great deal has been written about independent living skills, and you would not reinvent that wheel. Have a look at some of these resources. They will more than give you food for thought about what to consider for yourself or yours, as will any local or state policy at work in your area.

INDEPENDENT LIVING CENTERS

One of the most useful resources in the independent living area is the nationwide network of independent living centers (ILCs; www.acces.nysed.gov/vr/independent-living-centers). ILCs are nonresidential, community-based agencies run by people with various disabilities. ILCs help people with disabilities achieve and maintain self-sufficient lives within the community. Operated locally, ILCs serve a particular region, meaning their services vary from place to place. ILCs may charge for classes, but advocacy services are available at no cost.

Chapter 44 | Information about Special Needs Trust

POLICY FOR SPECIAL NEEDS TRUSTS ESTABLISHED UNDER SECTION 1917(D)(4)(A) OF THE ACT
General Rules for Special Needs Trusts Established on or after December 13, 2016

Section 5007 of this act allows individuals to establish their special needs trusts and qualify for the exception of resource counting under Section 1917(d)(4)(A) of the Social Security Act.

The resource counting provisions of Section 1613(e) do not apply to a trust that:
- Contains the assets of an individual under age 65 and disabled.
- It was established for such individuals' benefit through the actions of the individual, a parent, a grandparent, a legal guardian, or a court.
- Provides that the state(s) will receive all amounts remaining in the trust upon the individual's death up to a sum equal to the total medical assistance paid on behalf of the individual under a state Medicaid plan.

Who Established the Trust?

The special needs trust exception applies to a trust established through the actions of:
- The individual
- The parent(s)

This chapter includes text excerpted from "Program Operations Manual System (POMS)," U.S. Social Security Administration (SSA), June 9, 2022.

- The grandparent(s)
- The legal guardian(s)
- The court

POWER OF ATTORNEY

A trust is established under a power of attorney (POA) for the disabled individual to be established through the actions of the disabled individual because the POA establishes an agency relationship.

USE OF A SEED TRUST

If the legally competent, disabled adult does not establish the trust, a parent or grandparent may establish a "seed" trust using a nominal amount of her or his own money or, if state law allows, an empty or dry trust. After the seed trust is established, the legally competent, a disabled adult may transfer her or his own assets into the trust, or another individual with legal authority (such as a power of attorney) may transfer the individual's assets into the trust.

Legal Authority and Trusts

The person or entity establishing the trust with the assets of the legally competent, disabled individual or transferring the individual's assets into the trust must have the legal authority to act for the individual's assets. Attempting to establish a trust with the assets of another individual without proper legal authority to act concerning the individual's assets will generally result in an invalid trust under state law.

For example, John, who is establishing a seed trust for his adult child with his assets, has legal authority over his own assets to establish the trust. He needs legal authority over his child's assets only if he takes action with them by transferring them into a previously established trust.

A POA can establish legal authority to act concerning an individual's assets. A trust established under a POA for the disabled individual will result in a trust that is considered to be established through the actions of the disabled individual herself or himself

Information about Special Needs Trust

because the POA establishes an agency relationship. A third party can use the POA for the trust beneficiary as the legal authority to establish a trust or to transfer assets of the beneficiary into the trust, as long as the POA provides the proper authority to do so.

POLICY FOR POOLED TRUSTS ESTABLISHED UNDER SECTION 1917(D)(4)(C) OF THE ACT
General Rules for Pooled Trusts

A pooled trust contains the assets of many different individuals, each held in separate trust accounts and established through the actions of individuals for separate beneficiaries. By analogy, the pooled trust is like a bank that holds the assets of individual account holders. A pooled trust is established and managed by a nonprofit organization. The pooled trust instruments usually consist of an overarching "master trust" and a joinder agreement that contains provisions specific to the individual beneficiary.

Whenever you are evaluating the trust, it is important to distinguish between the master trust, which is established through the actions of the nonprofit association, and the individual trust accounts within the master trust, which are established through the actions of the individual or another person or entity for the individual, through a joinder agreement.

The resource-counting provisions of Section 1613(e) of the act do not apply to a trust containing the assets of a disabled individual that meets the following conditions:

- The pooled trust is established and managed by a nonprofit association.
- Separate accounts are maintained for each beneficiary, but assets are pooled for investment and management purposes.
- Accounts are established solely for the benefit of disabled individuals.
- The account in the trust is established through the actions of the individual, a parent, a grandparent, a legal guardian, or a court.
- The trust provides that to the extent that any amounts remaining in the beneficiary's account, upon the

death of the beneficiary, are not retained by the trust, the trust will pay to the state(s) from such remaining amounts in the account an amount equal to the total amount of medical assistance paid on behalf of the beneficiary under state Medicaid plan(s).

Disabled

To qualify for the pooled trust exception, the individual whose assets were used to establish the trust account must be disabled for supplemental security income (SSI) purposes under Section 1614(a)(3) of the act as of the date on which the trust account's resource status could affect the individual's SSI eligibility. This also includes individuals aged 65 and older.

Nonprofit Association

The pooled trust must be established and maintained by the actions of a nonprofit association. For the pooled trust exception, a nonprofit association is an organization established and certified under a state nonprofit statute.

Separate Account

A separate account within the trust must be maintained for each beneficiary of the pooled trust. However, for purposes of investment and management of funds, the trust may pool the funds in individual accounts. The trust must be able to provide an individual accounting for each individual.

Established for the Sole Benefit of the Individual

Under the pooled trust exception, the individual trust account must be established for the sole benefit of the disabled individual. This exception does not apply if the trust account:
- Provides a benefit to any other individual or entity during the disabled individual's lifetime.
- Allows termination of the trust account before the individual's death and payment of the corpus to another individual or entity.

Information about Special Needs Trust

Who Established the Trust Account?
To qualify for the pooled trust exception, the trust account must have been established through the actions of:
- The disabled individual herself or himself
- The disabled individual's parent(s)
- The disabled individual's grandparent(s)
- The disabled individual's legal guardian(s)
- A court

A legally competent, disabled adult establishing or adding to a trust account with her or his own assets has the legal authority to act on her or his own behalf. A third party establishing a trust account on behalf of a disabled individual with that individual's assets must have the legal authority to act on the individual's assets. An attempt to establish a trust account by a third party with the assets of a disabled individual without the legal right or authority to act with respect to that individual's assets will generally result in an invalid trust under state law. If there is a question regarding authority, consult your precedents or regional chief counsel.

A POA is a legal authority to act concerning an individual's assets. A pooled trust account may be established under a POA given by the individual, a parent, or a grandparent.

Court-Established Trusts
In the case of a trust account established through the actions of a court, the creation of the trust account must be required by court order for the exception in Section 1917(d)(4)(C) of the act to apply. That is, the pooled trust exception can be met when courts approve petitions and establish trust accounts by court order, so long as the execution of the trust account joinder agreement and funding of the trust has not been completed before the court issues the order. Court approval of an already executed pooled trust account joinder agreement is not sufficient for the trust account to qualify for the exception. The court must specifically either establish the trust account or order the establishment of the trust account.
- **Example of a court ordering establishment of a trust account.** John is a legally competent adult who

inherited $250,000 and is an SSI recipient. His sister, Justine, petitioned the court to create and order an account in the Chesapeake Pooled Trust. Justine also provided the court with an unsigned draft of the trust document. A month later, the court approved the petition and issued an order requiring the creation and funding of the trust account. The fact that the trust beneficiary is a competent adult and could have established the trust account himself is not a factor in the resource determination.

- **Example of a court-established trust account**. Mary, a legally incompetent SSI recipient, wins a lawsuit in the amount of $50,000. As part of the settlement, the judge ordered the creation of a pooled trust account for Mary to receive the $50,000. As a direct result of this court order, a pooled trust account was created with Mary's settlement money. The pooled trust records and documentation of the initial deposit list $50,000 as the initial principal amount.
- **Example of a court-approved trust account**. Jane is ineligible for SSI benefits because she has a self-established pooled trust account that does not meet the requirements for exception in SI 01120.203D, stating the pooled trust has to be established and managed by a nonprofit association. A for-profit association is managing Jane's pooled trust. The pooled trust changed management to a nonprofit association to satisfy the requirement. Jane petitioned the court to establish an amended trust account joinder agreement and to make the order retroactive so that her original trust account would become exempt from resource counting from its creation. The court approved the petition and issued a nunc pro tunc order stating that the court established the trust account as of the date Jane had previously established the trust account herself.

Information about Special Needs Trust

State Medicaid Reimbursement Provision

To qualify for the pooled trust exception, the trust must contain specific language that provides that to the extent that amounts remaining in the individual's account upon the death of the individual are not retained by the trust, the trust will pay to the state(s) from such remaining amounts in the account an amount equal to the total amount of medical assistance paid on behalf of the individual under the state Medicaid plan(s).

The trust must provide payback to any state(s) that has provided medical assistance under the state Medicaid plan(s) and not be limited to any particular state(s). Medicaid payback also cannot be limited to any particular period of time; for example, payback cannot be limited to the period after the establishment of the trust.

If the trust does not have sufficient funds upon the beneficiary's death to reimburse each state that provided medical assistance, the trust may reimburse the states on a pro rata or proportional basis.

Chapter 45 | **Understanding Disability Inclusion**

WHAT IS DISABILITY INCLUSION?

Including people with disabilities in everyday activities and encouraging them to have roles similar to their peers who do not have a disability is disability inclusion. This involves more than simply encouraging people; it requires ensuring that adequate policies and practices are in effect in a community or organization.

Inclusion should lead to increased participation in socially expected life roles and activities—such as being a student, worker, friend, community member, patient, spouse, partner, or parent.

Socially expected activities may include social activities, using public resources such as transportation and libraries, moving about within communities, receiving adequate health care, having relationships, and enjoying other day-to-day activities.

DISABILITY INCLUSION AND THE HEALTH OF PEOPLE WITH DISABILITIES

Disability inclusion allows people with disabilities to take advantage of the same health promotion and prevention activities experienced by people who do not have a disability. These activities include:
- Education and counseling programs that promote physical activity, improve nutrition, and reduce tobacco, alcohol, or drug use

---

This chapter includes text excerpted from "Disability Inclusion," Centers for Disease Control and Prevention (CDC), September 16, 2020.

- Blood pressure and cholesterol assessment during annual health exams and screening for illnesses such as cancer, diabetes, and heart disease

Including people with disabilities in these activities begins with identifying and eliminating barriers to participation.

IMPORTANCE OF DISABILITY INCLUSION

Disability affects approximately 61 million, or nearly one in four (26%) people in the United States. Disability affects more than one billion people worldwide. According to the United Nations Convention on the Rights of Persons with Disabilities (CRPD), people with disabilities include those who have long-term physical, mental, intellectual, or sensory (such as hearing or vision) impairments that in interaction with various barriers may hinder their full and effective participation in society on an equal basis with others.

People with disabilities experience significant disadvantages when it comes to health, such as:

- Adults with disabilities are three times more likely to have heart disease, stroke, diabetes, or cancer than adults without disabilities.
- Adults with disabilities are more likely than adults without disabilities to be current smokers.
- Women with disabilities are less likely than women without disabilities to have received a breast cancer x-ray test (mammogram) during the past two years.

Although disability is associated with health conditions (such as arthritis, mental, or emotional conditions) or events (such as injuries), the functioning, health, independence, and engagement in the society of people with disabilities can vary depending on several factors:

- The severity of the underlying impairment
- Social, political, and cultural influences and expectations

Understanding Disability Inclusion

- Aspects of natural and built surroundings
- Availability of assistive technology and devices
- Family and community support and engagement

Disability inclusion means understanding the relationship between how people function and how they participate in society and ensuring everybody has the same opportunities to participate in every aspect of life to the best of their abilities and desires.

DISABILITY AND HEALTH INCLUSION STRATEGIES

The inclusion of people with disabilities into everyday activities involves practices and policies designed to identify and remove physical, communication, and attitudinal barriers that hamper individuals' ability to participate fully in society as people without disabilities. Inclusion involves:
- Getting fair treatment from others nondiscrimination).
- Making products, communications, and the physical environment more usable by as many people as possible (universal design).
- Modifying items, procedures, or systems to enable a person with a disability to use them to the maximum extent possible (reasonable accommodations).
- Eliminating the belief that people with disabilities are unhealthy or less capable of doing things (stigma, stereotypes).

Disability inclusion involves input from people with disabilities, generally through disability-focused and independent living organizations, in the program or structural design, implementation, monitoring, and evaluation.

National Policy and Legislation

The following three federal laws protect the rights of people with disabilities and ensure their inclusion in many aspects of society:
- Section 504 of the Rehabilitation Act of 1973

- The Americans with Disabilities Act (ADA) of 1990 that was followed by the ADA Amendments Act of 2008 to restore the legislation's original intent
- The Patient Protection and Affordable Care Act in 2010

SECTION 504 OF THE REHABILITATION ACT

Section 504 of the Rehabilitation Act of 1973 is a federal law that protects individuals from discrimination based on disability. The nondiscrimination requirements of the law apply to employers and organizations that receive financial assistance from federal departments or agencies. Section 504 forbids organizations and employers from denying individuals with disabilities an equal opportunity to receive program benefits and services. It defines the rights of individuals with disabilities to participate in and access program benefits and services.

AMERICANS WITH DISABILITIES ACT

As amended, the Americans with Disabilities Act (ADA) of 1990 protects the civil rights of people with disabilities and has helped remove or reduce many barriers for people with disabilities. The legislation required the elimination of discrimination against people with disabilities. The ADA has expanded opportunities for people with disabilities by reducing barriers, changing perceptions, and increasing participation in community life.

The ADA guarantees equal opportunity for individuals with disabilities in several areas:
- Employment
- Public accommodations such as restaurants, hotels, theaters, doctor's offices, pharmacies, retail stores, museums, libraries, parks, private schools, and day-care centers
- Transportation
- State and local government services
- Telecommunications such as telephones, televisions, and computers

Understanding Disability Inclusion

PEOPLE WITH DISABILITIES AND THE PATIENT PROTECTION AND AFFORDABLE CARE ACT

On March 23, 2010, President Obama signed the Patient Protection and Affordable Care Act, commonly called "ACA."

For people with disabilities, the ACA:
- Provides more health-care choices and enhanced protection for Americans with disabilities.
- Provides new health-care options for long-term support and services.
- Improves the Medicaid home- and community-based services option.
- Provides access to high-quality, affordable health care for many people with disabilities.
- Mandates accessible preventive screening equipment.
- Designates disability status as a demographic category and mandates data collection to assess health disparities.

Universal Design

The universal design intends to simplify life for everyone by making products, communications, and the physical environment more usable by as many people as possible at little or no extra cost. Universal design benefits people of all ages and abilities. The Center for Universal Design (CUD) at North Carolina State University (NCSU) has developed seven principles for universal design:

- **Equitable use**. The design is useful and marketable to people with diverse abilities. For example:
  - Power doors with sensors at entrances that are convenient for all users
- **Flexibility in use**. The design accommodates a wide range of individual preferences and abilities. For example:
  - An automated teller machine (ATM) that enhances how it looks, feels, or sounds so that people with vision or hearing impairments can use it
  - A tapered card opening for ease in inserting or removing a bank card

- A palm rest to aid those with arm mobility or strength limitations
- **Simple and intuitive use**. The design is easy to understand, regardless of the user's experience, knowledge, language skills, or current concentration level. For example:
  - Including an instruction manual with clear drawings and no text.
- **Perceptible information**. The design communicates necessary information effectively to the user, regardless of the current light, visual, or sound conditions or the person's abilities to read, see, or hear. For example:
  - Alarm systems that can be both seen and heard
  - Routinely making captioning available in all television or video presentations
- **Tolerance for error**. The design minimizes hazards and the harmful consequences of accidental or unintended actions. For example:
  - Ground-fault interrupter (GFI) electrical outlet that reduces the risk of shock in bathrooms and kitchens
- **Low physical effort.** The design can be used efficiently and comfortably with minimum fatigue. For example:
  - Easy-to-use handles that make opening doors easier for people of all ages and abilities
- **Size and space for approach and use**. Appropriate size and space are provided for approach, reach, manipulation, and use regardless of a person's body size, posture, or mobility. For example:
  - Counters and service windows that are low enough for everyone to reach, including people who use wheelchairs
  - Curb cuts or sidewalk ramps that are essential for people in wheelchairs but are used by all people and are also convenient for people pushing baby strollers

Understanding Disability Inclusion

Accessibility

Accessibility is when the needs of people with disabilities are specifically considered, and products, services, and facilities are built or modified so that people of all abilities can use them. Here are a few examples of accessibility:
- Parking spaces are close to entrances.
- Floor spaces and hallways are free of equipment and other barriers.
- Staff and health-care professionals can use sign language or have access to someone who can use sign language.

Reasonable Accommodations

Accommodations are alterations made to items, procedures, or systems that enable a person with a disability to use them to the maximum extent possible. Accommodation can also be a modification to an existing environment or process to increase an individual's participation with an impairment or activity limitation. Braille, large print, or audiobooks are examples of accommodations for people who are blind or who have visual limitations otherwise. For people who are deaf or have difficulty hearing, accommodations may take the form of having an American Sign Language interpreter available during meetings or presentations or exchanging written messages. Communication accommodations do not have to be elaborated, but they must be able to convey information effectively.

Assistive Technology

Assistive technologies are devices or equipment that can be used to help a person with a disability fully engage in life activities. Assistive technology can help enhance functional independence and make daily living tasks easier through aids that help people travel, communicate with others, learn, work, and participate in social and recreational activities. An example of assistive technology can be anything from a low-tech device, such as a magnifying glass, to a high-tech device, such as a computer that talks and helps someone communicate.

Other examples are wheelchairs, walkers, and scooters, which are mobility aids that persons with physical disabilities can use. Smartphones have greatly expanded the availability of assistive technology for people with vision or hearing difficulties or who have problems communicating their thoughts effectively because of mental or physical limitations.

Independent Living

Independent living is about people with disabilities having a voice, choice, and control over their everyday lives. The person may not need any assistance or might need help with only complex issues, such as managing money, rather than day-to-day living skills. Whether an adult with disabilities continues to live at home or moves into the community depends largely on her or his ability to manage everyday tasks with little or no help.

Assisted Living

Assisted living is for adults who need help with everyday tasks. They may need help dressing, bathing, eating, or using the bathroom, but they do not need full-time nursing care. Some assisted living facilities are part of retirement communities. Others are near nursing homes, so a person can move easily if needs change.

Communicating with and about People with Disabilities

Disability is part of the human experience. Still, sometimes people use words or phrases that are insensitive and do not promote understanding, dignity, and respect for people with disabilities. More often than not, this is not intentional but can be hurtful. Learn how to communicate with and about people with disabilities using people-first language and other helpful tips. For some general tips on supporting people with disabilities with people-first language, refer to Table 45.1.

Understanding Disability Inclusion

Table 45.1. People with Disabilities Using People-First Language and Other Helpful Tips

Tips	Use	Do not use
Emphasize abilities, not limitations	Person who uses a wheelchair	Confined or restricted to a wheelchair, wheelchair-bound
	Person who uses a device to speak	Not able to talk, mute
Not using language that suggests the lack of something	Person with a disability	Disabled, handicapped
	Person of short stature	Midget
	Person with cerebral palsy	Cerebral palsy victim
	Person with epilepsy or seizure disorder	Epileptic
	Person with multiple sclerosis	Afflicted by multiple sclerosis
Emphasize the need for accessibility, not the disability	Accessible parking or bathroom	Handicapped parking or bathroom
Not using offensive language	Person with a physical disability	Crippled, lame, deformed, invalid, spastic
	Person with an intellectual, cognitive, developmental disability	Slow, simple, moronic, defective, afflicted, special person
	Person with and emotional or behavioral disability, a mental health impairment, or a psychiatric disability	Insane, crazy, psycho, maniac, nuts
Avoid language that implies negative stereotypes	Person without a disability	Normal person, healthy person
Not portraying people with disabilities as inspirational only because of their disabilities	Person who is successful, productive	Overcoming her/his disability, being courageous

Chapter 46 | Parenting a Child When You Have a Disability

People with disabilities face significant barriers to creating and maintaining families. These obstacles—created by the child welfare system, the family law system, adoption agencies, assisted reproductive technology providers, and society as a whole—result from perceptions concerning the child-rearing abilities of people with disabilities. But are these views informed? Does disability affect one's ability to parent?

Social science research examining the effect of disability on parenting is scarce. Historically, the absence of data has encouraged bias against parents with disabilities. Dr. Ora Prilleltensky, Ph.D., professor at the University of Miami and a person with a disability, says, "Despite the growing numbers of disabled adults who are having children, parents with disabilities continue to be primarily ignored by research and social policy. The sparse literature that can be found on the topic typically focuses on the relationship between parental disability and children's well-being. In some cases, a negative impact is hypothesized, studied, and verified; in other cases, the correlation between indices of dysfunction in children and parental disability is explored; and in others yet, the negative impact on children and the need to counsel them is taken as a given."

This chapter includes text excerpted from "Chapter 12: The Impact of Disability on Parenting," National Council on Disability (NCD), September 30, 2012. Reviewed November 2022.

Dr. Megan Kirshbaum, Ph.D., and Dr. Rhoda Olkin, Ph.D., of Through the Looking Glass (TLG), a disability community based nonprofit organization, write, "Much of the research on parents with disabilities has been driven by a search for problems in these families. The pathologizing assumptions framing such research presuppose the negative effects of the parents' disabilities on their children. The perennial pairing of parents with disabilities and problems in children perpetuates the belief in the deleterious effects of parental disability on children. Research reveals the widespread belief among professionals that disability severely limits parenting ability and often leads to maladjustment in children." Kirshbaum and Olkin believe such research may perpetuate negative beliefs in the general population. Correlation and causation are often confused in the research, resulting in an impression that parents' disabilities cause children's problems. Contextual problems—such as poverty, the parent's history of abuse, substance use, and a lack of adequate support—are frequently ignored, so any problems researchers find are attributed to disability.

However, high-quality studies indicate that disability alone is not a predictor of problems or difficulties in children and that problem parenting predictors are often the same for disabled and nondisabled parents. According to Dave Shade, J.D., an associate scientist in epidemiology at the Johns Hopkins Bloomberg School of Public Health, "The available evidence suggests that although parents with disabilities may have a very different approach to parenting, the presence of a disability (physical or mental) is a poor correlate of long-term maladjustment in children. Thus, although the data are far from clear, it seems safe to conclude that many parents with disabilities previously thought unable to raise a child at all may be able to do so and that many more parents with disabilities may succeed in raising their children if provided appropriate support services."

Echoing Shade, Dr. Paul Preston, Ph.D., director of the National Center for Parents with Disabilities at TLG, says, "The implications of being raised by a disabled parent have been the source of numerous studies, public conjectures, and professional scrutiny—all of which touch upon the fundamental rights of disabled people to be parents as well as the fundamental rights of children to be raised in an environment conducive to maximal development. Despite the lack of appropriate resources for most disabled parents and their children and persistent negative assumptions about these families, most children of disabled parents have been shown to have typical development and functioning and often enhanced life perspectives and skills." Clinical experience proposes that predictors of problem parenting may be the same as those for nondisabled parents, particularly a history of physical, sexual, or substance abuse in the parent's family.

PARENTS WITH INTELLECTUAL OR DEVELOPMENTAL DISABILITIES

Parents with intellectual or developmental disabilities face similarly significant and detrimental discrimination, which raises the following question: Do intellectual and developmental disabilities affect parenting ability? According to Preston, research has historically been focused on the pathological bias against parents with intellectual and developmental disabilities, "pointing out that much of the literature on parents with intellectual disabilities has failed to distinguish between characteristics that facilitate and inhibit parenting abilities. Most of these studies have focused only on identifying parents with intellectual disabilities who provide inadequate childcare, rather than identifying predictors of adequate childcare such as coping and skill acquisition—even though many parents with intellectual disabilities have provided adequate care."

According to professors at the University of Minnesota School of Social Work, "Despite disproportionately greater involvement in the child welfare system, a growing body of research on the outcomes for children of parents with disabilities does not necessarily support the assumption that parents with disabilities are more likely to abuse or neglect their children. Studies have found that children of parents with intellectual and developmental disabilities can have successful outcomes."

Dr. Chris Watkins, Ph.D., professor in computer science, Royal Holloway, notes, "Almost all studies have found a sizeable percentage of parents with developmental disabilities functioning within or near normal limits. In addition, many studies have found that parents labeled mentally retarded can benefit from training and support. Even researchers and commentators who have reached the most negative conclusions about cognitively disabled parents caution that such parents must be evaluated as individuals before reaching conclusions about their parental adequacy or ability to benefit from training and support."

Several researchers have used qualitative methods to investigate the life experiences and outcomes of children of parents with intellectual disabilities. In Denmark, J. Faureholm, M.Ed., worked for a number of years as a psychologist for the Ministry of Social Affairs and the Ministry for Refugees, Immigrants, and Integration, interviewed 20 young adult children of mothers with intellectual disabilities. Despite the difficult circumstances of their growing up, including being bullied and ostracized by their peers, most of the children discovered an underlying personal strength that enabled them to overcome these experiences, and all but one maintained a close and warm relationship with their parents.

Similarly, in England, internationally recognized researchers Dr. Tim Booth, Ph.D., and Dr. Wendy Booth, Ph.D., also interviewed adult children of parents with "learning difficulties." They said, "The majority recalled happy, if not carefree, childhoods. Only three regarded their childhoods as wholly unhappy." Significantly, most interviewees expressed positive feelings of love and affection toward their parents, and all maintained close contact with their parents. Tellingly, those who the child welfare system had removed had subsequently reestablished and maintained contact with their birth parents. "In both studies, family bonds endured despite time and circumstance intervening." Some of the research further demonstrates the absence of a clear correlation between low intelligence quotient (IQ) and parental unfitness. Studies have indicated that it is impossible to predict parenting outcomes oriented on intelligence testing results.

Thus, Chris Watkins says, "The available research suggests that factors unrelated to disability often have a more significant impact on parental fitness than the disability itself. The research also suggests a tremendous variance in the impact that disability has on parental fitness. Importantly, parenting services have been shown

Parenting a Child When You Have a Disability

to make a difference for many parents with insufficient parenting skills. While few conclusions can be drawn about the parenting abilities of developmentally disabled parents as a group, it is clear that individual inquiry is required before decisions are made to remove children from parents."

Chapter 47 | Employment for People with Learning Disabilities

JOB HELP FOR PEOPLE WITH DISABILITIES
If you have a disability and are looking for work, the following resources can help.

Develop Your Work and Job-Seeking Skills
- Get in-person counseling, training, support, and services to help you find and keep a job. Contact:
  - Your state vocational rehabilitation agency
  - The American Job Center in your area
- The Workers with Disabilities section at CareerOneStop.org (www.careeronestop.org) has resources to help you:
  - Develop job skills.
  - Conduct a job search.
  - Prepare for interviews.
- Find job tips and resources from the Campaign for Disability Employment's "What Can You Do?" website (www.whatcanyoudocampaign.org). There is information for families, educators, and employers too.
- Your local Independent Living Center can help you live on your own. They also offer job training and coaching.

This chapter includes text excerpted from "Jobs and Education for People with Disabilities," USA.gov, June 21, 2022.

Find a Job
- Ticket to Work trains Social Security disability recipients aged 18–64 who want to work. It is free and voluntary.
- AbilityOne.gov helps people who are blind or have significant disabilities find jobs. Job openings are with nonprofit agencies nationwide.
- The federal government has many jobs open to people with disabilities.

Job Help for Young Workers
- Find resources to help you move from school to work.
- Check out Job Corps. It is a free residential education and job training program for young adults. It accommodates participants aged 18–24 with disabilities.

Job Help for Veterans
- Take advantage of the veterans' Veteran Readiness and Employment (VR&E) program. It offers help with the following:
  - Job training
  - Employment accommodations
  - Resume development
  - Job-seeking skills
- Find more job help programs for veterans. These include:
  - Helping start your own business.
  - Qualifying for a hiring preference with the federal government.

Learn about Your Rights
- The Job Accommodation Network (JAN; askjan.org) helps you:
  - Get answers to your questions about workplace accommodations.
  - Learn about your rights under the Americans with Disabilities Act (ADA).

Employment for People with Learning Disabilities

- Visit the Office of Disability Employment Policy website (www.usa.gov/federal-agencies/office-of-disability-employment-policy). It explains the laws that protect workers with disabilities from job discrimination.
- Learn about your rights from the Equal Employment Opportunity Commission (EEOC; www.eeoc.gov/youth/disability-discrimination-01). Topics include:
  - Accommodation for your disability
  - Protection against harassment and discrimination

FEDERAL JOBS FOR PEOPLE WITH DISABILITIES
If you are looking for a job and have a disability, you might consider working for the federal government.

Advantages of Government Jobs for People with Disabilities
The federal government:
- Uses Schedule A, a noncompetitive hiring process. It is faster and easier than the competitive process.
- Provides reasonable accommodations to qualified employees.

You can also apply for jobs through the competitive hiring process.

Finding and Applying for Federal Jobs
You can search and apply online for most jobs at USAJOBS.gov (www.usajobs.gov).
- Check out USAJOBS' tips for individuals with disabilities. It covers Schedule A and other factors in applying for a job.

Apply for a job through an agency. Contact the agency's selective placement program coordinator (SPPC) for help.

College Students and Recent Graduates with Disabilities
Find summer jobs, internships, and permanent positions through the workforce recruitment program.

Veterans with Disabilities
Special hiring authorities let agencies appoint vets with service-connected disabilities to jobs.

DISCRIMINATION AND HARASSMENT AT YOUR JOB
If you are experiencing discrimination or harassment at your employment, first inform your manager or the human resources department.

The Equal Employment Opportunity Commission enforces federal laws prohibiting employment discrimination.

Protections Included under the Law
These laws protect employees and job applicants against the following:
- Discrimination, harassment, and unfair treatment in the workplace by anyone because of:
  - Race
  - Color
  - Religion
  - Sex (including gender identity, transgender status, and sexual orientation)
  - Pregnancy
  - National origin
  - Age (40 or older)
  - Disability
  - Genetic information
- Being denied reasonable workplace accommodations for a disability or religious beliefs
- Retaliation because they:
  - Complained about job discrimination.
  - Helped with an investigation or lawsuit.

How to File an Employment Discrimination Complaint

To file a complaint, contact your EEOC field office. Many state and local governments have antidiscrimination laws. These laws may offer extra protection beyond federal law. Some state laws:
- Apply to businesses with only five or six employees.
- Prohibit discrimination oriented on whether you are married or have children.
- Have different deadlines for filing a charge.
- Have different standards for deciding whether you are covered.

Many state laws have more protections for nursing mothers than federal law requires. State labor offices enforce these laws.

Filing a Lawsuit

You can file a lawsuit if you are a victim of job discrimination or harassment. If the discrimination violates federal law, you must file a charge with the EEOC first. (This does not apply to cases of unequal pay between men and women.)

You may decide to sue if the EEOC cannot help you. In either case, look for an attorney who specializes in employment law. You can check with:
- Your EEOC field office
- The American Bar Association
- The National Employment Lawyers Association

Not All Employers Are Subject to Equal Employment Opportunity Commission Laws

Only employers with a certain number of employees are subject to EEOC laws. The number of employees changes depending on the type of employer and the kind of discrimination alleged.
- Businesses, state, and local governments must follow most EEOC laws if they have 15 or more employees.
- Federal agencies must follow all EEOC laws, regardless of the number of their employees.

Laws That the Equal Employment Opportunity Commission Enforces
Federal employment discrimination laws include:
- **The Americans with Disabilities Act (ADA)**—which prohibits discrimination against workers with disabilities and mandates reasonable accommodations
- **The Age Discrimination in Employment Act of 1967 (ADEA)**
- **Title VII of the Civil Rights Act of 1964 (Title VII)**—which prohibits discrimination oriented on:
  - Race
  - Color
  - Religion
  - National origin
  - Sex (including sexual orientation and gender identity)
- **The Equal Pay Act (EPA)**—which requires equal pay for equal work by men and women

What Is Harassment?
Harassment is unwelcome conduct oriented on:
- Race
- Color
- Religion
- Sex
- National origin
- Age
- Pregnancy
- Disability
- Genetic information

It can include:
- Offensive jokes
- Physical assaults or threats
- Ridicule or insults
- Display of offensive objects or pictures

Sexual harassment may include:
- Unwelcome sexual advances
- Requests for sexual favors
- Other verbal or physical harassment of a sexual nature
- Offensive remarks about a person's sex

Harassment becomes illegal when:
- It creates a hostile or abusive work environment.
- The victim gets fired or demoted for refusing to put up with it.

Protection from Retaliation

The EEOC laws protect employees and job applicants from retaliation. For example, it is unlawful to punish people for:
- Filing or being a witness in an equal employment opportunity (EEO) charge or investigation.
- Talking to a supervisor or manager about discrimination or harassment.
- Refusing to follow orders that would result in discrimination.
- Resisting sexual advances or intervening to protect others.

Part 6 | Additional Help and Information

Chapter 48 | Glossary of Terms Related to Learning Disabilities

accommodations: Techniques and materials that allow individuals with various disabilities to complete school or work tasks with greater ease and effectiveness. Examples include spellcheckers, tape recorders, and expanded time for completing assignments.

assistive technology: Equipment that enhances the ability of students and employees to be more efficient and successful. For individuals with disabilities, computer grammar checkers, an overhead projector used by a teacher, or the audio/visual information delivered through a compact disk read-only memory (CD-ROM) would be typical examples.

attention deficit disorder (ADD): A severe difficulty in focusing and maintaining attention. Often leads to learning and behavior problems at home, school, and work. Also called attention deficit hyperactivity disorder (ADHD).

autism spectrum disorder (ASD): A neurological and developmental disorder that affects how people interact with others, communicate, learn, and behave.

axon: The fiber-like extension of a neuron through which the cell carries information to target cells.

basal ganglia: Deeply placed masses of gray matter within each cerebral hemisphere that assist in voluntary motor functioning.

biopsy: A procedure in which tissue or other materials is removed from the body and studied for signs of disease.

This glossary contains terms excerpted from documents produced by several sources deemed reliable.

brain injury: The physical damage to brain tissue or structure that occurs before, during, or after birth that is verified by electroencephalography (EEG), magnetic resonance imaging (MRI), computerized axial tomography (CAT), or a similar examination, rather than by observation of performance. When caused by an accident, the damage may be called traumatic brain injury (TBI).

brainstem: The structure at the base of the brain through which the forebrain sends information to, and receives information from, the spinal cord and peripheral nerves.

cerebellum: A portion of the brain that helps regulate posture, balance, and coordination.

cerebral cortex: The intricately folded surface layer of gray matter of the brain that functions chiefly in coordination of sensory and motor information. It is divided into four lobes: frontal, parietal, temporal, and occipital.

chromosomes: Genetic structures that contain DNA.

collaboration: A program model in which the learning disabilities (LD) teacher demonstrates for or team-teaches with the general classroom teacher to help a student with LD be successful in a regular classroom.

developmental aphasia: A severe language disorder that is presumed to be due to brain injury rather than because of a developmental delay in the normal acquisition of language.

Down syndrome: A genetic condition caused by having an extra chromosome 21 in some or all of the body's cells.

dyscalculia: A severe difficulty in understanding and using symbols or functions needed for success in mathematics.

dysgraphia: A severe difficulty in producing handwriting that is legible and written at an age-appropriate speed.

dyslexia: A severe difficulty in understanding or using one or more areas of language, including listening, speaking, reading, writing, and spelling.

epilepsy: A person is diagnosed with epilepsy when they have had two or more seizures. Also called a "seizure disorder."

executive functioning: A group of skills that help people focus on multiple streams of information at the same time and revise plans as necessary.

free appropriate public education (FAPE): A term used in the elementary and secondary school context; for purposes of Section 504, refers to

Glossary of Terms Related to Learning Disabilities

the provision of regular or special education and related aids and services that are designed to meet individual educational needs of students with disabilities as adequately as the needs of students without disabilities are met and is based upon adherence to procedures that satisfy the Section 504 requirements pertaining to educational setting, evaluation and placement, and procedural safeguards.

frontal lobe: One of the four divisions of each cerebral hemisphere. The frontal lobe is important for controlling movement, thinking, and judgment.

gray matter: Neural tissue, especially of the brain and spinal cord, that contains cell bodies as well as some nerve fibers, has a brownish gray color and forms most of the cortex and nuclei of the brain, the columns of the spinal cord, and the bodies of ganglia.

hippocampus: A component of the limbic system that is involved in learning and memory.

individualized education program (IEP): A written statement of the educational program designed to meet a child's individual needs. Every child who receives special education services must have an IEP.

limbic system: A set of brain structures that regulates our feelings, emotions, and motivations and that is also important in learning and memory. Includes the thalamus, hypothalamus, amygdala, and hippocampus.

mental disability: Conditions that include a learning disability, an intellectual disability, developmental disability, Alzheimer disease, senility, dementia or some other mental or emotional condition that seriously interferes with daily activity. Used in the Americans with disabilities report series.

midbrain: The upper part of the brainstem, which controls some reflexes and eye movements.

myelin: Fatty material that surrounds and insulates axons of some neurons.

neuron: A unique type of cell found in the brain and body that is specialized to process and transmit information.

neurotransmitter: A chemical produced by neurons to carry messages to other neurons.

Parkinson disease (PD): A progressive disorder of the nervous system marked by muscle tremors, muscle rigidity, decreased mobility, stooped posture, slow voluntary movements, and a mask-like facial expression.

perceptual handicap: Difficulty in accurately processing, organizing, and discriminating among visual, auditory, or tactile information. A person with a perceptual handicap may say that "cap" and "cup" sound the same or that "b" and "d" look the same. However, glasses or hearing aids do not necessarily indicate a perceptual handicap.

placement: A term used in the elementary and secondary school context refers to regular and/or special educational program in which a student receives educational and/or related services.

plasticity: The capacity of the brain to change its structure and function within certain limits. Plasticity underlies brain functions, such as learning, and allows the brain to generate normal, healthy responses to long-lasting environmental changes.

prefrontal cortex: A highly developed area at the front of the brain that plays a role in executive functions such as judgment, decision-making, and problem-solving, as well as emotional control and memory.

receptor: A protein that recognizes specific chemicals (e.g., neurotransmitters, hormones) and transmits the message carried by the chemical into the cell on which the receptor resides.

related services: A term used in the elementary and secondary school context to refer to developmental, corrective, and other supportive services, including psychological, counseling, and medical diagnostic services and transportation.

self-advocacy: The development of specific skills and understandings that enable children and adults to explain their specific learning disabilities to others and cope positively with the attitudes of peers, parents, teachers, and employers.

sensitive period: Windows of time in the developmental process when certain parts of the brain may be most susceptible to particular experiences.

sensory disability: Conditions that include blindness, deafness, or a severe vision or hearing impairment. Used in the Americans with disabilities report series.

specific learning disability (SLD): The official term used in federal legislation to refer to difficulty in certain areas of learning, rather than in all areas of learning. It is synonymous with learning disabilities.

stroke: In medicine, a loss of blood flow to part of the brain, which damages brain tissue. Strokes are caused by blood clots and broken blood vessels in the brain. Symptoms include dizziness, numbness, weakness on one side of the body, and problems with talking, writing, or understanding language.

Glossary of Terms Related to Learning Disabilities

synapse: The site where presynaptic and postsynaptic neurons communicate with each other.

temporal lobe: One of the four major subdivisions of each hemisphere of the cerebral cortex that assists in auditory perception, speech, and visual perceptions.

transition: Commonly used to refer to the change from secondary school to postsecondary programs, work, and independent living typical of young adults. Also used to describe other periods of major change such as from early childhood to school or from more specialized to mainstreamed settings.

traumatic brain injury (TBI): A form of acquired brain injury occurs when a sudden trauma causes damage to the brain. TBI can result when the head suddenly and violently hits an object or when an object pierces the skull and enters brain tissue.

white matter: Neural tissue, especially of the brain and spinal cord, that consists largely of myelinated nerve fibers bundled into tracts that help transmit signals between areas of the brain. It gets its name from the white color of the myelin.

x-ray: A type of high-energy radiation. In low doses, x-rays are used to diagnose diseases by making pictures of the inside of the body. In high doses, x-rays are also used to treat cancer.

yoga: An ancient system of practices used to balance the mind and body through exercise, meditation (focusing thoughts), and control of breathing and emotions.

Chapter 49 | Sources of College Funding for Students with Disabilities

In addition to scholarships available to the general public, minorities, and people pursuing a particular field of study, there are many scholarships specifically for students with disabilities. Below are some examples.

GENERAL

INCIGHT. Since 2004, INCIGHT has awarded more than 940 scholarships to students with disabilities pursuing higher education. These scholars are enrolled in community college, university, vocational school, and graduate programs. Students who demonstrate outstanding service to their community and overcome personal obstacles are awarded scholarships from INCIGHT. These scholars spread the message of INCIGHT far and wide. After graduation and throughout their life, INCIGHT scholars volunteer, support, and participate in INCIGHT.

INCIGHT
P.O. Box 82056
Portland, OR 97282
Phone: 971-244-0305
Website: www.incight.org
E-mail: piag@incight.org

Resources in this chapter were compiled from several sources deemed reliable; all contact information were verified and updated in November 2022.

Newcombe Scholarships for Students with Disabilities support completion of degrees by students with disabilities who need financial assistance at selected colleges and universities.

The Charlotte W. Newcombe Foundation
35 Park Pl.
Princeton, NJ 08542-6918
Phone: 609-924-7022
Website: www.newcombefoundation.org
E-mail: info@newcombefoundation.org

The Ability Center works to ensure that people with disabilities have opportunities to achieve higher education. In partnership with The Ability Center Auxiliary, they provide critical college scholarships to area students with disabilities.

The Ability Center Auxiliary
5605 Monroe St.
Sylvania, OH 43560
Toll-Free: 866-885-5733
Phone: 419-885-5733
Fax: 419-882-4813
Website: www.abilitycenter.org

BUSINESS PLAN SCHOLARSHIP FOR STUDENTS WITH DISABILITIES

The scholarship is open to students with any type of disability, including but not limited to physical disabilities, medical conditions, mental and psychiatric conditions, speech and language, learning disabilities, behavioral conditions, and all other disabling conditions.

Fit Small Business
228 Park Ave. S., Ste. 20702
New York, NY 10003-1502
Website: www.fitsmallbusiness.com
E-mail: info@fitsmallbusiness.com

Sources of College Funding for Students with Disabilities

FOR STUDENTS WHO ARE BLIND

The **American Council of the Blind (ACB)** and the **American Foundation for the Blind (AFB)** have now partnered together to offer educational scholarships ranging from $2,000 to $7,500 for those attending a technical college or as an entering freshman or an undergraduate or graduate student.

American Council of the Blind
1703 N. Beauregard St., Ste. 420
Alexandria, VA 22311
Toll-Free: 800-424-8666
Phone: 202-467-5081
Fax: 703-465-5085
Website: www.acb.org/scholarships
E-mail: scholarships@acb.org

American Foundation for the Blind
1401 S. Clark St., Ste. 730
Arlington, VA 22202
Toll-Free: 800-232-5463
Phone: 212-502-7600
Website: www.afb.org/about-afb/events-and-awards/afb-scholarships
E-mail: info@aph.org

The **Association of Blind Citizens** will offer $3,000 in college scholarships to legally blind individuals seeking a college degree.

Association of Blind Citizens
P.O. Box 246
Holbrook, MA 02343
Phone: 781-961-1023
Website: www.blindcitizens.org/abc_scholarship.htm
E-mail: scholarship@blindcitizens.org

The **Christian Record Services** for the blind offers the Anne Lowe scholarship. The scholarship is awarded to college students based on academic achievement, need, and future goals that are supported by an essay, reference letters, a projected budget, and proof that the student is blind.

Christian Record Services, Inc.
P.O. Box 6097
Lincoln, NE 68506-0097
Phone: 402-488-0981
Fax: 402-488-7582
Website: www.christianrecord.org
E-mail: info@christianrecord.org

Since 1991, the **Learning Ally** awards the Mary P. Oenslager Scholastic Achievement Awards (SAA) to outstanding college students who are blind or visually impaired. The students' Learning Ally supports are examples and role models for the many students we support. Three top winners receive awards of $6,000 each; three special honors winners receive awards of $2,000 each; and one honors winner receives a $1,000 award.

Learning Ally
20 Roszel Rd.
Princeton, NJ 08540
Toll-Free: 800-221-4792
Website: www.learningally.org
E-mail: CustomerCare@learningally.org

The **Lighthouse Guild** scholarship program offers up to 20 scholarships for outstanding high school students who are legally blind from across the United States. We also provide an annual scholarship to at least one qualifying graduate student. The award is unrestricted, so it can be used as needed: for tuition, room and board, books, supplies, or travel.

Lighthouse Guild
250 W. 64th St.
New York, NY 10023
Toll-Free: 800-284-4422
Phone: 212-769-6200
Website: www.lighthouseguild.org

The **National Federation of the Blind's** annual scholarship program is the largest of its kind in the nation. Every year, we award more than $250,000 in cash and prizes to blind scholars across the 50 states, the District of Columbia, and Puerto Rico in recognition of their achievements and professional aspirations.

Sources of College Funding for Students with Disabilities

National Federation of the Blind
200 E. Wells St.
Baltimore, MD 21230
Phone: 410-659-9314
Fax: 410-685-5653
Website: www.nfb.org
E-mail: nfb@nfb.org

The **U.S. Association of Blind Athletes (USABA)** has initiated the 2021 USABA Scholarship Program, including the I C You Foundation Valor Achievement Award. The Valor Achievement Award is awarded to one male and one female athlete, each in the amount of $500.

U.S. Association of Blind Athletes
1 Olympic Plaza
Colorado Springs, CO 80909
Phone: 719-866-3224
Website: www.usaba.org

FOR STUDENTS WHO ARE DEAF OR HARD OF HEARING

The **Alexander Graham Bell Association for the Deaf and Hard of Hearing (AG Bell)** offers several scholarships for full-time students who are deaf and hard of hearing and who are pursuing an undergraduate degree at an accredited mainstream college or university.

Alexander Graham Bell Association for the Deaf and Hard of Hearing
3417 Volta Place N.W.
Washington, DC 20007
Phone: 202-337-5220
TTY: 202-337-5221
Fax: 202-337-8314
Website: www.agbell.org
E-mail: info@agbell.org

Cochlear Americas offers several prestigious scholarships in honor of the amazing innovators who developed our hearing solutions. The Cochlear Graeme Clark Scholarship is an achievement award open to Cochlear Nucleus Implant recipients, and the Cochlear Anders Tjellström Scholarship is an achievement award open to Baha and Osia recipients; applicants must be a citizen of the United States or Canada.

Cochlear Americas
10350 Park Meadows Dr.
Lone Tree, CO 80124
Toll-Free: 800-523-5798
Phone: 303-790-9010
Fax: 303-790-1157
Website: www.cochlear.com/us

The **Graduate Fellowship Fund (GFF)** provides financial assistance to deaf and hard of hearing graduates of accredited colleges and universities who are studying full-time in terminal degree programs.

Graduate Fellowship Fund (GFF)
800 Florida Ave., N.E.
Chapel Hall, Ste. 102
Washington, DC 20002
Phone: 202-651-5000
TTY: 202-250-2453
Fax: 202-651-5062
Website: www.gallaudet.edu

FOR STUDENTS WITH LEARNING DISABILITIES

The **LD Resources Foundation** award program was created to help students diagnosed with dyslexia, ADHD, and other learning disabilities.

LD Resources Foundation, Inc.
14 Horatio St., Ste. 5H
New York, NY 10014
Phone: 646-701-0000
Website: www.ldrfa.org/award
E-mail: info@ldrfa.org

The **National Center for Learning Disabilities (NCLD)** offers annual scholarships and awards that celebrate the work and achievements of those students and leaders working to improve the lives of the one in five with learning and attention issues.

Sources of College Funding for Students with Disabilities

The National Center for Learning Disabilities
1220 L St., N.W., Ste. 100
P.O. Box 168
Washington, DC 20005
Phone: 301-966-2234
Website: www.ncld.org/what-we-do-2/scholarships-awards
E-mail afscholarship@ncld.org

P. Buckley Moss Foundation scholarships and awards offer financial assistance to high school seniors with learning disabilities who are getting a higher education or are planning a career in the visual arts.

P. Buckley Moss Foundation
74 Poplar Grove Ln.
Mathews, VA 23109
Toll-Free: 800-430-1320
Phone: 804-725-7378
Website: www.mossfoundation.org
E-mail: foundation@mossfoundation.org

The **Western Illinois University** offers the Chad Stovall Memorial Scholarship to incoming freshmen who have been diagnosed with Tourette syndrome, obsessive compulsive disorder, or attention deficit disorder. Eligible applicants must be enrolled full-time and remain in good academic standing.

Western Illinois University
1 University Cir.
Macomb, IL 61455
Phone: 309-298-1414; 309-298-4444
Website: www.wiu.edu
E-mail: info@wiu.edu

The **Learning Disabilities Association of Iowa** has a long history of offering scholarships to qualifying individuals impacted by learning disabilities.

Learning Disabilities Association of Iowa
5665 Greendale Rd., Ste. D
Johnston, IA 50131
Phone: 515-209-2290
Fax: 515-243-1902
Website: www.ldaiowa.org
E-mail: LearningDisabilitiesofIowa@gmail.com

Chapter 50 | Directory of Resources Related to Learning Disabilities

GENERAL—GOVERNMENT ORGANIZATIONS

Centers for Disease Control and Prevention (CDC)
1600 Clifton Rd.
Atlanta, GA 30329-4027
Toll-Free: 800-232-4636 (800-CDC-INFO)
Toll-Free TTY: 888-232-6348
Website: www.cdc.gov

Child Welfare Information Gateway
330 C St. S.W.
Washington, DC 20201
Toll-Free: 800-394-3366
Website: www.childwelfare.gov
E-mail: info@childwelfare.gov

Eunice Kennedy Shriver National Institute of Child Health and Human Development (NICHD)
NICHD Information Resource Center
P.O. Box 3006
Rockville, MD 20847
Toll-Free: 800-370-2943
Fax: 866-760-5947
Website: www.nichd.nih.gov
E-mail: NICHDInformationResourceCenter@mail.nih.gov

Genetic and Rare Diseases Information Center (GARD)
P.O. Box 8126
Gaithersburg, MD 20898-8126
Toll-Free: 888-205-2311
Website: www.rarediseases.info.nih.gov
E-mail: GARDinfo@nih.gov

Resources in this chapter were compiled from several sources deemed reliable; all contact information were verified and updated in November 2022.

MedlinePlus
8600 Rockville Pike
Bethesda, MD 20894
Website: www.medlineplus.gov

National Center for Education Statistics (NCES)
550 12th St. S.W.
Potomac Center Plaza
Washington, DC 20202
Phone: 202-403-5551
Website: www.nces.ed.gov

National Council on Disability (NCD)
1331 F St. N.W., Ste. 850
Washington, DC 20004
Phone: 202-272-2004
Fax: 202-272-2022
Website: www.ncd.gov
E-mail: ncd@ncd.gov

National Eye Institute (NEI)
Information Office
31 Center Dr., MSC 2510
Bethesda, MD 20892-2510
Phone: 301-496-5248
Website: www.nei.nih.gov
E-mail: 2020@nei.nih.gov

National Human Genome Research Institute (NHGRI)
Communications and Public Liaison Branch (CPLB)
9000 Rockville Pike
Bldg. 31, Rm. 4B09, 31 Center Dr., MSC 2152
Bethesda, MD 20892-2152
Phone: 301-402-0911
Fax: 301-402-2218
Website: www.genome.gov
E-mail: nhgripressoffice@mail.nih.gov

National Institute of Mental Health (NIMH)
Office of Science Policy, Planning, and Communications (OSPPC)
6001 Executive Blvd.
Rm. 6200, MSC 9663
Bethesda, MD 20892-9663
Toll-Free: 866-615-6464
Phone: 301-443-4513
TTY: 301-443-8431; 866-415-8051
Fax: 301-443-4279
Website: www.nimh.nih.gov
E-mail: nimhinfo@nih.gov

National Institute of Neurological Disorders and Stroke (NINDS)
NIH Neurological Institute
P.O. Box 5801
Bethesda, MD 20824
Toll-Free: 800-352-9424
Website: www.ninds.nih.gov

Directory of Resources Related to Learning Disabilities

National Institute on Alcohol Abuse and Alcoholism (NIAAA)
Bethesda, MD 20892-9304
Phone: 301-443-3860
Website: www.niaaa.nih.gov
E-mail: AskNIAAA@nih.gov

National Institute on Deafness and Other Communication Disorders (NIDCD)
NIDCD Office of Health Communication and Public Liaison (OHPL)
31 Center Dr., MSC 2320
Bethesda, MD 20892-2320
Toll-Free: 800-241-1044
Phone: 301-827-8183
Toll-Free TTY: 800-241-1055
Website: www.nidcd.nih.gov
E-mail: nidcdinfo@nidcd.nih.gov

National Science Foundation (NSF)
2415 Eisenhower Ave.
Alexandria, VA 22314
Phone: 703-292-5111
TDD: 703-292-5090; 800-281-8749
Website: www.nsf.gov
E-mail: info@nsf.gov

Substance Abuse and Mental Health Services Administration (SAMHSA)
5600 Fishers Lane
Rockville, MD 20857
Toll-Free: 877-SAMHSA-7 (877-726-4727)
TTY: 800-487-4889
Website: www.samhsa.gov
E-mail: SAMHSAInfo@samhsa.hhs.gov

U.S. Bureau of Labor Statistics (BLS)
Office of Occupational Statistics and Employment
PSB Ste. 2135
2 Massachusetts Ave. N.E.
Washington, DC 20212-0001
Phone: 202-691-5700
Website: www.bls.gov/ooh

U.S. Department of Education (ED)
400 Maryland Ave. S.W.
Washington, DC 20202
Toll-Free: 800-872-5327
Phone: 202-401-2000
Website: www2.ed.gov

U.S. Department of Health & Human Services (HHS)
Administration for Children & Families
330 C St. S.W.
Mary E. Switzer Bldg.
Washington, DC 20201
Toll-Free: 877-696-6775
Website: www.acf.hhs.gov

U.S. National Library of Medicine (NLM)
8600 Rockville Pike
Bethesda, MD 20894
Toll-Free: 888-FIND-NLM (888-346-3656)
Phone: 301-594-5983
Website: www.nlm.nih.gov
E-mail: NLMCommunications@nih.gov

GENERAL—PRIVATE ORGANIZATIONS

American Speech-Language-Hearing Association (ASHA)
ASHA Action Center
2200 Research Blvd.
Rockville, MD 20850-3289
Phone: 301-296-5700
TTY: 301-296-5650
Fax: 301-296-8580
Website: www.asha.org
E-mail: actioncenter@asha.org

Center for Parent Information and Resources (CPIR)
Statewide Parent Advocacy Network (SPAN)
35 Halsey St.
4th Fl.
Newark, NJ 07102
Phone: 973-642-8100
Website: parentcenterhub.org
E-mail: mrodriguez@spanadvocacy.org

Childhood Education International
1100 15th St., N.W.
4th Fl.
Washington DC 20005
Toll-Free: 800-423-3563
Phone: 202-372-9986
Website: www.ceinternational1892.org

Cleveland Clinic
9500 Euclid Ave.
Cleveland, OH 44195
Toll-Free: 800-223-2273
Phone: 216-444-2200
Website: my.clevelandclinic.org

Council for Exceptional Children (CEC)
3100 Clarendon Blvd., Ste. 600
Arlington, VA 22201
Toll-Free: 888-232-7733
Phone: 888-232-7733;
703-620-3660
Fax: 703-264-9494
Website: www.exceptionalchildren.org
E-mail: service@exceptionalchildren.org

Council for Learning Disabilities
11184 Antioch Rd.
P.O. Box 405
Overland Park, KS 66210
Phone: 913-491-1011
Fax: 913-491-1011
Website: www.council-for-learning-disabilities.org

DO-IT (Disabilities, Opportunities, Internetworking, and Technology)
University of Washington (UW)
P.O. Box 354842
Seattle, WA 98195-4842
Toll-Free: 888-972-DOIT (888-972-3648)
Phone: 206-685-3648
Fax: 206-221-4171
Website: www.washington.edu/doit
E-mail: doit@uw.edu

Directory of Resources Related to Learning Disabilities

FRAXA Research Foundation
10 Prince Pl, Ste. 203
Newburyport, MA 01950
Phone: 978-462-1866
Website: www.fraxa.org
E-mail: info@fraxa.org

GreatSchools
2201 Bdwy.
4th Fl.
Oakland, CA 94612
Website: www.greatschools.org

LD OnLine
WETA Public Television
3939 Campbell Ave.
Arlington, VA 22206
Website: www.ldonline.org
E-mail: ldonline@weta.org

Learning Disabilities Association of America (LDA)
4068 Mount Royal Blvd., Ste. 224B
Allison Park, PA 15101
Phone: 412-341-1515
Website: www.ldaamerica.org
E-mail: info@ldaamerica.org

Learning Disabilities Worldwide (LDW)
179 Bear Hill Rd., Ste. 104
Waltham, MA 02451
Phone: 978-897-5399
Website: www.ldworldwide.org
E-mail: help@ldworldwide.org

National Center for Learning Disabilities (NCLD)
1220 L St. N.W., Ste. 100
P.O. Box 168
Washington, DC 20005
Phone: 301-966-2234
Website: www.ncld.org
E-mail: info@ncld.org

PACER Center, Inc.
8161 Normandale Blvd.
Bloomington, MN 55437
Toll-Free: 800-537-2237
Phone: 952-838-9000
Fax: 952-838-0199
Website: www.pacer.org

St. Louis Learning Disabilities Association
13537 Barrett Parkway Dr., Ste. 110
Ballwin, MO 63021
Phone: 314-966-3088
Website: www.ldastl.org
E-mail: info@ldastl.org

APHASIA

Aphasia Hope Foundation (AHF)
750 Woodlands Pkwy.
Ridgeland, MS 39157
Phone: 913-484-8302
Website: www.aphasiahope.org
E-mail: jstradinger.2007@comcast.net

National Aphasia Association (NAA)
P.O.Box 87
Scarsdale, NY 10583
Website: www.aphasia.org
E-mail: naa@aphasia.org

ATTENTION DEFICIT HYPERACTIVITY DISORDER

Attention Deficit Disorder Association (ADDA)
P.O. Box 7557
Wilmington, DE 19803
Toll-Free: 800-939-1019
Fax: 800-939-1019
Website: www.add.org
E-mail: info@add.org

Children and Adults with Attention-Deficit/Hyperactivity Disorder (CHADD)
4221 Forbes Blvd., Ste. 270
Lanham, MD 20706
Phone: 301-306-7070
Fax: 301-306-7090
Website: www.chadd.org
E-mail: customer_service@chadd.org

AUTISM AND PERVASIVE DEVELOPMENTAL DISORDERS

Association for Science in Autism Treatment (ASAT)
P.O. Box 1447
Hoboken, NJ 07030
Website: www.asatonline.org
E-mail: info@asatonline.org

Autism Research Institute (ARI)
4182 Adams Ave.
San Diego, CA 92116
Toll-Free: 833-281-7165
Website: www.autism.com
E-mail: info@autism.org

Autism Network International (ANI)
P.O. Box 35448
Syracuse, NY 13235
Website: www.autreat.com

Directory of Resources Related to Learning Disabilities

Autism Society
6110 Executive Blvd., Ste. 305
Rockville, MD 20852
Toll-Free: 800-328-8476
Website: www.autism-society.org
E-mail: info@autism-society.org

Autism Speaks, Inc.
1060 State Rd.
2nd Fl.
Princeton, NJ 08540
Phone: 646-385-8500
Fax: 609-430-9163
Website: www.autismspeaks.org
E-mail: help@autismspeaks.org

Center for Autism and Related Disorders (CARD)
5850 Granite Pkwy., Ste. 600
Plano, TX 75024
Toll-Free: 877-448-4747
Phone: 469-694-1754
Fax: 818-758-8015
Website: www.centerforautism.com
E-mail: info@centerforautism.com

DYSLEXIA

International Dyslexia Association (IDA)
1829 Reisterstown Rd., Ste. 350
Pikesville, MD 21208
Phone: 410-296-0232
Fax: 410-321-5069
Website: dyslexiaida.org
E-mail: info@dyslexiaida.org

HEARING DISORDERS

The Children's Hearing Institute
575 8th Ave., Ste. 1201
New York, NY 10018
Phone: 212-257-6138
Website: www.childrenshearing.org
E-mail: Mwillis@childrenshearing.org

VISION DISORDERS

AAV Media, LLC
5215 N. O'Connor Blvd.
11th Fl.
Irving, TX 75039
Website: www.allaboutvision.com
E-mail: admin@allaboutvision.com

American Optometric Association
243 N. Lindbergh Blvd.
St. Louis, MO 63141-7881
Toll-Free: 800-365-2219
Phone: 314-991-4100
Fax: 314-991-4101
Website: www.aoa.org

INDEX

INDEX

Page numbers followed by 'n' indicate a footnote. Page numbers in *italics* indicate a table or illustration.

A

AAV Media, LLC, contact information 482
The Ability Center Auxiliary, contact information 468
ACA *see* Affordable Care Act
academic performance
 auditory processing disorder (APD) 55
 early intervention 285
 learning disabilities evaluation 48
 nonverbal learning disorder (NVLD) 84
accessible instructional materials (AIM)
 individualized education plan (IEP) 410
 learning disabilities evaluation 49
acquired immunodeficiency syndrome (AIDS), neurological disorders 11
AD *see* Alzheimer disease
ADA *see* Americans with Disabilities Act
ADD *see* attention deficit disorder
ADHD *see* attention deficit hyperactivity disorder
Administration for Children and Families (ACF)
 publication
  executive functions of brain 21n
adulthood
 attention deficit hyperactivity disorder (ADHD) 119
 brain development 13
 employment 387
 hearing loss 194
 hyperlexia 79
 individualized education program (IEP) 313
 Klinefelter syndrome 154
 specific language impairment (SLI) 101
 Tourette syndrome (TS) 216
 transition planning 340
Affordable Care Act (ACA), Section 504 299
aggressive behavior, bullying 411
alcohol use
 overview 181–187
 see also fetal alcohol spectrum disorders (FASDs)
alcohol-related neurodevelopmental disorder (ARND), fetal alcohol spectrum disorders (FASDs) 185
Alexander Graham Bell Association for the Deaf and Hard of Hearing, contact information 471

485

Alzheimer disease (AD),
    neurotransmitters 10
American Council of the Blind,
    contact information 469
American Foundation for the Blind,
    contact information 469
American Optometric Association,
    contact information 482
American Sign Language (ASL)
    disability inclusion 441
    voice, speech, and language
        program 109
American Speech-Language-Hearing
    Association (ASHA), contact
    information 478
Americans with Disabilities Act
    (ADA)
    bullying 414, 451
    disability inclusion 438
    employment 392
    high school 363
    Section 504 299
amniocentesis
    chromosomal disorders 147
    Turner syndrome (TS) 167
amyotrophic lateral sclerosis (ALS),
    voice, speech, and language
        program 124
anticoagulants, traumatic brain injury
    (TBI) 230
anxiety disorders, Tourette syndrome
    (TS) 220
APD *see* auditory processing disorder
Apgar score, cerebral palsy (CP) 128
aphasia
    Gerstmann syndrome 189
    IDEA 48
    overview 94–96
    see also epilepsy-aphasia spectrum
Aphasia Hope Foundation (AHF),
    contact information 480
approximate number system (ANS),
    developmental dyscalculia (DD) 64

apraxia of speech (AOS)
    overview 97–100
    speech and language development
        milestones 30
articulation disorders, voice, speech,
    and language disorders 92
AS *see* Asperger syndrome
ASD *see* autism spectrum disorder
ASL *see* American Sign Language
Asperger syndrome (AS)
    nonverbal learning disorder
        (NVLD) 88
    overview 206–207
assistive devices
    cerebral palsy (CP) 134
    hearing loss 198
assistive listening devices (ALDs),
    auditory processing disorder
        (APD) 59
assistive technology (AT)
    disability inclusion 437
    Rehabilitation Act of 1973 301
    visual impairment 243
Association for Science in Autism
    Treatment (ASAT), contact
    information 480
Association of Blind Citizens, contact
    information 469
attention deficit disorder (ADD),
    Williams syndrome (WS) 171
Attention Deficit Disorder Association
    (ADDA), contact information 480
attention deficit hyperactivity disorder
    (ADHD)
    auditory processing disorder
        (APD) 58
    autism spectrum disorder
        (ASD) 208
    brain 23
    fetal alcohol spectrum disorders
        (FASDs) 186
    47,xyy syndrome 148
    overview 119–122

486

Index

attention deficit hyperactivity disorder (ADHD), *continued*
    parenting 408
    Tourette syndrome (TS) 217
audiologists
    auditory processing disorder (APD) 57
    speech disorder and language disorders 31
auditory brainstem implant, hearing disabilities 198
auditory processing disorder (APD)
    language disorders 106
    overview 55–60
auditory stimulus, central auditory processing disorder (CAPD) 55
auditory system
    central auditory processing disorder (CAPD) 57
    hearing loss 193
Autism Network International (ANI), contact information 480
Autism Research Institute (ARI), contact information 480
Autism Society, contact information 481
Autism Speaks, Inc., contact information 481
autism spectrum disorder (ASD)
    executive function (EF) 23
    fragile X syndrome (FXS) 152
    hyperlexia 79
    language or speech disorders 106
    overview 208–209
    speech-language therapy 329
automated teller machine (ATM), disability inclusion 439
autonomic functions, brain development 12
autosomes, chromosomal disorder 139
axon, nervous system 9

B

baclofen, cerebral palsy (CP) 133
bacterial meningitis, cerebral palsy (CP) 125
basal ganglia, inner brain 9
behavioral disorders
    conduct disorder (CD) 219
    language or speech disorders 106
    neurotransmitters 11
behavioral therapists, hyperlexia 79
bilirubin, cerebral palsy (CP) 129
blood pressure
    cerebral palsy (CP) 127, 133
    disability inclusion 436
    Klinefelter syndrome 155
    traumatic brain injury (TBI) 230
    Turner syndrome (TS) 168
body mass index (BMI), Prader-Willi syndrome (PWS) 161
bone-anchored hearing aids, defined 199
botulinum toxin (BT-A), cerebral palsy (CP) 133
Braille
    Americans with Disabilities Act (ADA) 441
    educational considerations 241
    IDEA 317
    Sections 504 and 508 302
    transition to high school 369
brain imaging studies
    developmental dyscalculia (DD) 63
    science of learning disabilities 261
brain injury
    aphasia 95
    attention deficit hyperactivity disorder (ADHD) 120
    dyslexia 76
    emotional disturbance 254
    IDEA 48
    speech-language pathologists 330
    see also traumatic brain injury (TBI) 223

brain plasticity
    adolescent brain development 15
    speech and language problems 31
brain stem, architecture of the brain 6
brain tumors, neurological
    disorders 11
brain–computer interface (BCI), voice,
    speech, and language program 108
breech position, cerebral palsy
    (CP) 128
bullying
    early intervention 269
    overview 411–415
    see also cyberbullying

C

cancer, disability inclusion 436
CAPD *see* central auditory processing
    disorder
caregivers
    children with disabilities 407
    detecting problems with language
        or speech 104
    early and adolescent brain
        development 15
    emotional disturbance 248
    fragile X syndrome (FXS) 153
    Individualized Family Service Plan
        (IFSP) 277
    special education 397
    visual impairment 235
    visual processing disorders 114
Cayler cardiofacial syndrome,
    velocardiofacial syndrome (VCFS)
CBT *see* cognitive behavioral therapy
CD *see* conduct disorder
CDKL5 deficiency disorder, Rett
    syndrome 211
Center for Autism and Related
    Disorders (CARD), contact
    information 481

Center for Parent Information and
    Resources (CPIR)
    contact information 478
    evaluating children 44
    publications
        early intervention 269n, 278n
        evaluating children for learning
            disabilities 41n
        independent living 423n
        Individualized Education
            Program (IEP) 311n
        Individualized Family Service
            Plan (IFSP) 274n
        intellectual disability 339n
        learning disabilities 47n, 405n
        special education 291n
        students with disabilities 315n
        transition to adulthood 417n
        visual impairment 235n
Centers for Disease Control and
    Prevention (CDC)
    contact information 475
    publications
        attention deficit hyperactivity
            disorder (ADHD) 119n
        autism spectrum disorder
            (ASD) 208n
        bullying and learning
            disabilities 411n
        disability inclusion 435n
        Down syndrome 144n
        early brain development and
            health 18n
        early intervention 267n
        fetal alcohol spectrum disorders
            (FASDs) 181n, 184n
        fragile X syndrome (FXS) 150n
        hearing loss in children 193n,
            196n
        IDEA 303n
        language and speech disorders
            in children 104n

Index

Centers for Disease Control and
    Prevention (CDC)
    publications, *continued*
        parenting a child with a
            learning disability 405n
        Tourette syndrome (TS) 215n,
            217n
central auditory processing disorder
    (CAPD), language acquisition 55
cerebellum, brain 6
cerebral cortex
    auditory processing disorder
        (APD) 55
    brain 8
    cerebral palsy (CP) 123
cerebral hemisphere, brain 8
cerebral palsy (CP)
    disability inclusion 443
    IDEA 306
    overview 123–135
cerebrospinal fluid, brain 5
cerebrum
    brain 6
    epilepsy-aphasia spectrum 176
CHADD *see* Children and Adults with
    Attention Deficit Hyperactivity
    Disorder
The Charlotte W. Newcombe
    Foundation, contact
    information 468
Child Welfare Information
    Gateway
    contact information 475
    publication
        brain development 12n
childhood apraxia of speech (CAS) *see*
    apraxia of speech (AOS)
childhood disintegrative disorder,
    pervasive developmental disorders
    (PDD) 205
Childhood Education International,
    contact information 478

Children and Adults with
    Attention-Deficit/Hyperactivity
    Disorder (CHADD), contact
    information 480
children with disabilities
    bullying 411
    evaluating children 41
    free appropriate public education
        (FAPE) 363
    IDEA 304
    Individualized Family Service Plan
        (IFSP) 277
    parenting a child with a learning
        disability 408
    preparing for adulthood 418
    special education process 291
    special education supports 396
    supplementary aids and
        services 339
The Children's Hearing Institute,
    contact information 481
chorionic villus sampling (CVS),
    Down syndrome 147
choroid plexus, depicted 6
Christian Record Services, Inc.,
    contact information 470
chromosomes
    47,XYY syndrome 149
    Klinefelter syndrome 156
    Rett syndrome 211
    Turner syndrome (TS) 166
    velocardiofacial syndrome
        (VCFS) 169
chronic medical illness, emotional
    disturbance 248
chronic poverty, emotional
    disturbance 248
Cleveland Clinic, contact
    information 478
clinodactyly
    47,XYY syndrome 148
    Klinefelter syndrome 155

489

coagulation disorders, cerebral palsy (CP) 130
Cochlear Americas, contact information 472
cochlear implant, hearing loss 198
cognitive behavioral therapy, Asperger syndrome (AS) 207
cognitive therapy, rehabilitation therapy 232
coloboma, visual impairment 236
communication disorders
   aphasia 95
   auditory processing disorder (APD) 56
communication skills
   assistive devices 134
   early intervention 268
   Glasgow Coma Scale (GCS) 228
   pervasive developmental disorders (PDD) 205
   specific language impairment (SLI) 103
computed tomography (CT), neuroimaging 129
computer software *see* assistive devices
concussions, traumatic brain injury (TBI) 224
conduct disorder (CD), Tourette syndrome (TS) 217
conductive hearing loss, hearing loss treatment and intervention services 200
congenital cataracts, visual impairments 236
convulsions, traumatic brain injury (TBI) 225
coprolalia, Tourette syndrome (TS) 216
cortex
   auditory processing disorder (APD) 55
   brain 8
   cerebral palsy (CP) 123

cortical visual impairment (CVI), brain damage 236
cortisol, brain development and stress 18
Council for Exceptional Children (CEC), contact information 478
Council For Learning Disabilities, contact information 478
counseling
   depression 220
   disability coordinators 377
   disability inclusion 435
   early intervention services 306
   fragile X syndrome (FXS) 153
   job-seeking skills 451
   rehabilitation therapy 231
   speech-language pathologists 331
   velocardiofacial syndrome (VCFS) 171
CP *see* cerebral palsy
CT *see* computed tomography
CVI *see* cortical visual impairment
CVS *see* chorionic villus sampling
cyberbullying, child with disabilities 414
cytomegalovirus (CMV)
   brain 20
   cerebral palsy (CP) 127
cytosine-guanine-guanine (CGG), fragile X syndrome (FXS) 150

D

DAS *see* developmental apraxia of speech
delinquency prevention programs, early intervention 268
dendrites, brain functions 9
deoxyribonucleic acid (DNA), chromosomal disorders 140
depression
   attention deficit hyperactivity disorder (ADHD) 121

Index

depression, *continued*
  neurotransmitters 10
  nonverbal learning disorder (NVLD) 88
  self-esteem 399
  Tourette syndrome (TS) 217
  velocardiofacial syndrome (VCFS) 170
developmental aphasia, learning disability 48
developmental apraxia of speech, dysarthria 98
developmental delay
  cerebral palsy (CP) 124
  learning disability 50
  oppositional defiant disorder (ODD) 221
  speech-language pathologists 330
  velocardiofacial syndrome (VCFS) 170
developmental dyscalculia (DD), overview 61–66
developmental language disorder (DLD), specific language impairment (SLI) 101
developmental milestones
  autism spectrum disorder (ASD) 208
  brain development 20
  Prader-Willi syndrome (PWS) 163
  problems with language or speech 105
developmental psychologist, speech and language development milestones 31
diagnostic tests
  Down syndrome 146
  speech and language problems 31
DiGeorge syndrome, velocardiofacial syndrome (VCFS) 169
digital versatile discs (DVDs), assistive devices hearing 199

diplegia, cerebral palsy (CP) 131
discrimination
  auditory processing disorder (APD) 57
  child's legal rights 414
  equal employment opportunity 454
  nonverbal learning disorder (NVLD) 87
  parents with intellectual or developmental disabilities 447
  posttraumatic stress disorder (PTSD) 248
  Section 504 of the Rehabilitation Act 107, 438
  transition to high school 363
  visual processing disorders 112
distorting sounds, voice, speech, and language disorders 98
diuretics, traumatic brain injury (TBI) 230
DNA *see* deoxyribonucleic acid
documentation of a disability, transition to high school 369–379
DO-IT (Disabilities, Opportunities, Internetworking, and Technology), contact information 478
dopamine, serotonin 11
Down syndrome
  chromosome abnormalities 140
  developmental dyscalculia (DD) 63
  overview 144–148
  Usher syndrome 194
drug use, disability inclusion 435
DVDs *see* digital versatile discs
dysarthria
  apraxia of speech (AOS) 97
  speech sound disorders 92
dyscalculia
  approximate number system (ANS) 63
  coping with a learning disability 398

dyscalculia, *continued*
   Gerstmann syndrome 189
   math disability 262
dysgraphia
   coping with a learning
     disability 397
   Gerstmann syndrome 189
   overview 67–71
dyslexia
   coping with a learning
     disability 397
   decoding learning disabilities
     interventions 262
   overview 75–76
   specific language impairment (SLI) 31
dysphagia, speech therapy 231

E

ear infection
   auditory processing disorder
     (APD) 56
   Down syndrome 147
   Turner syndrome (TS) 165
Early Childhood Learning and
   Knowledge Center (ECLKC)
   publication
     Individualized Family Service
       Plans (IFSPs) 274n
Early Childhood Technical Assistance
   Center (ECTA), IDEA 396
early hearing detection and
   intervention (EHDI), defined 197
early intervention
   described 153
   hearing loss treatment 196
   IDEA 239
   nonverbal learning disorder
     (NVLD) 88
   overview 267–269
early learning, Individualized Family
   Service Plan (IFSP) 276

eating disorders, self-esteem 399
ECTA *see* Early Childhood Technical
   Assistance Center
EEG *see* electroencephalogram
EF *see* executive function
EHDI *see* early hearing detection and
   intervention
electroencephalogram (EEG)
   cerebral palsy (CP) 130
   epilepsy-aphasia spectrum 175
Elementary and Secondary Education
   Act (ESEA), described 309–310
emotional and behavioral disorders
   (EBDs), executive function (EF) 24
emotional challenges, learning
   disabilities 259
emotional disturbance
   IDEA 48
   overview 245–255
   transition planning 368
emotional strain, posttraumatic stress
   disorder (PTSD) 248
employment services, summary of
   performance (SOP) 386
epilepsy-aphasia spectrum
   IDEA 50
   overview 175–178
ESSA *see* Every Student Succeeds Act
Eunice Kennedy Shriver National
   Institute of Child Health and
   Human Development (NICHD)
   contact information 475
   publications
     learning disabilities 39n,
       259n, 395n
     Prader-Willi syndrome
       (PWS) 159n
     reading disorders 75n
     speech-language therapy for
       autism 329n
     traumatic brain injury
       (TBI) 223n

Index

Every Student Succeeds Act (ESSA), overview 307–310
executive function (EF)
    auditory processing disorder (APD) 59
    Klinefelter syndrome 155
    overview 21–26
expressive language
    apraxia of speech (AOS) 99
    auditory processing disorder (APD) 57
    Klinefelter syndrome 155

F

FAPE *see* free appropriate public education
FASD *see* fetal alcohol spectrum disorders
federal financial assistance
    Section 504 299
    transition to high school 363
fetal alcohol spectrum disorders (FASDs), overview 181–187
fetal growth, cerebral palsy (CP) 123
fidget, attention deficit hyperactivity disorder (ADHD) 119
Fit Small Business, contact information 468
FM *see* frequency modulation
FMR1 gene, fragile X syndrome (FXS) 150
FMR1 protein (FMRP), chromosomal disorders 150
folic acid, brain development 20
forebrain, brain architecture 5
47,XYY syndrome, overview 148–149
FOXG1 syndrome, Rett syndrome 211
fragile X syndrome (FXS), overview 150–154
FRAXA Research Foundation, contact information 479
free appropriate public education (FAPE)
    IDEA 303
    transition planning 384
frequency modulation (FM) system, hearing loss treatment 199
frontal lobe, brain development 14
functional magnetic resonance imaging (fMRI), developmental dyscalculia (DD) 62
FXS *see* fragile X syndrome

G

Gallaudet University, contact information 472
gamma-aminobutyric acid (GABA), neurotransmitters 11
Gaucher disease (GD), neurological disorders 11
GCS *see* Glasgow Coma Scale
general education curriculum
    alternate high school diploma 383
    intellectual disability 339
Genetic and Rare Diseases Information Center (GARD), contact information 475
genetic disorder, fragile X syndrome (FXS) 150
German measles, cerebral palsy (CP) 127
Gerstmann syndrome, overview 189–190
GFAP *see* glial fibrillary acidic protein
girlshealth.gov
    publication
        self-esteem and learning disabilities 399n
Glasgow Coma Scale (GCS), traumatic brain injury (TBI) diagnosis 227

glial fibrillary acidic protein (GFAP), blood tests 228
gray matter, cerebral cortex 8
GreatSchools, contact information 479
growth hormone (GH) therapy, Prader-Willi syndrome (PWS) 162
gut reaction, adolescent brain development 14
gynecomastia, Klinefelter syndrome 154

H

harassment
   bullying and learning disability 411
   employment for people with learning disability 453
health-care professional
   language or speech disorders treatment 107
   parenting a child with learning disability 406
   speech or language delay 31
   surgical intervention for hearing disability 200
hearing aids
   assistive devices 134
   intervention services for hearing loss 195
hearing loss
   auditory processing disorder (APD) 56
   early intervention services for babies 306
   health problems with Down syndrome 147
   health problems with Tourette syndrome (TS) 220
   overview 193–201
   specific language impairment (SLI) 101
   speech and language development milestones 30

speech-language pathologists 330
   Turner syndrome (TS) 165
hearing test
   audiologist 57
   helping children learn language 104
   overview 193–196
   speech or language delay 30
heredity, brain development 12
herpes, cerebral palsy (CP) 127
hindbrain, architecture of the brain 5
hippocampus, inner brain 9
homeschooling, overview 345–352
homework
   attention deficit hyperactivity disorder (ADHD) 119
   educational concerns 221
   parenting 409
   talking to your child's teacher 336
   visual impairment 242
human body
   brain basics 5
   chromosomes 139
Huntington disease (HD), neurotransmitters 11
hyperactivity
   auditory processing disorder (APD) 58
   autism spectrum disorder (ASD) 208
   cerebral palsy (CP) 131
   fetal alcohol spectrum disorder (FASD) 186
   learning disability 37
   parenting 408
hyperlexia, overview 77–80
hypertonia, early signs of cerebral palsy (CP) 124
hypothalamic-pituitary-adrenocortical (HPA) system, responding to stress 18
hypothalamus, described 8

Index

hypotonia
    cerebral palsy (CP) 124
    chromosome abnormalities 140
    Klinefelter syndrome 155
    Prader-Willi syndrome (PWS) 159

I

ICP *see* intracranial pressure
IDEA *see* Individuals with Disabilities Education Act
IEE *see* independent educational evaluation
IEP *see* individualized education plan
INCIGHT, contact information 467
independent educational evaluation (IEE), special education and related services 293
independent living
    defined 442
    early intervention services 304
    overview 423–426
    transition services 382, 418
individualized education plan (IEP)
    assistive technology (AT) 410
    hyperlexia 80
    special education services 39, 307
individualized education program (IEP)
    child's educational program 45
    overview 311–313
    special education and related services 293
    transition planning 367, 417
    transition services 388
    visual impairment 240
Individualized Family Service Plan (IFSP)
    early intervention program 269
    overview 274–278
    visual impairment 240

Individuals with Disabilities Education Act (IDEA)
    autism spectrum disorder (ASD) 24
    disability harassment 414
    early intervention program 269
    intellectual disability 339
    overview 303–307
    special education and related services 43
    specific learning disability (SLD) 289
    visual impairments 238
    vocational rehabilitation (VR) 363, 382
inner brain, defined 8
intellectual disability
    cerebral palsy (CP) 128
    emotional disturbance 254
    fragile X syndrome (FXS) 152
    Rett syndrome 211
    special education and related services 339
    specific language impairment (SLI) 101
    specific learning disability (SLD) 48
    Williams syndrome (WS) 171
intellectual or developmental disabilities, parenting 447
intelligence quotient (IQ)
    child welfare system 448
    Down syndrome 144
    fetal alcohol spectrum disorders (FASDs) 181
intelligence test, child welfare system 448
International Dyslexia Association (IDA), contact information 481
interpreting services, students with disabilities 318
intracranial hematoma, traumatic brain injury (TBI) 223

intracranial pressure (ICP), traumatic brain injury (TBI) 230
intraparietal sulcus (IPS), developmental dyscalculia (DD) 64
IQ *see* intelligence quotient

J

Job Accommodation Network, job-seeking skills 452
job discrimination, Americans with Disabilities Act (ADA) 453
job opportunities, individualized learning plans (ILPs) 390
job-based training, workforce development system 390
joint problems, Williams syndrome (WS) 172

K

karyotype
   chromosomal disorders 140
   Klinefelter syndrome 158
Klinefelter syndrome, overview 154–159

L

language acquisition, epilepsy-aphasia spectrum 175
language comprehension
   auditory processing disorder (APD) 59
   hyperlexia 79
language delay
   early intervention services 153
   fetal alcohol spectrum disorders (FASDs) 184
   specific language impairment (SLI) 101

language disorder
   language disorder statistics 93
   speech and language development 30
   speech-language pathologists 331
   Tourette syndrome (TS) 217
language impairment
   emotional disturbance 254
   executive function (EF) 24
   IDEA 51
language module, language learning 33
language problem
   epilepsy-aphasia spectrum 178
   language disorders statistics 92
   speech and language development 31
   speech-language pathologists 330
language skills
   Asperger syndrome (AS) 206
   cerebral palsy (CP) 131
   epilepsy-aphasia spectrum 175
   health inclusion strategies 440
   Klinefelter syndrome 155
   language disorders statistics 93
   learning disability in adulthood 395
   speech and language development 30
lawsuit
   court-established trusts 432
   employment discrimination complaint 455
LD *see* learning disabilities
LD OnLine, contact information 479
LD Resources Foundation, Inc., contact information 472
LDRC *see* Learning Disabilities Research Centers
Learning Ally, contact information 470
learning disabilities (LD)
   choosing a tutor 353
   executive function (EF) 23
   fetal alcohol spectrum disorders (FASDs) 184

Index

learning disabilities (LD), *continued*
   Klinefelter syndrome 157
   learning disabilities
      interventions 259
   learning disability in adulthood 395
   nonverbal learning disorder
      (NVLD) 84
   overview 37–38
Learning Disabilities Association
   of America (LDA), contact
   information 479
Learning Disabilities Association of
   Iowa, contact information 473
Learning Disabilities Research Centers
   (LDRC), learning disabilities
   interventions 259
Learning Disabilities Worldwide
   (LDW), contact information 479
learning styles
   hyperlexia 80
   students with disabilities 315
least restrictive environment (LRE),
   IDEA 305
letter and symbol reversal, visual
   processing disorders 113
Lighthouse Guild, contact
   information 470
limbic system, early brain
   development 12
Literacy Information and
   Communication System (LINCS)
   publication
      differentiated instruction 325n
lobes
   adolescent brain development 14
   architecture of the brain 7
   developmental dyscalculia
      (DD) 63
local educational agencies (LEAs)
   IDEA 48
   transition to college and vocational
      programs 381

locked-in syndrome (LIS), voice,
   speech, and language program 108
LRE *see* least restrictive environment

M

magnetic resonance imaging (MRI)
   aphasia 95
   brain development 13
   cerebral palsy (CP) 129
   developmental dyscalculia
      (DD) 62
   traumatic brain injury (TBI) 227
maladjustment
   nonverbal learning disorder
      (NVLD) 88
   parenting 446
maternal age, chromosomal
   disorders 142
math disability, emotional
   challenges 262
MECP2 duplication syndrome, Rett
   syndrome 210
mediation, individualized education
   program (IEP) 295
Medicaid
   Affordable Care Act (ACA) 439
   special needs trusts 427
medical exam
   attention deficit hyperactivity
      disorder (ADHD) 121
   response to intervention
      (RTI) 40
   see also neurological exam
medications
   cerebral palsy (CP) 124, 133
   emotional disturbance 246
   hearing loss treatment 200
   neurotransmitters 11
   Prader-Willi syndrome
      (PWS) 161
   traumatic brain injury (TBI) 230

MedlinePlus
   contact information 476
   publications
      aphasia 94n
      chromosomal disorders 139n
      epilepsy-aphasia spectrum 175n
      47, XYY syndrome 148n
      Klinefelter syndrome 154n
      learning disabilities 37n
      Prader–Willi syndrome (PWS) 159n
      Rett syndrome 209n
      Turner syndrome (TS) 164n
      Williams syndrome (WS) 171n
meiosis, chromosomal disorders 142
memory aids, dyscalculia 398
meninges, depicted 6
mental health
   early brain development 20
   emotional disturbance 245
   self-esteem 399
   special education 38
   tabulated *443*
   Tourette syndrome (TS) 217
   transition planning 367
mental illness, velocardiofacial syndrome (VCFS) 170
midbrain, early brain development 12
minimal brain dysfunction, IDEA 48
mitosis, chromosomal disorders 142
mnemonics, auditory processing disorder (APD) 59
mood disorders, Tourette syndrome (TS) 219
mood instability, traumatic brain injury (TBI) 230
mosaicism
   Klinefelter syndrome 158
   Turner syndrome (TS) 166
   velocardiofacial syndrome (VCFS) 170

motor area
   brain basics 7
   cerebral palsy (CP) 123
MRI *see* magnetic resonance imaging
muscle coordination, cerebral palsy (CP) 123
myelin sheath, depicted 10
myelination, brain development 13

N

National Aphasia Association (NAA), contact information 480
National Center for Education Statistics (NCES), contact information 476
National Center for Learning Disabilities (NCLD), contact information 479
National Council on Disability (NCD)
   contact information 476
   publication
      disability on parenting 445n
National Eye Institute (NEI), contact information 476
National Federation of the Blind, contact information 471
National Human Genome Research Institute (NHGRI)
   contact information 476
   publications
      chromosome abnormalities 139n
      Klinefelter syndrome 154n
      Turner syndrome (TS) 164n
      velocardiofacial syndrome (VCFS) 168n
National Institute of Mental Health (NIMH), contact information 476

Index

National Institute of Neurological
Disorders and Stroke (NINDS)
contact information 476
publications
Asperger syndrome (AS) 206n
brain basics 5n
cerebral palsy (CP) 123n
dysgraphia 67n
dyslexia 75n
Gerstmann syndrome 189n
pervasive developmental
disorders (PDDs) 205n
National Institute on Alcohol Abuse
and Alcoholism (NIAAA), contact
information 477
National Institute on Deafness and
Other Communication Disorders
(NIDCD)
contact information 477
publications
apraxia of speech (AOS) 97n
specific language impairment
(SLI) 101n
speech and language
developmental
milestones 29n
voice, speech, and language
disorders statistics 91n
voice, speech, and language
program 107n
National Science Foundation (NSF)
contact information 477
publication
language acquisition 32n
native language
disabilities 317
early intervention 271
speech and language development
milestones 30
natural environments, early
intervention strategies 277

NCLB see No Child Left Behind Act
neonatal encephalopathy, Rett
syndrome 210
neonatal intensive care unit (NICU),
hearing loss 194
neurodevelopmental disorders,
attention deficit hyperactivity
disorder (ADHD) 119
neuroimaging
cerebral palsy (CP) 129
developmental dyscalculia (DD) 62
neurological exam, diagnosing
learning disabilities 40
neurons
brain basics 9
epilepsy-aphasia spectrum 177
neurotransmitters 10
Rett syndrome 210
neuroplasticity, decoding learning
disabilities 261
neuropsychological assessments,
traumatic brain injury (TBI) 228
neurotransmitters, brain functions 10
No Child Left Behind Act (NCLB),
child's right to special education
services 310
nonverbal learning disorders
(NVLDs), overview 83–88

O

obesity
Prader-Willi syndrome (PWS) 159
Williams syndrome (WS) 172
object tracking system (OTS),
dyscalculia 64
obsessive-compulsive disorder (OCD),
Tourette syndrome (TS) 217
occipital lobes
brain basics 7
developmental dyscalculia (DD) 63

499

occupational therapy (OT),
  hyperlexia 80
OCD *see* obsessive-compulsive
  disorder
OCR *see* Office for Civil Rights
ODD *see* oppositional defiant disorder
Office for Civil Rights (OCR)
  Section 504 99
  transition to high school 363
Office of Juvenile Justice and
  Delinquency Prevention (OJJDP),
  early intervention 269
OJJDP *see* Office of Juvenile Justice
  and Delinquency Prevention
Omnigraphics
  publications
    hyperlexia 77n
    visual processing disorders 111n
oppositional defiant disorder (ODD),
  Tourette syndrome (TS) 217
orientation and mobility services
  students with disabilities 318
  transition planning 382
orthopedic impairment
  disability type 254
  students with disabilities 50
orthotic devices, cerebral palsy
  (CP) 132
osteoporosis
  Klinefelter syndrome 155
  Turner syndrome (TS) 167
OT *see* occupational therapy

P

P. Buckley Moss Foundation, contact
  information 473
PACER Center, Inc., contact
  information 479
parental consent
  early intervention 269
  IDEA 292

parenting
  attention deficit hyperactivity
    disorder (ADHD) 121
  disability 445
  emotional distress 248
  learning disability 405
parietal lobes, brain basics 7
Parkinson disease (PD)
  brain basics 9
  speech-language therapy 330
PDD *see* pervasive developmental
  disorders
PDD-NOS *see* pervasive
  developmental disorder not
  otherwise specified
percutaneous umbilical blood
  sampling (PUBS), Down
  syndrome 147
peripheral auditory system, auditory
  processing disorder (APD) 55
peripheral hearing loss, auditory
  processing disorder (APD) 56
periventricular leukomalacia (PVL),
  cerebral palsy (CP) 126
persistent developmental stuttering,
  voice, speech, and language
  disorders 93
pervasive developmental disorder not
  otherwise specified (PDD-NOS),
  Asperger syndrome (AS) 206
pervasive developmental disorder
  (PDD)
  nonverbal learning disorder
    (NVLD) 88
  overview 205–211
pes planus
  47,XYY syndrome 148
  Klinefelter syndrome 155
phenylketonuria (PKU), brain
  development 20
philtrum, fetal alcohol spectrum
  disorders (FASDs) 184

Index

phonological awareness activities, auditory processing disorder (APD) 59
physical assaults, employment discrimination 456
physical therapy
    cerebral palsy (CP) 132
    Down syndrome 147
    early intervention 267
    Prader-Willi syndrome (PWS) 163
    transition to high school 367
    traumatic brain injury (TBI) 231
pineal gland, depicted 6
plasticity, brain development 14
pooled trust, special needs 129
positive stress, brain development 17
posttraumatic stress disorder (PTSD)
    emotional disturbance 248
    Tourette syndrome (TS) 220
power of attorney (POA), special needs trust 428
PPM-X syndrome, pervasive developmental disorders (PDD) 210
Prader-Willi syndrome (PWS), overview 159–164
pregnancy
    alcohol use 181
    attention deficit hyperactivity disorder (ADHD) 120
    brain development 19
    cerebral palsy (CP) 135
    employment discrimination 454
    fragile X syndrome (FXS) 152
    hearing loss 194
    learning disability 37
    Turner syndrome (TS) 167
premature
    attention deficit hyperactivity disorder (ADHD) 121
    brain development 20
    visual impairment 236

preschool program, executive function (EF) 22
problem-based learning (PBL), differentiated instruction 327
psychiatric
    disability inclusion *443*
    nonverbal learning disorder (NVLD) 84
psychological counseling, traumatic brain injury (TBI) 231
psychological disorders, emotional disturbance 248
PTSD *see* posttraumatic stress disorder
puberty
    brain development 14
    Klinefelter syndrome 154
    Turner syndrome (TS) 164
PUBS *see* percutaneous umbilical blood sampling

Q

quadriplegia, cerebral palsy (CP) 130

R

reading disability
    diagnosing learning disabilities 40
    genes associated with learning disabilities 261
receptive language
    auditory processing disorder (APD) 56
    chromosomal disorders 155
    detecting problems 105
rehabilitation
    disability 437
    employment 451
    postadmission 372
    Section 508 301
    transition to high school 363
    traumatic brain injury (TBI) 231
    see also physical therapy

reimbursement, Medicaid 433
residual hearing, hearing loss
    treatment 198
response to intervention (RTI)
    described 39
    overview 283–289
    visual processing disorder 114
retinitis pigmentosa, visual
    impairment 236
retinopathy, visual impairment 236
Rett syndrome
    overview 209–211
    pervasive developmental disorders
        (PDD) 205
rhesus (Rh), cerebral palsy (CP) 127
rheumatoid arthritis (RA), Klinefelter
    syndrome 158
RTI see response to intervention

S

safety equipment, childcare 406
St. Louis Learning Disabilities
    Association, contact
    information 479
schizophrenia
    emotional disturbance 245
    velocardiofacial syndrome
        (VCFS) 170
school health services, students with
    disabilities 318
school psychologists
    diagnosing learning disabilities 40
    nonverbal learning disorder
        (NVLD) 83
    transition to high school 374
scoliosis
    cerebral palsy (CP) 131
    47,XYY syndrome 148
    Prader-Willi syndrome
        (PWS) 162
    Rett syndrome 210

screening tests
    Down syndrome 146
    response to intervention (RTI) 288
Section 504 of the Rehabilitation Act
    disability inclusion 437
    discrimination on disability 299
    transition to high school 363
seed trust, special needs trust 428
seizures
    cerebral palsy (CP) 124
    47,XYY syndrome 148
    neurotransmitters 10
    Rett syndrome 210
    traumatic brain injury (TBI) 225
    velocardiofacial syndrome
        (VCFS) 169
self-esteem
    bullying 412
    cerebral palsy (CP) 133
    Klinefelter syndrome 158
    overview 399–404
    peer tutoring 353
    visual processing disorder 111
sensitive periods, brain
    development 15
separation anxiety, Tourette syndrome
    (TS) 220
serotonin reuptake inhibitors (SRIs),
    Prader-Willi syndrome (PWS) 163
sex hormones, Prader-Willi syndrome
    (PWS) 163
sheath, brain learning 13
short-term memory, auditory
    processing disorder (APD) 57
SLD see specific learning disability
SLI see specific language impairment
social networks, teaching
    technique 328
social skills
    bullying 413
    early intervention 268
    executive function (EF) 24

Index

social skills, *continued*
  hearing loss 193
  hyperlexia 77
  Klinefelter syndrome 155
  nonverbal learning disorder (NVLD) 88
  parental involvement 341
  pervasive developmental disorders (PDD) 205
  response to intervention (RTI) 287
  speech-language therapy 329
social workers
  hyperlexia 79
  Individualized Family Service Plan (IFSP) 274
  speech-language therapy 331
socialization
  pervasive developmental disorders (PDD) 205
  postsecondary education 389
  visual processing disorder 111
sound field amplification system, auditory processing disorder (APD) 59
spasticity, cerebral palsy (CP) 123
special education services
  learning disability in adulthood 396
  response to intervention (RTI) 39
  services for school-aged children 307
  speech development problem 107
special needs trusts, overview 427–433
specific language impairment (SLI)
  executive function (EF) 24
  overview 101–103
  see also reading disorder
specific learning disability (SLD)
  developmental dyscalculia (DD) 61
  IDEA 47
  response to intervention (RTI) 289

speech therapy
  early intervention services 153
  IDEA 306
  traumatic brain injury (TBI) 231
  velocardiofacial syndrome (VCFS) 171
speech-language pathologist
  aphasia 95
  response to intervention (RTI) 40
  speech and language development 30
  speech-language therapy 329
spike-and-wave during sleep syndrome (ECSWS), epilepsy-aphasia spectrum 175
SSI *see* supplemental security income
stiff muscles, cerebral palsy (CP) 131
StopBullying.gov
  publication
    bullying and learning disabilities 411n
strabismus, visual impairment 236
stroke
  aphasia 94
  brain development 5
  cerebral palsy (CP) 126
  disability inclusion 436
  speech and language problems 330
  traumatic brain injury (TBI) 224
students with disabilities
  emotional disturbance 249
  parental involvement 340
  peer tutoring 353
  postsecondary education 391
  support for education 317
  transition planning 366
substance abuse
  disabled parents 447
  nonverbal learning disorder (NVLD) 88

Substance Abuse and Mental
    Health Services Administration
    (SAMHSA)
    contact information 477
    publication
        emotional disturbance 245n
suicide
    bullying 411
    depression 220
supplemental security income (SSI),
    special needs trust 430
supplementary aids and services
    parental involvement 339
    special education services 307
    support for education 319
supravalvular aortic stenosis (SVAS),
    Williams syndrome (WS) 172
synapses
    brain development 12
    Rett syndrome 210

T

TBI *see* traumatic brain injury
TDDs *see* telecommunications devices
    for deaf persons
telecommunications devices for deaf
    persons (TDDs), Section 504 302
temporal lobes
    auditory processing (APD) 55
    brain works 8
thalamus, inner brain 9
therapeutic recreation, students with
    disabilities 318
tinnitus, traumatic brain injury
    (TBI) 225
tiny nub, brain basics 9
Tourette syndrome (TS),
    overview 215–217
toxic stress, brain development 18
transition planning
    civil rights 363

IDEA 305
individualized learning plans
    (ILPs) 388
intellectual disability 340
learning disabilities 417
vocational programs 381
transition services
    individualized education programs
        (IEDs) 313
    learning disabilities 417
    special education staff 374
traumas, emotional distress 248
traumatic brain injury (TBI)
    overview 223–233
    visual processing disorder 111
trigger events, emotional
    distress 246
trisomy 21, Down syndrome 141
TS *see* Tourette syndrome
Turner syndrome (TS)
    chromosome abnormalities 114
    overview 164–168
tutor
    auxiliary aids 372
    differentiated instruction 326
    overview 353–359

U

U.S. Association of Blind Athletes,
    contact information 471
U.S. Bureau of Labor Statistics (BLS)
    contact information 477
    publication
        speech-language
            pathologists 329n
U.S. Department of Education (ED)
    contact information 477
    independent living 424
    publications
        auditory processing disorder
            (APD) 55n

Index

U.S. Department of Education (ED)
publications, *continued*
- brain executive functions 21n
- developmental dyscalculia (DD) 61n
- dysgraphia 67n
- emotional disturbance 245n
- Every Student Succeeds Act (ESSA) 307n
- IDEA 303n
- nonverbal learning disorders (NVLDs) 83n
- response to intervention (RTI) 283n
- self-esteem and children with learning disabilities 399n
- students with disabilities 47n, 363n
- transition of students with disabilities to postsecondary education 363n, 369n
- transition to college and vocational programs 381n
- tutoring students with learning disabilities 353n
- working with teachers and schools 335n

transition planning 363
visual impairment 238
workforce development system 390

U.S. Department of Health and Human Services (HHS)
contact information 477
publication
Sections 504 and 508 299n
Section 504 299
workforce development system 390

U.S. National Library of Medicine (NLM), contact information 477

U.S. Social Security Administration (SSA)
publication
Program Operations Manual System (POMS) 427n

ubiquitin c-terminal hydrolase L1 (UCH-L1), traumatic brain injury (TBI) 228

UCH-L1 *see* ubiquitin c-terminal hydrolase L1 (UCH-L1)

United States Census Bureau
publication
home schooling 345n

universal screening, response to intervention (RTI) 285

USA.gov
publication
jobs and education for people with disabilities 291n, 451n

V

velocardiofacial syndrome (VCFS), overview 168–171
verbal apraxia, overview 97–100
verbal skills, speech-language therapy 329
veterans, employment for people with learning disabilities 452
violence
- early intervention 269
- executive function (EF) 21
- fetal alcohol spectrum disorders (FASDs) 187

viral encephalitis, cerebral palsy (CP) 125
visual closure, visual processing disorder 113
visual discrimination, visual processing disorder 112

505

visual impairment
   emotional disturbance 254
   specific learning disability
      (SLD) 50
   overview 235–243
   transition planning 366
visual memory, visual processing
   disorder 113
visual processing disorders,
   overview 111–115
visual sequencing, visual processing
   disorder 113
visual system
   neurotransmitter 11
   visual impairment 236
visual techniques, dyscalculia 398
visual-motor processing, visual
   processing disorder 113
visual-spatial relationships, visual
   processing disorder 113
vocabulary
   Asperger syndrome (AS) 206
   auditory processing disorder
      (APD) 59
   differentiated instruction 326
   Klinefelter syndrome 155
   learning disabilities
      intervention 262
   specific language impairment
      (SLI) 103
vocal tics, Tourette syndrome
   (TS) 215
vocational counseling, traumatic brain
   injury (TBI) 232
vocational rehabilitation (VR)
   transition planning 381
   transition to high school 363
voice disorder
   speech-language therapy 330
   voice, speech, language, or
      swallowing disorder 92

W

webbed neck, Turner syndrome
   (TS) 164
webinars, differentiated
   instruction 328
Western Illinois University, contact
   information 473
white matter
   adolescent brain development 14
   cerebral palsy (CP) 126
Williams syndrome (WS),
   overview 171–174
word-level reading, learning
   disabilities intervention 260
writhing movements, cerebral palsy
   (CP) 130
writing disability, Gerstmann
   syndrome 189

X

x-ray
   cerebral palsy (CP) 130
   disability inclusion 436
   traumatic brain injury
      (TBI) 227

Y

young children
   brain development 13
   dysgraphia 71
   early intervention 267
   early intervention of hearing
      loss 197
   hyperlexia 80
   IDEA 305
   specific language impairment
      (SLI) 103
   speech and language
      development 29

Index

young children, *continued*
    traumatic brain injury (TBI) 224
    Turner syndrome (TS) 220
    voice, speech, and language disorders 92
    Williams syndrome (WS) 172
youth development, employment considerations 391

Youth.gov
    publications
        employment and postsecondary education 387n
        prevention and early intervention 267n

Z

Zika, early brain development 20